Cardiovascular

made
Incredibly
Easy! ®

Fifth Edition

Cardiovascular Care

made Incredibly Easy!

Fifth Edition

Clinical Editor

Mary Ann Siciliano McLaughlin, EdD, MSN, RN
Associate Dean, Undergraduate Nursing Program and
  Associate Professor of Nursing
Neumann University
Aston, PA

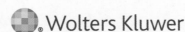

Philadelphia • Baltimore • New York • London
Buenos Aires • Hong Kong • Sydney • Tokyo

Not authorised for sale in United States, Canada, Australia, New Zealand, Puerto Rico, and U.S. Virgin Islands.

Vice President and Publisher: Julie K. Stegman
Senior Acquisitions Editor: Joyce Berendes
Director of Nursing Education and Practice Content: Jamie Blum
Senior Development Editor: Jacquelyn Saunders
Editorial Coordinator: Varshaanaa SM
Editorial Assistant: Sara Thul
Marketing Manager: Amy Whitaker
Production Project Manager: Kirstin Johnson
Manager, Graphic Arts & Design: Stephen Druding
Art Director, Illustration: Jennifer Clements
Manufacturing Coordinator: Bernard Tomboc
Prepress Vendor: TNQ TECH

Library of Congress Cataloging-in-Publication Data

ISBN-13: 978-1-975243-20-3

Cataloging in Publication data available on request from publisher.

shop.lww.com

QUADM0624

Dedication

I dedicate this book to my husband, James Joseph "Jimmy" McLaughlin. Thank you for believing in me and supporting my professional adventures over the years. Without your love and support, success in my professional nursing career would not have been possible.

All my love,
Mary Ann Siciliano McLaughlin

Contributors

Laraine Amoia-Watters, Ed.D, MSN, CRNP
Associate Professor
Francis M. Maguire School of Nursing and
    Health Professions
Gwynedd Mercy University
Gwynedd Valley, Pennsylvania

Kristen Evans, PhD, MSN, RN
Assistant Professor of Nursing
School of Nursing and Health Sciences
Neumann University
Aston, Pennsylvania

Stacy L. Lutter, D.Ed, RN
Department Chair and Associate
    Professor of Nursing
The Stabler Department of Nursing
York College of Pennsylvania
York, Pennsylvania

Mary Ann Siciliano McLaughlin, Ed.D, MSN, RN
Associate Dean, Undergraduate Nursing
    Program and Associate Professor of
    Nursing
School of Nursing and Health Sciences
Neumann University
Aston, Pennsylvania

Lori Ann Prol, PhD, APN, FNP-BC
Nursing Program Director & Associate
    Professor
Department of Health Sciences and
    Nursing
College of Arts and Sciences
Rider University
Lawrenceville, New Jersey

Carrie L. Pucino, D.Ed, RN
Director of Undergraduate Nursing
    Programs
The Stabler Department of Nursing
York College of Pennsylvania
York, Pennsylvania

Eileen Thomas, Ed.D, RN, CHSE
Adjunct Assistant Professor (retired)
Lienhard School of Nursing
Pace University
New York, New York

Mariann Ward, RN, DNP, CRNP
Nursing Content Tutor
School of Nursing and Health Sciences
Neumann University
Aston, Pennsylvania
Emergency Nurse Practitioner
Crozer Keystone Health System

Foreword

If you're like me, you're too busy to wade through a foreword that uses pretentious terms and umpteen dull paragraphs to get to the point. So let's cut right to the chase! Here's why this book is so terrific:

1. It will teach you all the important things you need to know about cardiovascular care. (And it will leave out all the fluff that wastes your time.)
2. It will help you remember what you've learned.
3. It will make you smile as it enhances your knowledge and skills.

This book has been updated and reviewed by a group of dedicated nursing professionals. We strive to ensure that you have the most up-to-date and easy-to-use information. This book combines the Cardiovascular Care Made Incredibly Easy and Made Visual texts to bring you the best of graphics and information in one text.

I hope you find this book helpful. Best of luck throughout your career!

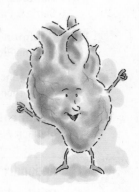

Contents

Chapter 1

Anatomy and physiology

Just the facts

In this chapter, you'll learn:

◆ components of the heart
◆ the way in which the heart contracts
◆ the heart's role in blood flow.

A look at the cardiovascular system

The cardiovascular system (sometimes called the *circulatory system*) consists of the heart, blood vessels, and lymphatics. This network brings life-sustaining oxygen and nutrients to the body's cells, removes metabolic waste products, and carries hormones from one part of the body to another.

Right to the lungs… and left to the body

The heart consists of muscular tissue that separates into two sides. The right side "pumps" or pushes forward the flow of blood from the right side of the heart to the pulmonary arteries and veins of the lungs. The blood then flows to the left side of the heart where it is "pumped" to the rest of the body.

Where the heart lies

About the size of a closed fist, the heart lies beneath the sternum in the mediastinum (the cavity between the lungs), between the second and sixth ribs. In most people, the heart rests obliquely or tilted, with its right side below and almost in front of the left. Because of its oblique angle, the heart's broad part (base) is at its upper right, and its pointed end (apex) is at its lower left (imagine an ice cream cone). The apex, also called the *PMI* or *point of maximal impulse*, is where heart sounds can be heard the loudest and also where the cardiac impulse can be felt or "palpated." This is due to its close proximity to the chest wall. Additionally, when a person is lying on their left side or leaning forward, gravity pushes the heart even closer to the anterior aspect of the chest, making it easier to hear the sounds of the heart and to palpate the PMI.

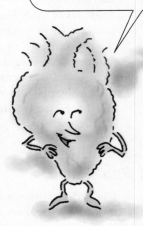

The cardiovascular system is a complex network that helps sustain life.

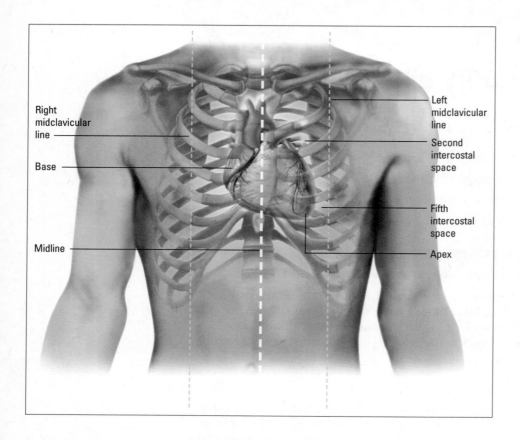

Right
midclavicular
line

Base

Midline

Left
midclavicular
line

Second
intercostal
space

Fifth
intercostal
space

Apex

Heart structure

Surrounded by a sac called the *pericardium*, the heart has a wall
made up of three layers: the endocardium (endo = inner), the myocardium (myo = middle), and the epicardium (epi = outer). Within
the heart lie four chambers (two atria, a right side and a left side,
and two ventricles, also a right side and a left side). Within these
chambers are structures known as valves. The primary function of
these valves is to move blood throughout the heart. By opening and
closing, blood is able to flow into the atria and ventricles at coordi-
nated times.

The pericardium

The pericardium is a fibroserous sac that surrounds the heart and the
roots of the great vessels (those vessels that enter and leave the heart).
It consists of the fibrous pericardium and the serous pericardium.

Inside the heart

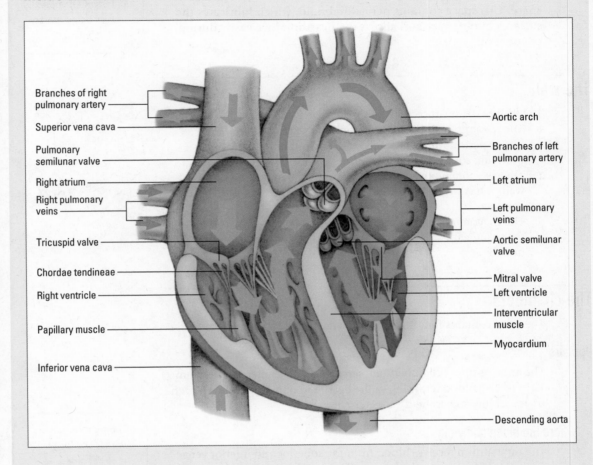

Branches of right pulmonary artery

Superior vena cava

Pulmonary semilunar valve

Right atrium

Right pulmonary veins

Tricuspid valve

Chordae tendineae

Right ventricle

Papillary muscle

Inferior vena cava

Aortic arch

Branches of left pulmonary artery

Left atrium

Left pulmonary veins

Aortic semilunar valve

Mitral valve

Left ventricle

Interventricular muscle

Myocardium

Descending aorta

Fibrous fits freely

The fibrous pericardium, composed of tough, white fibrous tissue, fits loosely around the heart, protecting it.

Serous is smooth

The serous pericardium, the thin, smooth inner portion, has two layers:
- The parietal layer lines the inside of the fibrous pericardium.
- The visceral layer adheres to the surface of the heart.

And fluid in between

Between the fibrous and serous pericardium is the pericardial space. This space contains pericardial fluid, which lubricates the surfaces of the space and allows the heart to move easily during contraction.

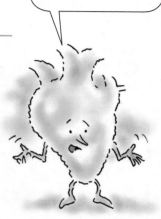

Sure, I have a wall up, but my myocardial layer helps me to contract.

The wall

The wall of the heart consists of three layers:
1. The *epicardium*, the outer layer (and the visceral layer of the serous pericardium), is made up of squamous epithelial cells overlying connective tissue.
2. The *myocardium*, the middle layer, forms most of the heart wall. It has striated muscle fibers that cause the heart to contract.
3. The *endocardium*, the heart's inner layer, consists of endothelial tissue with small blood vessels and bundles of smooth muscle.

The chambers

The heart contains four hollow chambers: two atria and two ventricles.

Upstairs...

The atria, or upper chambers, are separated by the interatrial septum. They receive blood returning to the heart and pump blood to the ventricles, or lower chambers.

...where the blood comes in

The right atrium receives blood from the superior and inferior venae cavae. The left atrium, which is smaller but has thicker walls than the right atrium, forms the uppermost part of the heart's left border. It receives blood from the two pulmonary veins.

The more a muscle works, the larger it becomes.

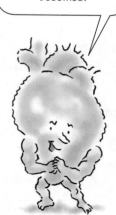

Downstairs...

The right and left ventricles, which are separated by the interventricular septum, make up the two lower chambers. The ventricles receive blood from the atria. Composed of highly developed musculature, the ventricles are larger and have thicker walls than the atria.

...where the blood goes out

The right ventricle pumps blood to the lungs. The left ventricle, which is larger than the right, pumps blood through all other vessels of the body.

The valves

In total, there are four valves (see *Heart valves*, page 6):

Tricuspid valve: located between the right atrium and the right ventricle

Pulmonary valve: located between the right ventricle and the pulmonary artery

Mitral valve: located between the left atrium and the left ventricle

Aortic valve: located between the left ventricle and the aorta

Forward flow only

The valves allow forward flow of blood through the heart and prevent backward flow, or regurgitation. The valves open and close in response to pressure changes caused by ventricular contraction and blood ejection. The two atrioventricular (AV) valves separate the atria from the ventricles. The tricuspid valve, or right AV valve, prevents backflow from the right ventricle into the right atrium. The mitral valve, or left AV valve, prevents backflow from the left ventricle into the left atrium. One of the two semilunar valves is the pulmonic valve, which prevents backflow from the pulmonary artery into the right ventricle. The other semilunar valve is the aortic valve, which prevents backflow from the aorta into the left ventricle.

On the cusps

The tricuspid valve has three triangular cusps, or leaflets. The mitral, or bicuspid, valve contains two cusps, a large anterior and a smaller posterior. Chordae tendineae (tendinous cords) attach the cusps of the AV valves to papillary muscles in the ventricles. The semilunar valves have three cusps that are shaped like half-moons. (See *Heart valves*.)

Conduction system

The heart's conduction system causes it to contract, moving blood throughout the body. For this system to work properly, the heart requires electrical stimulation as well as a mechanical response. (See *The cardiac conduction system*, page 7.)

Electrical stimulation

The conduction system contains pacemaker cells, which have three unique characteristics:
1. automaticity, the ability to generate an electrical impulse automatically

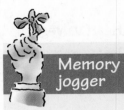

Memory jogger

If you can remember that there are two distinct heart sounds, you can recall that there are two sets of heart valves. Closure of these valves produces the heart sounds frequently known as the "lub-dub." The first heart sound is created when the atrioventricular valves close. Again, this valvular closure makes the first heart sound, the lub. Closure of the semilunar valves produces the second heart sound, the dub.

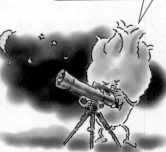

The semilunar valves, which prevent blood backflow into the ventricles, are shaped like half-moons.

Heart valves

The four valves of the heart are illustrated below. Note the number of cusps in each valve.

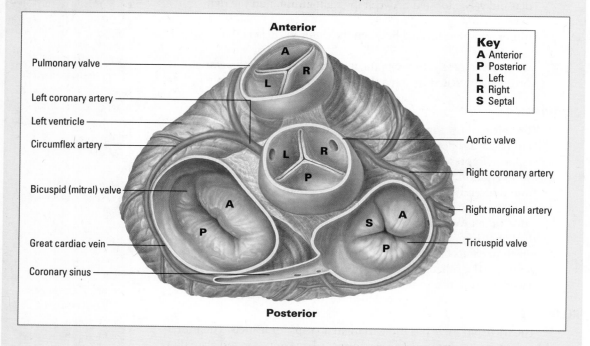

Anterior

Pulmonary valve

Left coronary artery

Left ventricle

Circumflex artery

Bicuspid (mitral) valve

Great cardiac vein

Coronary sinus

Aortic valve

Right coronary artery

Right marginal artery

Tricuspid valve

Key
A Anterior
P Posterior
L Left
R Right
S Septal

Posterior

2. conductivity, the ability to pass the impulse to the next cell
3. contractility, the ability to shorten the fibers in the heart when receiving the impulse.

Start with a bang

The sinoatrial (SA) node, located on the endocardial surface of the right atrium, near the superior vena cava, is the normal pacemaker of the heart, generating an impulse between 60 and 100 times per minute. The SA node's firing spreads an impulse throughout the right and left atria, resulting in atrial contraction.

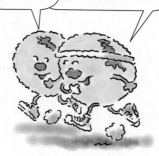

We have the qualities a properly functioning heart is looking for in pacemaker cells . . .

Automaticity, conductivity, and contractility.

The cardiac conduction system

Specialized fibers propagate electrical impulses throughout the heart's cells, causing the heart to contract. This illustration shows the elements of the cardiac conduction system.

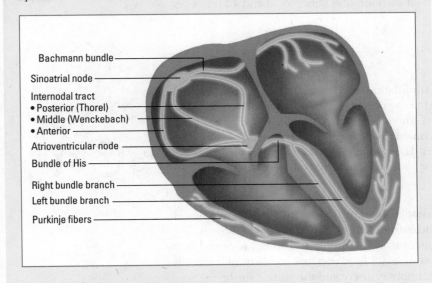

Bachmann bundle
Sinoatrial node
Internodal tract
• Posterior (Thorel)
• Middle (Wenckebach)
• Anterior
Atrioventricular node
Bundle of His
Right bundle branch
Left bundle branch
Purkinje fibers

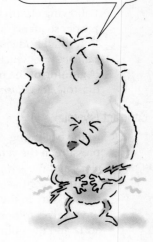

You might say that the heart has a firing squad. If the SA node doesn't fire, the AV node fires. If the SA node and the AV node fail, the ventricles fire their own impulse.

Slow and fill

The AV node, situated low in the septal wall of the right atrium, slows impulse conduction between the atria and ventricles. This "resistor" node allows the contracting atria to fill the ventricles with blood before the lower chambers contract.

Impulsive signal

From the AV node, the impulse travels to the bundle of His (modified muscle fibers), which branches off to the right and left bundles. Finally, the impulse travels to the Purkinje fibers, the distal portions of the left and right bundle branches. These fibers fan across the surface of the ventricles from the endocardium to the myocardium. As the impulse spreads, it signals the blood-filled ventricles to contract.

Just in case

The conduction system has two built-in safety mechanisms. If the SA node fails to fire, the AV node generates an impulse between 40 and 60 times per minute. If the SA node and the AV node fail, the ventricles can generate their own impulse between 20 and 40 times per minute.

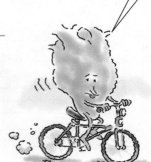

The cardiac cycle lasts from the start of one heartbeat all the way to the start of the next heartbeat.

Mechanical events

Following electrical stimulation, mechanical events must occur in the proper sequence and to the proper degree to provide adequate blood flow to all body parts. These events are collectively known as the *cardiac cycle*, which consists of the period from one heartbeat to the beginning of the next. The cardiac cycle has two phases—systole and diastole. (See *Events of the cardiac cycle*, page 9.)

Contract (systole)...

At the beginning of systole, the ventricles contract. Increasing blood pressure in the ventricles forces the AV valves (mitral and tricuspid) to close and the semilunar valves (pulmonic and aortic) to open. As the ventricles contract, ventricular blood pressure builds until it exceeds the pressure in the pulmonary artery and the aorta, causing the semilunar valves to open. This allows the ventricles to eject blood into the aorta and the pulmonary artery.

...and relax (diastole)

When the ventricles empty and relax, ventricular pressure falls below the pressure in the pulmonary artery and the aorta. At the beginning of diastole, the semilunar valves close to prevent the backflow of blood into the ventricles, and the mitral and tricuspid valves open, allowing blood to flow into the ventricles from the atria.

When the ventricles become full, near the end of this phase, the atria contract to send the remaining blood to the ventricles. Then a new cardiac cycle begins as the heart enters systole again.

Output = rate × volume

Cardiac output refers to the amount of blood the heart pumps in 1 minute. It's equal to the heart rate multiplied by the stroke volume, the amount of blood ejected with each heartbeat. Stroke volume, in turn, depends on three major factors: preload, contractility, and afterload. (See *Understanding preload, contractility, and afterload*.)

Events of the cardiac cycle

The cardiac cycle lasts from the start of one heartbeat all the way to the start of the next heartbeat. The cardiac cycle consists of the following five events.

1. Isovolumetric ventricular contraction

In response to ventricular depolarization, tension in the ventricles increases. This rise in pressure within the ventricles leads to closure of the mitral and tricuspid valves. The pulmonic and aortic valves stay closed during the entire phase.

2. Ventricular ejection

When ventricular pressure exceeds aortic and pulmonary arterial pressure, the aortic and pulmonic valves open and the ventricles eject blood.

3. Isovolumetric relaxation

When ventricular pressure falls below the pressure in the aorta and pulmonary artery, the aortic and pulmonic valves close. All valves are closed during this phase. Atrial diastole occurs as blood fills the atria.

4. Ventricular filling

Atrial pressure exceeds ventricular pressure, which causes the mitral and tricuspid valves to open. Blood then flows passively into the ventricles. About 70% of ventricular filling takes place during this phase.

5. Atrial systole

Known as the *atrial kick*, atrial systole (coinciding with late ventricular diastole) supplies the ventricles with the remaining 30% of the blood for each heartbeat.

1. Isovolumetric ventricular contraction
In response to ventricular depolarization, tension in the ventricles increases. This rise in pressure within the ventricles leads to closure of the mitral and tricuspid valves. The pulmonic and aortic valves stay closed during the entire phase.

2. Ventricular ejection
When ventricular pressure exceeds aortic and pulmonary arterial pressure, the aortic and pulmonic valves open and the ventricles eject blood.

3. Isovolumetric relaxation
When ventricular pressure falls below the pressure in the aorta and pulmonary artery, the aortic and pulmonic valves close. All valves are closed during this phase. Atrial diastole occurs as blood fills the atria.

5. Atrial systole
Known as the *atrial kick*, atrial systole (coinciding with late ventricular diastole) supplies the ventricles with the remaining 30% of the blood for each heartbeat.

4. Ventricular filling
Atrial pressure exceeds ventricular pressure, which causes the mitral and tricuspid valves to open. Blood then flows passively into the ventricles. About 70% of ventricular filling takes place during this phase.

Understanding preload, contractility, and afterload

If you think of the heart as a balloon, it can help you understand stroke volume.

Blowing up the balloon

Preload is the stretching of muscle fibers in the ventricles. This stretching results from blood volume in the ventricles at end diastole. According to *Starling law*, the more the heart muscles stretch during diastole, the more forcefully they contract during systole. Think of preload as the balloon stretching as air is blown into it. The more air being blown, the greater the stretch.

The balloon's stretch

Contractility refers to the inherent ability of the myocardium to contract normally. Contractility is influenced by preload. The greater the stretch, the more forceful the contraction—or, the more air in the balloon, the greater the stretch and the farther the balloon will fly when air is allowed to expel.

The knot that ties the balloon

Afterload refers to the pressure that the ventricular muscles must generate to overcome the higher pressure in the aorta to get the blood out of the heart. *Resistance* is the knot on the end of the balloon, which the balloon has to work against to get the air out.

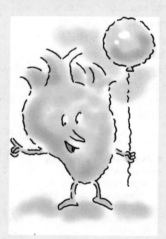

Blood flow

Blood flows through the body in five types of vessels, involving three methods of circulation.

Blood vessels

The five distinct types of blood vessels are:
- arteries
- arterioles
- capillaries
- venules
- veins.

The structure of each type of vessel differs according to its function in the cardiovascular system and the pressure exerted by the volume of blood at various sites within the system.

Built for high speed...

Arteries have thick, muscular walls to accommodate the flow of blood at high speeds and pressures. *Arterioles* have thinner walls than arteries. They constrict or dilate to control blood flow to the *capillaries*, which (being microscopic) have walls composed of only a single layer of endothelial cells.

...and low pressure

Venules gather blood from the capillaries; their walls are thinner than those of arterioles. *Veins* have thinner walls than arteries but have larger diameters because of the low blood pressure of venous return to the heart.

Frequent flyer miles

About 60,000 miles of arteries, arterioles, capillaries, venules, and veins keep blood circulating to and from every functioning cell in the body. (See *Major arteries*, page 12 and *Major veins*, page 13.)

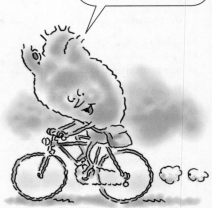

> Combined, the arterioles, venules, and capillaries equal nearly 60,000 miles of blood vessels.

Circulation

Three methods of circulation carry blood throughout the body: pulmonary, systemic, and coronary.

Pulmonary circulation

In pulmonary circulation, blood travels to the lungs to pick up oxygen and release carbon dioxide.

Returns and exchanges

As blood moves from the heart to the lungs and back again, it proceeds as follows:

* Unoxygenated blood travels from the right ventricle through the pulmonic valve into the pulmonary arteries.
* Blood passes through progressively smaller arteries and arterioles into the capillaries of the lungs.
* Blood reaches the alveoli and exchanges carbon dioxide for oxygen.
* Oxygenated blood then returns via venules and veins to the pulmonary veins, which carry it back to the heart's left atrium.

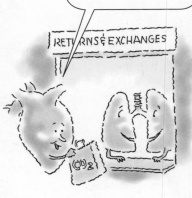

> I'd like to exchange this for some oxygen, please.

Systemic circulation

Systemic circulation begins when blood pumped from the left ventricle carries oxygen and other nutrients to body cells. This same circulation also transports waste products for excretion.

Major arteries

This illustration shows the body's major arteries.

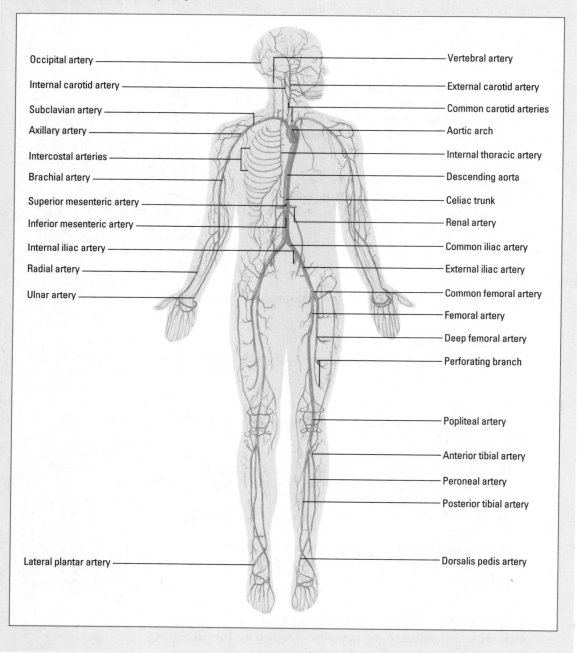

Occipital artery

Internal carotid artery

Subclavian artery

Axillary artery

Intercostal arteries

Brachial artery

Superior mesenteric artery

Inferior mesenteric artery

Internal iliac artery

Radial artery

Ulnar artery

Lateral plantar artery

Vertebral artery

External carotid artery

Common carotid arteries

Aortic arch

Internal thoracic artery

Descending aorta

Celiac trunk

Renal artery

Common iliac artery

External iliac artery

Common femoral artery

Femoral artery

Deep femoral artery

Perforating branch

Popliteal artery

Anterior tibial artery

Peroneal artery

Posterior tibial artery

Dorsalis pedis artery

Major veins

This illustration shows the body's major veins.

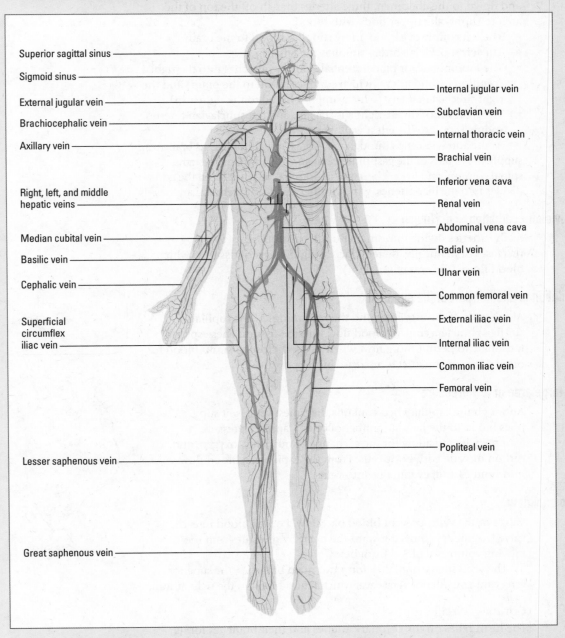

Superior sagittal sinus

Sigmoid sinus

External jugular vein

Brachiocephalic vein

Axillary vein

Right, left, and middle hepatic veins

Median cubital vein

Basilic vein

Cephalic vein

Superficial circumflex iliac vein

Lesser saphenous vein

Great saphenous vein

Internal jugular vein

Subclavian vein

Internal thoracic vein

Brachial vein

Inferior vena cava

Renal vein

Abdominal vena cava

Radial vein

Ulnar vein

Common femoral vein

External iliac vein

Internal iliac vein

Common iliac vein

Femoral vein

Popliteal vein

Branching out

The major artery, the aorta, branches into vessels that supply specific organs and areas of the body. As it arches out of the top of the heart and down to the abdomen, three arteries branch off the top of the arch to supply the upper body with blood:
- The left common carotid artery supplies blood to the brain.
- The left subclavian artery supplies the left arm.
- The innominate, or brachiocephalic, artery branches into the right common carotid artery (which supplies blood to the brain) and the right subclavian artery (which supplies blood to the right arm).
- The right innominate, right subclavian, and left subclavian arteries supply blood to the chest wall.

As the aorta descends through the thorax and abdomen, its branches supply the organs of the gastrointestinal and genitourinary systems, spinal column, and lower chest and abdominal muscles. Then the aorta divides into the iliac arteries, which further divide into femoral arteries.

Division = addition = perfusion

As the arteries divide into smaller units, the number of vessels increases dramatically, thereby increasing the area of tissue to which blood flows (the *area of perfusion*).

Dilation is another part of the equation

At the ends of the arterioles and the beginnings of the capillaries, strong sphincters control blood flow into the tissues. These sphincters dilate to permit more flow when needed, close to shunt blood to other areas, or constrict to increase blood pressure.

A large area of low pressure

Although the capillary bed contains the tiniest vessels, it supplies blood to the largest number of cells. Capillary pressure is extremely low to allow for the exchange of nutrients, oxygen, and carbon dioxide with body cells. From the capillaries, blood flows into venules and, eventually, into veins.

No backflow

Valves in the veins prevent blood backflow. Pooled blood in each valved segment is moved toward the heart by pressure from the moving volume of blood from below.

The veins merge until they form two main branches, the superior vena cava and inferior vena cava, which return blood to the right atrium.

Coronary circulation
The heart relies on the coronary arteries and their branches for its supply of oxygenated blood. It also depends on the cardiac veins to remove oxygen-depleted blood. (See *Vessels that supply the heart.*)

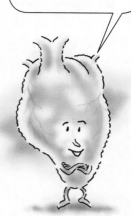

Valves in the veins prevent blood backflow.

Vessels that supply the heart

Coronary circulation involves the arterial system of blood vessels that supplies oxygenated blood to the heart and the venous system that removes oxygen-depleted blood from it. Think of it as "A = Away," meaning the "**A**rteries" carry oxygenated blood **away** from the heart to the rest of the body, whereas "V = Venue," meaning the "**V**eins" carry unoxygenated blood **back** to the **v**enue or the site of the exchange, which is the heart.

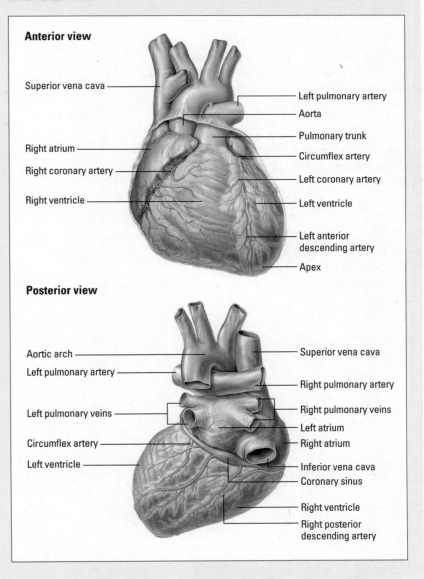

Anterior view

- Superior vena cava
- Right atrium
- Right coronary artery
- Right ventricle
- Left pulmonary artery
- Aorta
- Pulmonary trunk
- Circumflex artery
- Left coronary artery
- Left ventricle
- Left anterior descending artery
- Apex

Posterior view

- Aortic arch
- Left pulmonary artery
- Left pulmonary veins
- Circumflex artery
- Left ventricle
- Superior vena cava
- Right pulmonary artery
- Right pulmonary veins
- Left atrium
- Right atrium
- Inferior vena cava
- Coronary sinus
- Right ventricle
- Right posterior descending artery

The heart gets its part

During left ventricular systole, blood is ejected into the aorta. During diastole, blood flows out of the heart and then through the coronary arteries to nourish the heart muscle.

From the right...

The right coronary artery supplies blood to the right atrium, part of the left atrium, most of the right ventricle, and the inferior part of the left ventricle.

...and from the left

The left coronary artery, which splits into the anterior descending artery and circumflex artery, supplies blood to the left atrium, most of the left ventricle, and most of the interventricular septum.

Superficially speaking

The cardiac veins lie superficial to the arteries. The largest vein, the coronary sinus, opens into the right atrium. Most of the major cardiac veins empty into the coronary sinus; the anterior cardiac veins, however, empty into the right atrium.

Suggested references

Bickley, L. S., Szilagyi, P. G., Hoffman, R. M., & Soriano, R. P. (2023). *Bates' guide to physical examination and history taking* (13th ed.). Wolters Kluwer.

Jarvis, C., & Eckhardt, A. L. (2024). *Physical examination & health assessment* (9th ed.). Elsevier.

Chapter 2

Assessment

Just the facts

In this chapter, you'll learn:

◆ components of a cardiovascular health history
◆ techniques used in a physical examination of the cardiovascular system
◆ normal and abnormal cardiovascular findings.

Obtaining a health history

The first step in assessing the cardiovascular system is to obtain a health history. Begin by introducing yourself and explaining what will occur first during the health history and later during the physical examination. Then ask about the patient's chief complaint. Be sure to ask about the patient's personal *and* family health history. Remember, the health history interview is an interview with a purpose.

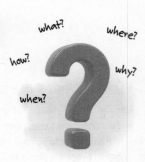

Chief complaint

You'll find that patients with cardiovascular problems typically cite specific complaints, such as chest pain, palpitations, syncope, intermittent claudication, and peripheral edema. Let's take a closer look at each of these chief complaints as well as some other common signs and symptoms.

Chest pain

Many patients with cardiovascular problems complain, at some point, of chest pain. Chest pain can arise suddenly or gradually and can radiate to the arms, neck, jaw, or back. It can be steady, intermittent, or even chronic; mild or acute; and can range, in character, from a sharp, shooting sensation to a feeling of heaviness, fullness, or even indigestion. At times, patients may deny pain but will describe chest discomfort, which presents in diverse ways.

RX
• Why are you here today?
• What does your problem feel like?
• Where does it hurt?
• When did your problem begin?
• When did the problem get worse?
• How is the problem relieved?
• What other family members have had this problem?

A full menu of causes

The cause of chest pain may be difficult to determine at first. Chest pain can be provoked or aggravated by stress, anxiety, exertion, deep breathing, or consumption of certain foods. (See *Understanding chest pain*, page 19.)

Pinpointing pain

If the patient's chest pain isn't severe, proceed with obtaining the history. Ask if the patient feels diffuse pain or can point to the painful area. Ask if they have any discomfort that radiates to their neck, jaw, arms, or back. If they do, ask them to describe it. Is it a dull, aching, pressurelike sensation? A sharp, stabbing, knifelike pain? Do they feel it on the surface or deep inside? Ask them to rate the pain on a scale of 1 to 10 in which 1 means negligible and 10 means the worst imaginable.

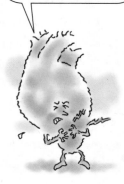

The pain I'm experiencing is sudden, radiating, steady, acute, and sharp. Does that help?

PQRST: What's the story?

Use the PQRST mnemonic to fully explore your patient's chest pain. When you ask the questions below, you'll encourage them to describe their symptom in greater detail.

*Remember to streamline your questions according to the patient's pain severity so that emergency care can be initiated promptly when indicated.

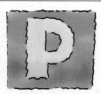 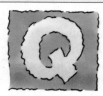 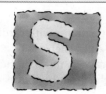

Provocative or palliative	**Quality or quantity**	**Region or radiation**	**Severity**	**Timing**
• What provokes or relieves the chest pain? • What makes the pain worsen or subside?	• What does the pain feel like? • Are you having the pain right now? If so, is it more or less severe than usual? • To what degree does chest pain affect your normal activities?	• Where in the chest does the pain occur? • Does the pain appear in other regions as well? If so, where?	• How severe is the chest pain? How would you rate it on a scale of 0 to 10, with 10 being the most severe? • Does the pain seem to be diminishing, intensifying, or staying about the same?	• When did the pain begin? • Was the onset sudden or gradual? • How often does the pain occur? • How long does it last?

Understanding chest pain

Use this table to help you more accurately assess chest pain and its possible causes.

What it feels like	Where it's located	What makes it worse	What causes it	What makes it better
Aching, squeezing, pressure, heaviness, burning pain; usually subsides within 10 minutes	Substernal; may radiate to jaw, neck, arms, and back	Eating, physical effort, smoking, cold weather, stress, anger, hunger, supine position	Angina pectoris	Rest, nitroglycerin (Note: Unstable angina appears even at rest.)
Tightness or pressure; burning, aching pain; possibly accompanied by shortness of breath, diaphoresis, weakness, anxiety, or nausea; sudden onset; lasts 30 minutes to 2 hours	Typically across chest but may radiate to jaw, neck, arms, and back	Exertion, anxiety	Acute coronary syndromes, which include acute myocardial infarction and unstable angina	Opioid analgesics such as morphine and nitroglycerin
Chest pain associated with diaphoresis, shortness of breath, extreme fatigue, palpitations, nausea, or dizziness	Across chest and may radiate to jaw, arms, or shoulders	Emotional stress, uncontrolled high blood pressure, and extreme physical exercise	Spontaneous coronary artery dissection	Nitroglycerin and calcium channel blockers; coronary stenting or surgery may be needed.
Sharp and continuous pain; may be accompanied by friction rub; sudden onset	Substernal; may radiate to neck and left arm	Deep breathing, supine position	Pericarditis	Sitting up, leaning forward, anti-inflammatory drugs
Excruciating, tearing pain; may be accompanied by blood pressure difference between right and left arm; sudden onset	Retrosternal, upper abdominal, or epigastric; may radiate to back, neck, and shoulders	Not applicable	Dissecting aortic aneurysm	Opioid analgesics, surgery
Sudden, stabbing pain; may be accompanied by cyanosis, dyspnea, or cough with hemoptysis	Anterior and posterior thorax	Inspiration	Pulmonary embolus	Analgesics
Sudden and severe pain; sometimes accompanied by dyspnea, increased pulse rate, decreased breath sounds, or deviated trachea	Lateral thorax	Normal respiration	Pneumothorax	Analgesics, chest tube insertion

(Continued)

Understanding chest pain (continued)

What it feels like	Where it's located	What makes it worse	What causes it	What makes it better
Dull, pressurelike, squeezing pain	Substernal, epigastric areas	Food, cold liquids, exercise	Esophageal spasm	Nitroglycerin, calcium channel blockers
Sharp, severe pain	Lower chest or upper abdomen	Eating a heavy meal, bending, supine position	Hiatal hernia	Antacids, walking, semi-Fowler position
Burning feeling after eating; sometimes accompanied by hematemesis or tarry stools; sudden onset that generally subsides within 15–20 minutes	Epigastric area	Lack of food, eating highly acidic foods	Peptic ulcer	Food, antacids
Gripping, sharp pain; may be accompanied by nausea and vomiting	Right epigastric or abdominal areas; may radiate to shoulders	Eating fatty foods, supine position	Cholecystitis	Rest and analgesics, surgery
Continuous or intermittent sharp pain; possibly tender to touch; gradual or sudden onset	Anywhere in chest	Movement, palpation	Chest wall syndrome/ costochondritis	Time, analgesics, heat applications
Dull or stabbing pain; usually accompanied by hyperventilation or breathlessness; sudden onset; can last less than a minute or as long as several days	Anywhere in chest	Increased respiratory rate, stress, anxiety	Acute anxiety	Slowing of respiratory rate, stress relief

Going steady?

Then find out whether the pain is constant or intermittent. If it's intermittent, how long does it last? Ask if movement, exertion, breathing, position changes, or eating certain foods worsens or helps relieve the pain. Does anything in particular seem to bring it on? Find out what medications the patient is taking, if any, and ask about recent dosage or schedule changes.

Palpitations

Defined as a conscious awareness of one's heartbeat, palpitations are usually felt over the precordium or in the throat or neck. The patient may describe them as pounding, jumping, turning, fluttering, or flopping. They may also describe a sensation of missed or skipped beats. Palpitations may be regular or irregular, fast or slow, paroxysmal or sustained.

Don't skip this beat

To help characterize the palpitations, ask the patient to simulate their rhythm by tapping their finger on a hard surface. An irregular "skipped beat" rhythm points to premature ventricular contractions, whereas an episodic racing rhythm that ends abruptly suggests paroxysmal atrial tachycardia (brief periods of tachycardia alternating with normal sinus rhythm).

> A racing rhythm that suddenly stops can mean paroxysmal atrial tachycardia. No slamming on the brakes for me!

Maybe it was that triple shot of espresso

Next, ask if the patient has a history of hypertension or if they have recently started digoxin therapy. Be sure to obtain a drug history and ask about caffeine, tobacco, and alcohol consumption and use of herbal supplements or illicit drugs. Do not forget to ask about energy drinks, as palpitations may accompany use of these substances.

No big deal—unless...

Palpitations are typically insignificant and are relatively common. However, they can be caused by such cardiovascular disorders as arrhythmias, hypertension, mitral prolapse, and mitral stenosis. Additionally, short circuits in the electrical conduction can lead to waves of abnormal firing.

Syncope

Syncope is a brief, self-limiting loss of consciousness caused by a lack of blood flow to the brain. It usually occurs abruptly and lasts for seconds to minutes. It may result from such cardiovascular disorders as aortic arch syndrome, aortic stenosis, arrhythmias, and postural orthostatic tachycardia syndrome.

Barely breathing

When syncope occurs, the patient typically lies motionless, with their skeletal muscles relaxed. The depth of unconsciousness varies—some patients can hear voices or see blurred outlines; others are unaware of their surroundings. Often the patient is strikingly pale

RX

Ask the patient the following questions about their palpitations:
- What are your palpitations like? For example, are they pounding, jumping, fluttering, or flopping or bopping?
- Do you have a sensation of missed or skipped beats?
- Do you have a history of hypertension?
- Have you recently started digoxin therapy?
- What medications do you take?
- Do you smoke, drink caffeinated beverages, or consume alcohol? If so, how much?

with a slow, weak pulse; is hypotensive; and has almost imperceptible breathing.

Fainting facts

If the patient reports a fainting episode, gather information about the episode from the patient and their family. Did the patient feel weak, light-headed, nauseated, or diaphoretic just before they fainted? Did the patient change position quickly getting up from a chair or from lying down? Any visual changes, such as blurring or narrow visual field? During the fainting episode, did the patient have muscle spasms or incontinence? How long were they unconscious? When they regained consciousness, was the patient alert or confused? Did they have a headache? Have they fainted before? If so, how often do the episodes occur?

Intermittent claudication

Intermittent claudication is cramping limb pain that's brought on by exercise and relieved by 1 or 2 minutes of rest. It most commonly occurs in the legs and is a prominent symptom of peripheral arterial disease. This pain may be acute or chronic. When pain is acute and not relieved by rest, it may signal acute arterial occlusion.

Midlife crisis

Intermittent claudication is most common in males ages 50 to 60 who have a history of diabetes mellitus, hyperlipidemia, hypertension, or tobacco use. It typically results from such cardiovascular disorders as aortic arteriosclerotic occlusive disease, acute arterial occlusion, or arteriosclerosis obliterans.

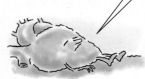

Hmm...
The patient is pale and motionless; has a slow, weak pulse; and is hypotensive. They are barely breathing. I'd say they are not getting enough blood to their brain.

RX

Ask the patient the following questions about their syncope:
• Did you feel weak, light-headed, nauseous, or sweaty just before you fainted?
• Did you get up quickly from a chair or from lying down?
• During the fainting episode, did you have muscle spasms or incontinence?

• How long were you unconscious?
• When you regained consciousness, were you alert or confused? Did you have a headache?
• Have you fainted before? If so, how often do the episodes occur?

Claudication interrogation

If the legs are affected, ask the patient how far they can walk before pain occurs and how long they must rest before it subsides. Can the patient walk as far as they could before, or do they need to rest longer? Does the pain–rest pattern vary? Is the pain in one leg or both? Where is the pain located? Has the pain affected the patient's lifestyle?

Peripheral edema

Peripheral edema results from excess interstitial fluid in the arms or legs. It may be unilateral or bilateral, slight or dramatic, pitting or nonpitting.

In your face (and arm and leg)

Arm and facial edema may be caused by superior vena cava syndrome or thrombophlebitis. Leg edema is an early sign of heart failure, especially if it's bilateral. It can also signal thrombophlebitis and chronic venous insufficiency.

Since when?

Ask the patient how long they have had the edema. Did it develop suddenly or gradually? Does the edema decrease if the patient elevates their arms or legs? Is it worse in the mornings, or does it get progressively worse during the day? Did the patient recently injure the affected extremities or have surgery or an illness that may have immobilized them? Does the patient have a history of any cardiovascular disease? What medications, if any, is the patient currently taking? What medications has the patient taken in the past?

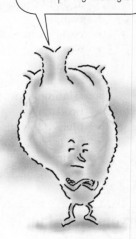

Intermittent claudication really cramps my lifestyle.

RX

Ask the patient the following questions about their intermittent claudication:
- How far can you walk before pain occurs?
- How long must you rest before it subsides?
- Can you walk as far as you could before, or must you rest more often?
- Does the pain–rest pattern vary?
- Has this symptom affected your lifestyle?

RX

Ask the patient the following questions about their peripheral edema:
- How long have you had the edema?
- Did it develop suddenly or gradually?
- Does the edema decrease if you elevate your extremity?
- Is it worse in the mornings, or does it progressively worsen during the day?
- Did you recently injure the affected extremity or have surgery or an illness that caused you to be immobile?
- Do you have a history of cardiovascular disease?
- Are you taking prescription or over-the-counter medications?

Other signs and symptoms

Other common signs and symptoms to ask the patient about include:

- shortness of breath on exertion, when lying down (orthopnea), or at night (paroxysmal nocturnal dyspnea)
- cough
- cyanosis or pallor
- weakness
- fatigue
- unexplained weight change
- fainting (syncope)
- headache
- high or low blood pressure
- nocturia
- peripheral skin changes, such as decreased hair distribution; skin color changes; or a thin, shiny appearance to the skin.

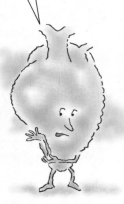

Yeah, yeah. Blame me. Shortness of breath and coughing can be heart-related.

Personal and family health

After you've asked about the patient's chief complaint, then inquire about their family history and past medical history, including heart disease; diabetes; and chronic lung, kidney, or liver disease. (See *Recognizing cardio risk*.)

Recognizing cardio risk

As you analyze a patient's condition, remember that age, sex, and race are important considerations in identifying patients at risk for cardiovascular disorders.

Most common

For example, coronary artery disease most commonly affects White males between ages 40 and 60. Hypertension is most common in Black people.

Also at risk

Females are also vulnerable to heart disease. Postmenopausal females and those with diabetes mellitus are at particular risk and are more likely to present with atypical symptoms.

We aren't getting any younger

Overall, older people have a higher incidence of cardiovascular disease than do younger people. Many older people have increased systolic blood pressure because blood vessel walls become increasingly rigid with age.

All in the family

Ask if any family members have had heart disease, a history of myocardial infarction (MI); heart failure; cerebrovascular accident; or an unexplained, sudden death. Find out at what age the MIs occurred.

Getting personal

In addition to obtaining information about the patient's family history, be sure to ask the patient about their:

- stress level and coping mechanisms
- current health habits, such as smoking and exercise habits, alcohol and caffeine intake, and dietary intake of fat and sodium
- drug use, including over-the-counter drugs, illicit drugs, and herbal supplements
- previous surgeries
- environmental or occupational hazards
- activities of daily living.

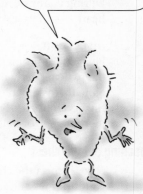

Remember to ask about a patient's occupational risks. Standing for long periods at work can be problematic.

Also related

Also ask the patient these questions:

- Are you ever short of breath? If so, what activities cause you to be short of breath?
- How many pillows do you use for sleep?
- Do you sleep sitting up?
- Do you feel dizzy or light-headed?
- Has your energy level decreased, or are you unable to do things you used to?
- Do your rings or shoes feel tight?
- Do your ankles swell?
- Have you noticed changes in color or sensation in your legs? If so, what are those changes?
- If you have sores or ulcers, how quickly do they heal?
- Do you stand or sit in one place for long periods at work?

Performing a physical assessment

The key to accurate assessment is regular practice, which helps improve technique and efficiency. A consistent, methodical approach to your assessment can help you identify abnormalities.

Shopping list

For the physical assessment, you'll need a stethoscope with a bell and a diaphragm, an appropriate-sized blood pressure cuff, a ruler, and a penlight or other flexible light source. Make sure the room is quiet.

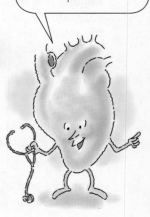

I have my stethoscope. Now, all I need is a patient!

Dressed down

Ask the patient to remove all clothing except their underwear and to put on an examination gown. Have the patient lie on their back, with the head of the examination table at a 30° to 45° angle. Stand on the patient's right side for the exam because you may need the patient to assume a left lateral recumbent position to move the heart closer to the chest wall.

Assessing the heart

During your assessment, inspect, palpate, percuss, and auscultate the heart.

Inspection

First, take a moment to assess the patient's general appearance. Is the patient overly thin? Is the patient overweight? Alert? Anxious? Note their skin color, temperature, turgor, and texture. Are their fingers clubbed? If the patient is dark-skinned, inspect their mucous membranes for pallor.

Checking out the chest

Next, inspect the chest. Note landmarks you can use to describe your findings and to identify structures underlying the chest wall. (See *Identifying cardiovascular landmarks*.) Also, look for pulsations, symmetry of movement, retractions, or heaves (a strong outward thrust of the chest wall that occurs during systole).

Location, location

Position a light source, such as a flashlight or gooseneck lamp, so that it casts a shadow on the patient's chest. Note the location of the apical impulse. You should find it in the fifth intercostal space, medial to the left midclavicular line. Because it corresponds to the apex of the heart, the apical pulse helps indicate how well the left ventricle is working. The apical pulse is usually the point of maximal impulse (PMI). In patients with an enlarged heart (cardiomegaly), the PMI may be displaced laterally toward the axilla.

Remember, though, that the apical impulse can only be seen in about 50% of adults. You'll notice it more easily in children and in patients with thin chest walls. To find the apical impulse in a female with large breasts, displace the breasts during the examination.

Palpation

Maintain a gentle touch when you palpate so that you don't obscure pulsations or similar findings. Using the ball of your hand, then your

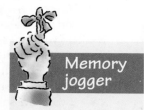

Memory jogger

To remember the order in which you should perform assessment of the cardiovascular system, just think, "I'll Properly Perform Assessment":

Inspection

Palpation

Percussion

Auscultation

Identifying cardiovascular landmarks

These views show where to find critical landmarks used in cardiovascular assessment.

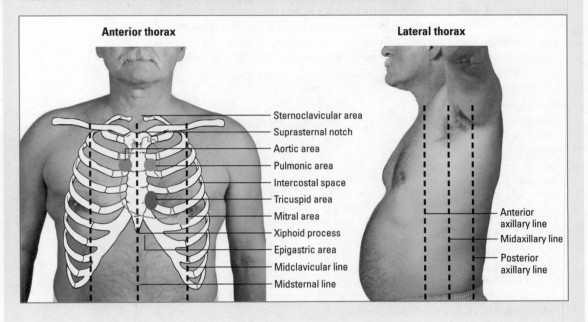

Anterior thorax

- Sternoclavicular area
- Suprasternal notch
- Aortic area
- Pulmonic area
- Intercostal space
- Tricuspid area
- Mitral area
- Xiphoid process
- Epigastric area
- Midclavicular line
- Midsternal line

Lateral thorax

- Anterior axillary line
- Midaxillary line
- Posterior axillary line

fingertips, palpate over the precordium to find the apical impulse. Note heaves or thrills (fine vibrations that feel like the purring of a cat). (See *Palpating the apical impulse*, page 27.)

The apical impulse may be difficult to palpate in a pregnant patient, a patient who carries extra weight, or a patient with a thick chest wall. If it's difficult to palpate with the patient lying on their back, have them lie on their left side or sit upright. It may also be helpful to have the patient exhale completely and hold their breath for a few seconds.

Not normally there

Palpate the sternoclavicular, aortic, pulmonic, tricuspid, and epigastric areas for pulsations, which normally aren't felt in those areas. In thin patients, an aortic arch pulsation in the sternoclavicular area or an abdominal aorta pulsation in the epigastric area may be a normal finding.

Palpating the apical impulse

The apical impulse is associated with the first heart sound and carotid pulsation. To ensure that you're feeling the apical impulse and not a muscle spasm or some other pulsation, use one hand to palpate the patient's carotid artery and the other to palpate the apical impulse. Then compare the timing and regularity of the impulses. The apical impulse should roughly coincide with the carotid pulsation. The point of maximal impulse (PMI) may be laterally displaced toward the anterior axillary line in a patient with cardiomegaly.

Note the amplitude, size, intensity, location, and duration of the apical impulse. You should feel a gentle pulsation in an area about ½" to ¾" (1.5 to 2 cm) in diameter.

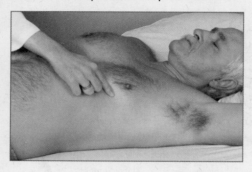

Percussion

Although percussion isn't as useful as other assessment techniques, it may help you locate cardiac borders.

From resonance to dullness

Begin percussing at the anterior axillary line and percuss toward the sternum along the third, fourth, and fifth intercostal spaces. The sound changes from resonance to dullness over the left border of the heart, normally at the midclavicular line. The right border of the heart is typically aligned with the sternum and can't be percussed.

Borderline trouble

Percussion may be difficult in a patient who carries a lot of extra weight (because of the fat overlying the chest) or in a female patient (because of breast tissue). In this case, a chest x-ray can be used to provide information about the heart border.

Auscultation

You can learn a great deal about the heart by auscultating for heart sounds. Cardiac auscultation requires a methodical approach and lots of practice. Begin by warming the stethoscope in your hands and then identify the sites where you'll auscultate: over the four cardiac valves, at Erb point, and the third intercostal space at the left sternal border. Use the bell to hear low-pitched sounds and the diaphragm to hear high-pitched sounds. (See *Sites for heart sounds*.)

Have a plan

Auscultate for heart sounds with the patient in three positions: lying on their back with the head of the bed raised 30° to 45°, sitting up, and lying on their left side. You can start at the base and work downward or start at the apex and work upward. Whichever approach you use, be consistent. (See *Auscultation tips*, page 30.)

Use the diaphragm to listen as you go in one direction; use the bell as you come back in the other direction. Be sure to listen over the entire precordium, not just over the valves.

Determine the *dub*

As you proceed, note the heart rate and rhythm. Always identify normal heart sounds (S_1 and S_2) and then listen for adventitious sounds, such as third and fourth heart sounds (S_3 and S_4), murmurs, and rubs.

Start auscultating at the aortic, over the second intercostal space, along the right sternal border, where S_2 is loudest. The S_2 is best heard at the base of the heart at the end of ventricular systole. This sound corresponds to closure of the pulmonic and aortic valves and is generally described as sounding like "dub." It's a shorter, louder, higher pitched sound than S_1. When the pulmonic valve closes later than the

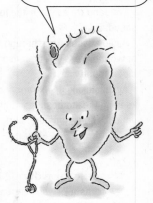

Now hear this: Auscultation is one of the most important—and difficult—parts of the assessment.

Sites for heart sounds

When auscultating for heart sounds, place the stethoscope over the **five** different sites illustrated at right.

Normal heart sounds indicate events in the cardiac cycle, such as the closing of heart valves, and are reflected to specific areas of the chest wall. Auscultation sites are identified by the names of heart valves but aren't located directly over the valves. Rather, these sites are located along the pathway blood takes as it flows through the heart's chambers and valves.

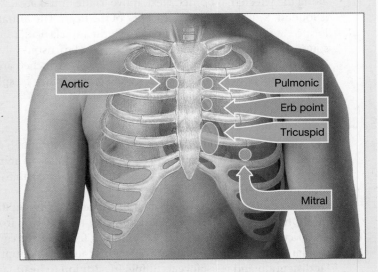

Auscultation tips

Follow these tips when you auscultate a patient's heart:
• Concentrate as you listen for each sound.
• Avoid auscultating through clothing or wound dressings because they can block sound.
• Avoid picking up extraneous sounds by keeping the stethoscope tubing off the patient's body and other surfaces.

• Until you gain proficiency at auscultation and can examine a patient quickly, explain to them that even though you may listen to their chest for a long period, it doesn't necessarily mean anything is wrong.
• Ask the patient to breathe normally and to hold their breath periodically to enhance sounds that may be difficult to hear.

aortic valve during inspiration, you'll hear a split S_2, which is referred to as a physiological split. A fixed split of S_2 does not change with respiration and may be indicative of right ventricular failure or an atrial septal defect.

Listen for the *lub*

From the base of the heart, move to the pulmonic area, at the second intercostal space, at the left sternal border, and then down to the tricuspid area, which lies over the fourth and fifth intercostal spaces, along the left sternal border. Next, move to the mitral area, where S_1 is loudest. S_1 is best heard at the apex of the heart. The mitral area is located at the fifth intercostal space near the midclavicular line. This sound corresponds to closure of the mitral and tricuspid valves and is generally described as sounding like "lub." Low-pitched and dull, S_1 occurs at the beginning of ventricular systole. It may be split if the mitral valve closes just before the tricuspid valve.

S_3: Classic sign of heart failure

S_3 is commonly heard in children and in patients with high cardiac output (CO). Called a *ventricular gallop* when it occurs in adults, S_3 may be a cardinal sign of heart failure. But don't worry, an S_3 is common in children.

S_3 is best heard at the apex when the patient is lying on their left side. Often compared to the *y* sound in "Ken-tuck-y," S_3 is low-pitched and occurs when the ventricles fill rapidly. It follows S_2 in early ventricular diastole and results from vibrations caused by abrupt ventricular distention and resistance to filling. In addition to heart failure, S_3

may also be associated with such conditions as pulmonary edema, atrial septal defect, and acute MI. It may also be heard during the last trimester of pregnancy.

S₄: An MI aftereffect

Also called an *atrial gallop*, S_4 is an adventitious heart sound that's heard over the tricuspid or mitral area when the patient is on their left side. You may hear an S_4 in patients who are older or those with hypertension, aortic stenosis, or history of MI.

S_4, commonly described as sounding like "Ten-nes-see," occurs just before S_1, after atrial contraction. The S_4 sound indicates increased resistance to ventricular filling. It results from vibrations caused by the forceful atrial ejection of blood into ventricles, that don't move or expand as much as they should.

Auscultating for murmurs

Murmurs occur when structural defects in the heart's chambers or valves cause turbulent blood flow. Turbulence may also be caused by changes in blood viscosity or the speed of blood flow. Listen for murmurs over the same precordial areas used in auscultation for heart sounds.

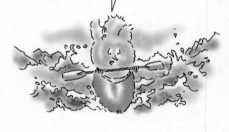

Whoa! A murmur is turbulent blood flow caused by a structural defect in the heart.

Making the grade

Murmurs can occur during systole or diastole and are described by several criteria. (See *Tips for describing murmurs*.) Their pitch can be high, medium, or low. They can vary in intensity, growing louder or softer. (See *Grading murmurs*.) Murmurs can vary by location, sound pattern (blowing, harsh, or musical), radiation (to the neck or axillae), and the time period during which they occur within the cardiac cycle (pansystolic or midsystolic).

For more information, see "Murmurs," page 41.

Grading murmurs

Use the system outlined below to describe the intensity of a murmur. When recording your findings, use Roman numerals as part of a fraction, always with VI as the denominator. For instance, a grade III murmur would be recorded as "grade III/VI."
- Grade I is a barely audible murmur.
- Grade II is audible but quiet and soft.
- Grade III is moderately loud, without a thrust or thrill.
- Grade IV is loud, with a thrill.
- Grade V is very loud, with a thrust or a thrill.
- Grade VI is loud enough to be heard before the stethoscope comes into contact with the chest.

Advice from the experts

Tips for describing murmurs

Describing murmurs can be tricky. After you've auscultated a murmur, list the terms you would use to describe it. Then check the patient's chart to see how others have described it or ask an experienced colleague to listen and describe the murmur. Compare the descriptions and then auscultate for the murmur again, if necessary, to confirm the description.

Differentiating murmurs

What you'll hear	Where you'll hear it	What causes it
• Medium pitch • Harsh quality • Possibly musical at apex • Loudest with expiration • Grade IV or higher		Aortic stenosis
• Medium pitch • Harsh quality • Variable-grade intensity		Hypertrophic cardiomyopathy
• High pitch • Blowing quality • Grade I–III intensity		Aortic insufficiency
• Medium to high pitch • Blowing quality • Soft to loud grade intensity		Mitral insufficiency
• Medium to high pitch • Blowing quality • Variable intensity • Increases slightly with inspiration		Tricuspid insufficiency
• High pitch • Harsh quality • Grade V or VI intensity		Ventricular septal defect
• Low pitch • Rumbling quality • Grade I–IV intensity		Mitral stenosis

= Bell
= Diaphragm

Sit up, please

The best way to hear murmurs is with the patient sitting up and leaning forward. You can also have them lie on their left side. (See *Positioning the patient for auscultation*, page 33.)

Auscultating for pericardial friction rub

Listening for a pericardial friction rub is also an important part of your assessment. To do this, have the patient sit upright, lean forward, and exhale. Listen with the diaphragm of the stethoscope over the third intercostal space on the left side of the chest. A pericardial friction rub has a scratchy, rubbing quality. If you suspect a rub but have trouble hearing one, ask the patient to hold their breath.

Peak technique

Positioning the patient for auscultation

If heart sounds are faint or undetectable, try listening to them with the patient seated and leaning forward or lying on their left side, which brings the heart closer to the surface of the chest. These illustrations show how to position the patient for high- and low-pitched sounds.

Forward leaning

The forward-leaning position is best suited for hearing high-pitched sounds related to semilunar valve problems, such as aortic and pulmonic valve murmurs. To auscultate for these sounds, place the diaphragm of the stethoscope over the aortic and pulmonic areas in the right and left second intercostal spaces, as shown at right.

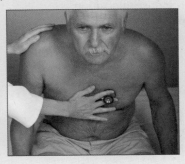

Left lateral recumbent

The left lateral recumbent position is best suited for hearing low-pitched sounds, such as mitral valve murmurs and extra heart sounds. To hear these sounds, place the bell of the stethoscope over the apical area, as shown at right.

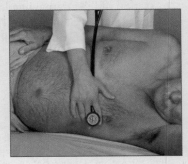

Assessing the vascular system

Assessing the vascular system is important because it can reveal arterial and venous disorders. Examine the patient's arms when you assess their vital signs. Check the patient's legs later during the physical examination, when they are lying on their back. Remember to evaluate leg veins when the patient is standing.

Inspection

Start your assessment of the vascular system the same way you start an assessment of the cardiac system—by making general observations. Are the arms equal in size? Are the legs symmetrical?

Inspect the skin color. Note how body hair is distributed. Also note lesions, scars, cyanosis, clubbing, and edema of the extremities. If the patient is confined to bed, check the sacrum for swelling. Examine the fingernails and toenails for abnormalities such as pulsations or transverse lines.

Start at the top

Next, move on to a closer inspection. Start by observing the vessels in the patient's neck. Inspection of these vessels can provide information about blood volume and pressure in the right side of the heart.

The carotid artery should appear to have a brisk, localized pulsation. This pulsation does not decrease when the patient is upright, when they inhale, or during palpation. Note whether the pulsations are weak or bounding.

Inspect the jugular veins. The internal jugular vein has a softer, undulating pulsation. Unlike the pulsation of the carotid artery, pulsation of the internal jugular vein changes in response to position, breathing, and palpation. The vein normally protrudes when the patient is lying down and flattens when the patient stands.

RX

- Are the patient's arms equal in size?
- Are the patient's legs symmetrical?
- When the patient stands, what do their leg veins look like?
- How would you describe the patient's skin color?
- How is the patient's body hair distributed?
- Does the patient have lesions or scars?
- Do you see signs of clubbing or edema of the extremities?
- If the patient is confined to bed, is their sacrum swollen?
- Do the patient's fingernails or toenails have any abnormalities?

Take this lying down

To check the jugular venous pulse, have the patient lie on their back. Elevate the head of the bed 30° to 45° and turn the patient's head slightly away from you. Normally, the highest pulsation occurs no more than 1.5″ (about 4 cm) above the sternal notch. Pulsations above that point indicate central venous pressure elevation and jugular vein distention (See *Assessing jugular vein distention*).

Assessing jugular vein distention

Now inspect the jugular veins. The internal jugular vein has a softer, undulating pulsation. Unlike the pulsation of the carotid artery, pulsation of the internal jugular vein changes in response to position, breathing, and palpation. The vein normally protrudes when the patient is lying down and lies flat when they stand.

When jugular vein distention is detected, place the patient at a 45° angle and then measure the distention with a horizontal straight edge aligned with the top of the pulsations. Then, read the vertical distance on a ruler. A measurement of 3 to 4 cm above the sternal angle is abnormal.

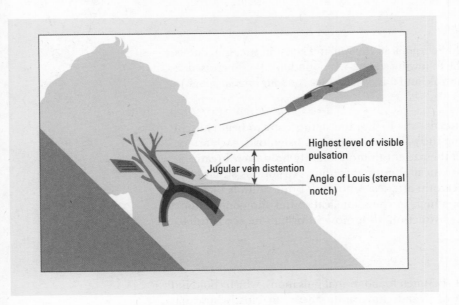

Highest level of visible pulsation

Jugular vein distention

Angle of Louis (sternal notch)

Palpation

The first step in palpation is to assess the patient's skin temperature, texture, and turgor. Palpate the patient's arms and legs for temperature and edema. Edema is graded on a 4-point scale. If your finger leaves a slight imprint, the edema is recorded as +1. If your finger leaves a deep imprint that only slowly returns to normal, the edema is recorded as +4.

Then check capillary refill by assessing the nail beds on the fingers and toes. Refill time should be no more than 3 seconds or the time it takes to say, "capillary refill."

Artery check!

Palpate for arterial pulses by gently pressing with the pads of your index and middle fingers. Start at the top of the patient's body with the temporal artery and work your way down. Check the carotid, brachial, radial, femoral, popliteal, posterior tibial, and dorsalis pedis pulses on each side of the body, comparing pulse volume and symmetry. *Don't palpate both carotid arteries at the same time or press too firmly. If you do, the patient may faint or become bradycardic.* If you haven't put on gloves for the examination, do so before you palpate the femoral arteries.

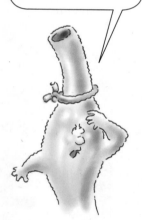

Pressing too firmly on the carotid artery may make the patient faint.

The pulses get pluses

All pulses should be regular in rhythm and equal in strength. Pulses are graded on the following scale: 4+ is bounding, 3+ is increased, 2+ is normal, 1+ is weak, and 0 is absent. (See *Assessing arterial pulses.*)

Auscultation

After you palpate, use the bell of the stethoscope to begin auscultation. Following the palpation sequence, listen over each artery. If necessary, ask the patient to momentarily hold their breath so you can clearly hear abnormal sounds. No sounds should be heard over the carotid arteries. A hum, or bruit, sounds like buzzing, blowing, or a high-pitched, musical sound and could indicate arteriosclerotic obstruction. (For more information, see "Bruits," page 44.)

Moving on up

Assess the upper abdomen for abnormal pulsations, which could indicate the presence of an abdominal aortic aneurysm. Finally, auscultate the femoral and popliteal pulses, checking for a bruit or other abnormal sounds.

Peak technique

Assessing arterial pulses

To assess arterial pulses, apply pressure with your index and middle fingers. The following illustrations show where to position your fingers when palpating various pulses.

Carotid pulse

Lightly place your fingers just medial to the trachea and below the jaw angle. *Never* palpate both carotid arteries at the same time.

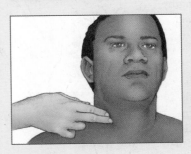

Brachial pulse

Position your fingers medial to the biceps tendon.

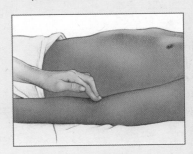

Radial pulse

Apply gentle pressure to the medial and ventral side of the wrist, just below the base of the thumb.

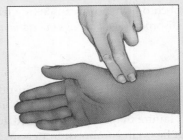

Femoral pulse

Press relatively hard at a point inferior to the inguinal ligament. For a patient who carries a lot of extra weight, palpate in the crease of the groin, halfway between the pubic bone and the hip bone.

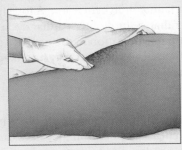

Popliteal pulse

Press firmly in the popliteal fossa at the back of the knee.

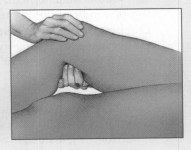

Posterior tibial pulse

Apply pressure behind and slightly below the malleolus of the ankle.

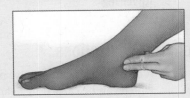

Dorsalis pedis pulse

Place your fingers on the medial dorsum of the foot while the patient points his toes down. The pulse is difficult to palpate here and may appear absent in healthy patients.

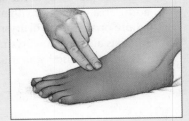

Recognizing abnormal findings

This section outlines some common abnormal cardiovascular system assessment findings and their causes.

Abnormal skin and hair findings

Cyanosis, pallor, or cool or cold skin may indicate poor CO and tissue perfusion. Conditions causing fever or increased CO may make the skin warmer than normal. An absence of body hair on the arms or legs may indicate diminished arterial blood flow to those areas. Clubbing of fingers is a sign of chronic hypoxia caused by a lengthy cardiovascular or respiratory disorder. (See *Findings in arterial and venous insufficiency*, page 39.)

How swell!

Swelling, or edema, may indicate heart failure or venous insufficiency. It may also be caused by varicosities or thrombophlebitis.

Chronic right-sided heart failure may cause ascites and generalized edema. If the patient has vein compression in a specific area, there may be localized swelling along the path of the compressed vessel. Right-sided heart failure may cause edema in the lower legs.

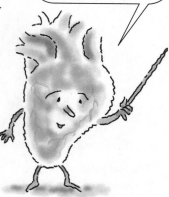

Hmmm . . . no body hair on the arms or legs. Could be a problem with arterial blood flow.

Abnormal pulsations

A displaced apical impulse may indicate an enlarged left ventricle, which can be caused by heart failure or hypertension. A forceful apical impulse, or one lasting longer than a third of the cardiac cycle, may point to increased CO. If you find a pulsation in the patient's aortic, pulmonic, or tricuspid area, their heart chamber may be enlarged, or they may have valvular disease.

Pulses here, there, everywhere

Increased CO or an aortic aneurysm may produce pulsations in the aortic area. A patient with an epigastric pulsation may have early heart failure or an aortic aneurysm. A pulsation in the sternoclavicular area suggests an aortic aneurysm. A patient with anemia, anxiety, increased CO, or a thin chest wall might have slight pulsations to the right and left of the sternum.

Findings in arterial and venous insufficiency

Assessment findings differ in patients with arterial insufficiency and those with chronic venous insufficiency. These illustrations show those differences.

Arterial insufficiency

In a patient with arterial insufficiency, pulses may be decreased or absent. The skin will be cool, pale, and shiny, and the patient may have pain in their legs and feet. Ulcerations typically occur in the area around the toes and heel, and the foot usually turns deep red when dependent. Nails may be thick and ridged.

Chronic venous insufficiency

In a patient with chronic venous insufficiency, check for ulcerations around the ankle. Pulses are present but may be difficult to locate because of edema. The patient's foot may become cyanotic when dependent.

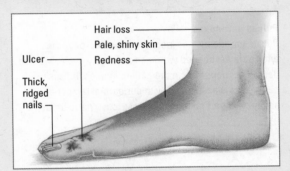

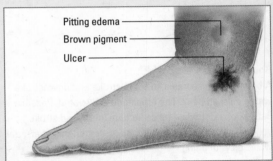

Weak ones, strong ones

A weak arterial pulse may indicate decreased CO or increased peripheral vascular resistance, both of which point to arterial atherosclerotic disease. Many older patients have weak pedal pulses.

Strong or bounding pulsations usually occur in patients with conditions that cause increased CO, such as hypertension, hypoxia, anemia, exercise, hyperthyroidism, or anxiety. (See *Pulse waveforms*, page 38.)

Heave ho! What a thrill!

A heave, lifting of the chest wall felt during palpation, along the left sternal border may mean right ventricular hypertrophy. A heave over the left ventricular area suggests a ventricular aneurysm. A thrill, which is a palpable vibration, usually suggests valvular dysfunction.

Pulse waveforms

To identify abnormal arterial pulses, check the waveforms below and see which one matches your patient's peripheral pulse.

Weak pulse

A weak pulse has a decreased amplitude with a slower upstroke and downstroke. Possible causes of a weak pulse include increased peripheral vascular resistance, as sometimes occurs in response to cold temperatures or with severe heart failure, and decreased stroke volume, as occurs with hypovolemia or aortic stenosis.

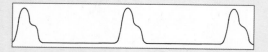

Bounding pulse

A bounding pulse has a sharp upstroke and downstroke with a pointed peak. The amplitude is elevated. Possible causes of a bounding pulse include increased stroke volume, as with aortic insufficiency, or stiffness of arterial walls, as with aging.

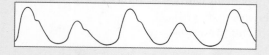

Pulsus alternans

Pulsus alternans has a regular, alternating pattern of a weak and strong pulse. This pulse is associated with left-sided heart failure.

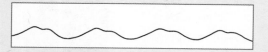

Pulsus bigeminus

Pulsus bigeminus is similar to pulsus alternans but occurs at irregular intervals. This pulse is caused by premature atrial or ventricular beats.

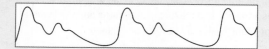

Pulsus paradoxus

Pulsus paradoxus has increases and decreases in amplitude associated with the respiratory cycle. Marked decreases occur when the patient inhales. Pulsus paradoxus is associated with pericardial tamponade, advanced heart failure, and constrictive pericarditis.

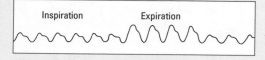

Pulsus bisferiens

Pulsus bisferiens shows an initial upstroke, a subsequent downstroke, and then another upstroke during systole. Pulsus bisferiens is caused by aortic stenosis and aortic insufficiency.

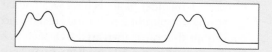

Abnormal auscultation findings

Abnormal auscultation findings include abnormal heart sounds (previously discussed), heart murmurs, and bruits. (See *Recognizing abnormal heart sounds*, page 41.)

Murmurs

Murmurs can result from several conditions and have widely varied characteristics. Here's a rundown on some of the more common murmurs.

Recognizing abnormal heart sounds

Whenever auscultation reveals an abnormal heart sound, try to identify the sound and its timing in the cardiac cycle. Knowing those characteristics can help you identify the possible cause for the sound. Use this table to put all that information together.

Abnormal heart sound	Timing	Possible causes
Accentuated S_1	Beginning of systole	• Mitral stenosis • Fever
Diminished S_1	Beginning of systole	• Mitral insufficiency • Heart block • Severe mitral insufficiency with a calcified, immobile valve
Split S_1	Beginning of systole	• Right bundle-branch block • Premature ventricular contractions
Accentuated S_2	End of systole	• Pulmonary or systemic hypertension
Diminished or inaudible S_2	End of systole	• Aortic or pulmonic stenosis
Persistent S_2 split	End of systole	• Delayed closure of the pulmonic valve, usually from overfilling of the right ventricle, causing prolonged systolic ejection time
Reversed or paradoxical S_2 split that appears during expiration and disappears during inspiration	End of systole	• Delayed ventricular stimulation • Left bundle-branch block • Prolonged left ventricular ejection time
S_3 (ventricular gallop)	Early diastole	• Overdistention of the ventricles during the rapid-filling segment of diastole or mitral insufficiency of ventricular failure (normal in children and young adults)
S_4 (atrial or presystolic gallop)	Late diastole	• Pulmonic stenosis • Hypertension • Coronary artery disease • Aortic stenosis • Forceful atrial concentration due to resistance to ventricular filling late in diastole (resulting from left ventricular hypertrophy)
Pericardial friction rub (grating or leathery sound at the left sternal border, usually muffled, high-pitched, and transient)	Throughout systole and diastole	• Pericardial inflammation

Murmur configurations

To help classify a murmur, begin by identifying its configuration (shape). The following are four basic patterns of murmurs:

Crescendo/decrescendo (diamond-shaped)
- Begins softly, peaks sharply, and then fades
- Examples: Pulmonic stenosis, aortic stenosis, mitral valve prolapse, mitral stenosis

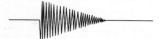

Decrescendo
- Starts loudly and then gradually diminishes
- Examples: Aortic insufficiency, pulmonic insufficiency

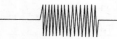

Pansystolic (holosystolic or plateau-shaped)
- Is uniform from beginning to end
- Examples: Mitral or tricuspid regurgitation

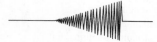

Crescendo
- Begins softly and then gradually increases
- Examples: Tricuspid stenosis, mitral valve prolapse

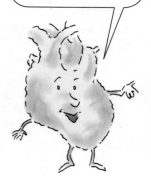

Listen up! You can tell what's causing a murmur by how it sounds.

Low-pitched

Aortic stenosis, a condition in which the aortic valve has calcified and restricts blood flow, causes a midsystolic, low-pitched, harsh murmur that radiates from the valve to the carotid artery. The murmur shifts from crescendo to decrescendo and back.

Crescendo describes a murmur that increases in intensity; a *decrescendo* murmur decreases in intensity. The crescendo–decrescendo murmur of aortic stenosis results from the turbulent, highly pressured flow of blood across stiffened leaflets and through a narrowed opening.

Medium-pitched

During auscultation, listen for a murmur near the pulmonic valve. This murmur might indicate pulmonic stenosis, a condition in which the pulmonic valve has calcified and interferes with the flow of blood out of the right ventricle. The murmur is medium pitched, systolic, and harsh and shifts from crescendo to decrescendo and back. The murmur is caused by turbulent blood flow across a stiffened, narrowed valve.

High-pitched

In a patient with aortic insufficiency, blood flows backward through the aortic valve and causes a high-pitched, blowing, decrescendo, diastolic murmur. The murmur radiates from the aortic valve area to the left sternal border.

In a patient with pulmonic insufficiency, blood flows backward through the pulmonic valve, causing a blowing, diastolic, decrescendo murmur at Erb point (at the left sternal border of the third intercostal space). If the patient has a higher-than-normal pulmonary pressure, the murmur is high pitched. If not, it's low-pitched.

High-pitched and blowing

In a patient with mitral insufficiency, blood regurgitates into the left atrium. This regurgitation produces a high-pitched, blowing murmur throughout systole (pansystolic or holosystolic). The murmur may radiate from the mitral area to the left axillary line. You can hear it best at the apex.

In a patient with tricuspid insufficiency, blood regurgitates into the right atrium. This backflow of blood through the valve also causes a high-pitched, blowing murmur, this time throughout systole in the tricuspid area. The murmur becomes louder when the patient inhales.

Low-pitched and rumbling

Mitral stenosis is a condition in which the mitral valve has calcified and is blocking blood flow out of the left atrium. Listen for a low-pitched, rumbling, crescendo–decrescendo murmur in the mitral valve area. This murmur results from turbulent blood flow across the stiffened, narrowed valve.

Tricuspid stenosis is a condition in which the tricuspid valve has calcified and is blocking blood flow through the valve from the right atrium. Listen for a low-pitched, rumbling, crescendo–decrescendo murmur in the tricuspid area. The murmur results from turbulent blood flow across the stiffened, narrowed valvular leaflets.

Bruits

A murmurlike sound of vascular (rather than cardiac) origin is called a *bruit*. If you hear a bruit during arterial auscultation, the patient may have occlusive arterial disease or an arteriovenous fistula. Various high CO conditions—such as anemia, hyperthyroidism, and pheochromocytoma—may also cause bruits.

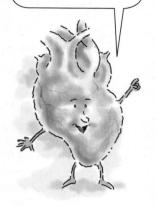

Bruits are of vascular, not cardiac, origin.

Suggested references

Ball, J., Dains, J., Flynn, J., Solomon, B., & Stewart, R. (2022). *Seidel's guide to physical examination: An interprofessional approach (Mosby's guide to physical examination)* (10th ed.). Elsevier.

Chang, A. M., Fischman, D. L., & Hollander, J. E. (2018). Evaluation of chest pain and acute coronary syndromes. *Cardiology Clinics, 36*(1), 1–12.

Roffi, M., Patrono, C., Collet, J. P., Mueller, C., Valgimigli, M., Andreotti, F., Bax, J. J., Borger, M. A., Brotons, C., Chew, D. P., Gencer, B., Hasenfuss, G., Kjeldsen, K., Lancellotti, P., Landmesser, U., Mehilli, J., Mukherjee, D., Storey, R. F., Windecker, S., ESC Scientific Document Group. (2016). 2015 ESC guidelines for the management of acute coronary syndromes in patients presenting without persistent ST-segment elevation: Task force for the management of acute coronary syndromes in patients presenting without persistent ST-segment elevation of the European Society of Cardiology (ESC). *European Heart Journal, 37*(3), 267–315. https://doi.org/10.1093/eurheartj/ehv320

Chapter 3

Prevention and risk reduction

Just the facts

In this chapter, you'll learn:

♦ the incidence of cardiovascular disease in the United States

♦ modifiable and nonmodifiable risk factors for cardiovascular disease

♦ strategies for preventing cardiovascular disease.

Understanding cardiovascular disease

Cardiovascular disease (CVD) is a term used to describe various conditions that affect the structure and function of the heart and blood vessels. Common types of CVD include the following:

- coronary artery disease (CAD)
- heart failure (HF)
- cerebrovascular disease
- peripheral artery disease
- ischemic heart disease
- rheumatic heart disease
- congenital heart disease

Heart–breaking numbers

- About 11% of American adults (that's more than one of every nine) have been diagnosed with heart disease (https://www.nhlbi.nih.gov/resources/know-differences-cardiovascular-disease-heart-disease-coronary-heart-disease).
- In the United States, someone has a heart attack every 40 seconds (https://www.cdc.gov/heartdisease/facts.htm).
- Every year, about 805,000 people in the United States have a heart attack.
  - 605,000 people are experiencing a first heart attack
  - 200,000 happen to people who have already had a heart attack.
  - About one in five heart attacks are silent—the damage is done, but the person is not aware of it (https://www.cdc.gov/heartdisease/facts.htm).

- Heart diseases cost the United States about $239.9 billion each year from 2018 to 2019. This includes the cost of healthcare services, medicines, and lost productivity due to death (https://www.cdc.gov/heartdisease/facts.htm).
- CVD is the leading cause of mortality and morbidity among males and females in the United States.
- One person dies every 33 seconds in the United States from cardiovascular disease (https://www.cdc.gov/heartdisease/facts.htm).
- About 695,000 people in the United States died from heart disease in 2021—that's one in every five deaths (https://www.cdc.gov/heartdisease/facts.htm).

Hocus focus

Prevention and risk reduction strategies for CVD tend to focus on atherosclerotic disease, or atherosclerosis. Atherosclerosis occurs when lipid deposits, thrombi, or calcifications cause inflammation and arterial wall changes.

Risk assessment

> Find out your patient's risk score. The more you know about a patient's risk, the more you can do to prevent disease from developing.

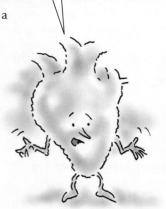

Atherosclerotic disease, which includes CAD, used to be considered a normal, inevitable part of the aging process. However, the Framingham Heart Study—which followed 5,209 healthy males and females for several years in search of characteristics shared by those who eventually developed CAD—identified factors to help assess a patient's risk of CAD. Now, a Framingham Risk Score is an important part of caring for patients who have or are at risk for CAD. Knowing a patient's risk can guide healthcare providers to plan interventions that may help prevent or reduce the patient's risk of developing atherosclerotic disease.

What's the score?

The Framingham Risk Score estimates a patient's risk of developing CAD by assigning a score to these patient factors:
- age
- total cholesterol level
- high-density lipoprotein (HDL) level
- low-density lipoprotein (LDL) level
- blood pressure
- presence or absence of diabetes mellitus
- smoking status.

Individual risk factor scores differ for males and females and may be based on total cholesterol level or LDL cholesterol level. A patient's total score (the sum of the individual risk factor scores) determines their 10-year risk of developing CAD. (Visit: https://www.nhlbi.nih.gov/health-topics/ischemic-heart-disease.) The patient's relative risk of developing disease can then be determined by comparing the patient's score with the total scores of individuals of the same sex and age whose risk of CAD is average or low.

Other applications

Researchers hope that ongoing research will provide evidence to support using the Framingham Risk Score for risk assessment of other atherosclerotic diseases, such as peripheral vascular arterial disease (associated with major limb loss) and cerebrovascular arterial disease.

Risk factors

Understanding the risk factors associated with CVD helps patients and healthcare providers develop strategies for prevention and risk reduction. Risk factors may be *modifiable* (controllable) or *nonmodifiable* (not controllable).

Nonmodifiable risk factors

Nonmodifiable risk factors for CVD include the following:
- advanced age
- sex
- heredity.

Advanced age

Although specific age-related changes may vary from person to person, individuals generally become more vulnerable to CVD with age. Complex organ systems start to decline, so other systems are forced to compensate.

With every beat of my heart

Age-related heart changes include the following:
- thickening and stiffening of the left ventricle
- fibrotic changes in the valves
- valve calcification
- increased reliance on atrial contractions to maintain cardiac output
- increased sensitivity to hypovolemia
- fibrotic changes in the bundle branches (a common cause of bundle-branch block in people older than age 65).

Vascular variations

Changes in the vascular system that tend to be age-related include the following:

- thickened intimal and medial layers of the arteries
- decreased arterial diameter
- stiffer, less elastic arterial walls due to calcium and lipid deposits. These changes cause hypertension to develop.

Sex

Research has shown that males are at greater risk for developing CAD at a younger age than females. In males, risk increases beginning at age 45, whereas the risk in females increases after menopause (around age 55, but it is still the number one killer of females (https://www. nhlbi.nih.gov/health/heart-healthy-living/risks). Additionally, the lifetime risk of developing CAD is one in two for males and one in three for females.

Hormones: Helpful or hurtful?

Hormone replacement therapy for postmenopausal females was once thought to protect females from CVD. However, studies have shown that the risk of stroke, myocardial infarction, and deep vein thrombosis increases with hormone replacement therapy.

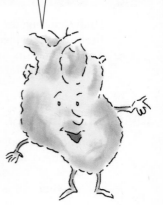

Inquiry and the patient interview: When assessing a postmenopausal female's risk of CVD, ask if they are receiving hormone replacement therapy.

Heredity

Researchers' understanding of the complex relationship between genes and environmental factors in the development of CVD is in its infancy. However, many researchers believe that one-half of CVD cases can be attributed to genetic causes.

Genes on the scene

Genetics play a huge role in hypertension, heart disease, and other vascular conditions.

For example, some individuals with familial hypercholesterolemia (an inherited metabolic disorder affecting LDL receptors) carry a genetic mutation that makes it difficult for their cells to remove LDL from their blood. Patients with familial hypercholesterolemia have high serum cholesterol levels and are at risk for developing atherosclerosis.

History lesson

Obtaining a patient's family history helps to identify patterns of early CVD and familial risk factors. For example, a patient has a higher risk of developing early CVD if they have a first-degree male relative who was diagnosed with CVD before age 55 or a female first-degree relative who was diagnosed with CVD before age 65. It is also likely that people with a family history of heart disease share common environments and risk factors that increase their risks. Approximately 4% to 10% of heart attacks occur in individuals younger than 45, and most of these heart attacks impact males (https://www.health.harvard.edu/topics/heart-disease).

Modifiable risk factors

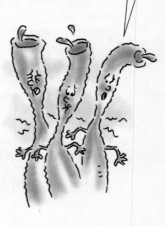

Unfortunately, early development of CVD is commonly the result of lifestyle choices involving modifiable risk factors. Risk reduction strategies aim to reduce or eliminate the impact of these factors.

Modifiable risk factors include the following:

- smoking
- dyslipidemia
- hypertension
- diabetes mellitus
- obesity/diet
- sedentary lifestyle
- excessive alcohol (ethanol [ETOH]) intake.

Smoking

Smoking is the most common modifiable risk factor for CVD. In the United States, smoking causes almost as many deaths from heart disease as it does from lung cancer. The more a patient smokes and the longer they smoke, the higher their risk of CVD (https://www.nhlbi.nih.gov/health/heart/smoking).

The damage done

Nicotine stimulates the sympathetic nervous system to constrict the arteries and raises blood pressure, which causes arterial wall damage. This damage promotes the formation of atherosclerotic plaque, causing tissues to become starved for oxygen. Exposure to second-hand smoke can increase the risk of heart disease for nonsmokers. Thirdhand smoke is residual nicotine and other chemicals left on indoor surfaces by tobacco smoke. People are exposed to this chemical by touching contaminated surfaces or breathing in the off gassing from these surfaces (https://www.mayoclinic.org/healthy-lifestyle/quit-smoking/expert-answers/third-hand-smoke/faq-20057791).

Stuck on you

Smoking also makes platelets stickier, making them more likely to adhere to artery walls.

Quitters wanted

All patients should be encouraged to quit smoking. Healthcare providers should educate patients about the risks of smoking and help develop an action plan for quitting. The best formal smoking cessation programs combine multiple approaches:
- behavioral modification therapies
- medications such as antidepressants
- nicotine replacement strategies, such as nicotine patches or gum.

Dyslipidemia

Dyslipidemia refers to abnormal lipoprotein levels in the blood. Lipoproteins, which are compounds that have proteins on the outside and lipids (fats) on the inside, carry cholesterol in the bloodstream.

Cholesterol: a waxy, fat-like substance found in your body and many foods. Too much can build up on your arteries, over time narrow them, and allow less blood to pass through.

High is good, low is bad

Types of lipoproteins include the following:
- LDL—considered the "bad cholesterol" because it carries cholesterol into the tissues
- HDL—considered the "good cholesterol" because it removes cholesterol from tissues and returns it to the liver.
  Therefore, the risk of developing CVD increases when a patient has:
- increased LDL levels
- decreased HDL levels
- abnormal lipid metabolism.

Tri this on for size

Triglycerides are lipids produced by the liver. They're also found in food. Elevated triglyceride levels increase the risk of CVD and may also lead to pancreatitis. Factors that contribute to elevated triglyceride levels include the following:
- obesity
- smoking
- excessive alcohol consumption.

Take it down a notch

Addressing dyslipidemia by reducing serum LDL levels helps prevent or slow the progression of atherosclerotic disease. Strategies for reducing serum LDL levels include the following:
- dietary changes, such as following a Mediterranean-style diet that replaces saturated fats with polyunsaturated fats (particularly omega-3 fatty acids) and avoiding trans fats, which increase LDL levels
- drug therapy if necessary. (See *Drugs that lower cholesterol.*)

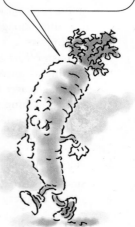

Diet plays a big role in modifying such risk factors as dyslipidemia, diabetes, and obesity.

Drugs that lower cholesterol

Drugs that lower cholesterol include various statins, the antilipemic ezetimibe (Zetia), bile acid resins, nicotinic acid, and fibrates.

Statins

Examples of statins include lovastatin (Advicor), pravastatin (Pravachol), simvastatin (Zocor), fluvastatin (Lescol), atorvastatin (Lipitor), and rosuvastatin (Crestor). These drugs inhibit the action of an enzyme that controls the rate at which the body produces cholesterol. They also lower triglyceride levels and raise high-density lipoprotein (HDL) levels. Statins are more effective in lowering low-density lipoprotein (LDL) levels than other types of drugs.

Ezetimibe

Ezetimibe reduces the amount of cholesterol absorbed by the body. It's sometimes used in combination with a statin to further reduce LDL levels.

Bile acid resins

Bile acid resins bind with cholesterol-containing bile acids in the intestines. The cholesterol is then eliminated from the body when the drug is excreted in the stool.

Nicotinic acid

Also called *niacin*, this water-soluble B vitamin improves levels of total cholesterol, LDLs, triglycerides, and HDLs when taken in doses above the recommended daily allowance.

Fibrates

Fibrates lower triglycerides and, to a lesser degree, raise HDL levels. Fibrates are less effective in lowering LDL levels.

Track progress (or lack thereof)

The National Cholesterol Education Program recommends obtaining a patient's lipid profiles every 5 years starting at age 20.

Hypertension

Hypertension (increased blood pressure) tends to be discovered incidentally because patients usually don't experience symptoms. A diagnosis of hypertension is confirmed when two or more elevated blood pressure readings are obtained on separate occasions. (See *Blood pressure categories*.)

Dangerous deposits

Hypertension causes inflammation and damages the lining of the arteries. This damage increases fat deposits, which leads to atherosclerosis. In addition, plaque deposits become unstable, leading to thromboses and emboli. Damage to the small, fragile arteries of the organs can lead to heart attacks, retinopathies, stroke, peripheral artery disease, and kidney failure.

Taking control

Treating hypertension includes the following:

- lifestyle modifications, such as smoking cessation, dietary changes, and regular physical activity
- medications to control blood pressure, such as beta-adrenergic blockers, calcium channel blockers, angiotensin receptor blockers, and thiazide diuretics.

Blood pressure categories

BP category	Systolic blood pressure (mm Hg)		Diastolic blood pressure (mm Hg)
	Upper number		Lower number
Normal	<120	and	<80
Elevated	120–129	and	<80
Hypertension, stage 1	130–139	or	80–89
Hypertension, stage 2	140 or higher	or	90 or higher

Source: Adapted from American College of Cardiology. (2017). New ACC/AHA high blood pressure guidelines: Lower definition of hypertension. Retrieved from https://www.acc.org/latest-in-cardiology/articles/2017/11/08/11/47/mon-5pm-bp-guideline-aha-2017; Journal of the American College of Cardiology. (2018). JACC instructions for authors. Retrieved from http://www.online-jacc.org/content/71/19; and Whelton, P. K., Carey, R. M., Aronow, W. S., Casey, D. E., Jr, Collins, K. J., Dennison Himmelfarb, C., DePalma, S., M., Gidding, S., Jamerson, K. A., Jones, D. W., MacLaughlin, E. J., Muntner, P., Ovbiagele, B., Smith, S. C. Jr, Spencer, C. C., Stafford, R. S., Taler, S. J., Thomas, R. J., Williams, K. A. Sr, Williamson, J. D., & Wright, J. T. Jr. (2018). 2017 ACC/AHA/AAPA/ABC/ACPM/AGS/APhA/ASH/ASPC/NMA/PCNA guideline for the prevention, detection, evaluation, and management of high blood pressure in adults: A report of the American College of Cardiology/American Heart Association Task Force on clinical practice guidelines. *Journal of the American College of Cardiology, 71*(19), e127–e248. https://doi.org/10.1016/j.jacc.2017.11.006

DASH into a proper diet

Following the Dietary Approaches to Stop Hypertension diet plan can significantly improve blood pressure. This plan involves eating a diet that's low in sodium (2,300 mg/day or less or 1,500 mg if you're age 51 or older; African American; or have high blood pressure, diabetes, or chronic kidney disease) but high in fruits, vegetables, and low-fat dairy. (See *Tips for reducing sodium intake*.)

Mighty meds

Drugs and drug classes used to help reduce blood pressure include, but are not limited to, the following:
- thiazide diuretics such as hydrochlorothiazide (HydroDIURIL), which increase sodium, chloride, and water excretion by the kidneys
- atenolol (Tenormin), which decreases the heart's excitability, cardiac output, and oxygen consumption and decreases the release of renin from the kidney
- angiotensin-converting enzyme inhibitors such as lisinopril (Zestril), which block the conversion of angiotensin I to angiotensin II (a potent vasoconstrictor).

Tips for reducing sodium intake

Only a small amount of sodium occurs naturally in foods. Most sodium is added to foods during processing. To help your patient cut down on sodium intake, offer these suggestions.

Read those labels
- Read food labels to determine sodium content.
- Use food products with reduced sodium or no added salt.
- Be aware that soy sauce, broth, sauces, and foods that are pickled or cured have high sodium contents.
  Examples: cold cuts, cheese, soups, fast foods, pizza, pasta dishes, and processed foods

Now you're cookin'
- Instead of cooking with salt, use herbs, spices, cooking wines, lemon, lime, or vinegar to enhance food flavors.
- Cook pasta and rice without salt.
- Rinse canned foods, such as tuna, to remove some sodium.
- Avoid adding salt to foods, especially at the table.

- Avoid condiments such as soy and teriyaki sauces and monosodium glutamate (MSG)—or use lower sodium versions.
- Fact: One tablespoon (15 mL) of soy sauce, for example, has about 1,000 mg of sodium.

You are what you eat
- Eat fresh poultry, fish, and lean meat rather than canned, smoked, or processed versions (which typically contain a lot of sodium).
- Whenever possible, eat fresh foods rather than canned or convenience foods.
- Limit intake of cured foods (such as bacon and ham), foods packed in brine (pickles, olives, and sauerkraut), and condiments (mustard, ketchup, horseradish, and Worcestershire sauce).
- When dining out, ask how food is prepared. Ask that your food be prepared without added salt or MSG.

It's cool to comply

Because the patient may not experience symptoms of their hypertension, they may have difficulty understanding why drug therapy is necessary. Stress to the patient the importance of complying with drug therapy to control blood pressure. Also, advise the patient to report adverse effects such as fatigue.

Diabetes mellitus

Diabetes mellitus is a chronic disease in which the body has trouble producing or using insulin (the hormone that enables the body to use glucose).

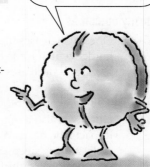

Remind patients that even though they may not feel the symptoms of hypertension, they may need medications to treat it.

What's your type?

With type 1 diabetes, the body can't produce enough insulin. With type 2 diabetes, the body can't use insulin efficiently. Type 2 diabetes accounts for 90% of all diabetes cases.

Diabetic disturbances

Diabetes causes disturbances in protein and fat metabolism, which can lead to weight problems. As a result, most patients with type 2 diabetes are overweight or obese. Maintaining a normal weight through diet and exercise and taking prescribed medications is crucial to maintaining adequate blood sugar control.

Diabetes also damages small- and medium-sized arteries, which can lead to heart attack, stroke, renal failure, and peripheral artery disease. It also accelerates the development of atherosclerosis.

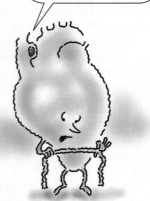

Is your patient's waist bigger than their hips? Then they are at risk for CVD.

Obesity and belly fat

Obesity is defined as a body mass index (BMI) of 30 or greater and can affect your ability to manage your diabetes. Excess belly fat around your waist can raise your chances of developing heart disease (https://www.niddk.nih.gov/health-information/diabetes/overview/preventing-problems/heart-disease-stroke). It develops, in part, as a result of dietary habits and a sedentary lifestyle. Basically, if an individual eats more calories than their body uses, the excess calories are stored in the body as adipose tissue (fat). Patients who have a larger waist measurement than hip measurement are at greater risk for developing CVD.

Putting a number on it

Researchers estimate that a male with a BMI of 45 in early adulthood may have a reduced life expectancy of up to 13 years. A female with a BMI of 45 may have a life expectancy reduced by 8 years.

Obesity outcomes

Obesity increases the risk of CVD by causing the heart to have to work harder, which leads to increased blood pressure. It also increases LDL levels and decreases HDL levels.

Nothing to snore at

Obesity is also a major contributing factor in sleep apnea, which impacts the heart. With sleep apnea, a person experiences multiple cycles during sleep in which they stop breathing, partially wakes, and then begins breathing again. These periods of apnea cause the oxygen level in the blood to drop, putting strain on the heart. This strain can lead to right-sided HR and pulmonary hypertension.

Sedentary lifestyle

Patients with sedentary lifestyles are more likely to be overweight or obese. Encouraging physical activity can help patients achieve and maintain target weight goals, thus decreasing the risk of CVD. The recommended amount of exercise is 30 minutes of moderate physical activity per day on most days of the week.

Reasons to move

Cardiovascular benefits of exercise include the following:
- improved lipid metabolism
- decreased blood pressure
- enhanced insulin sensitivity
- utilization of excess calories, which prevents them from being stored as fat.

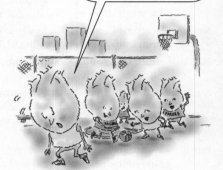

Phew! That was quite a workout. I can feel my lipid metabolism improving as we speak!

Suggested references

Agarwala, A., Patel, J., Stephens, J., Roberson, S., Scott, J., Beckie, T., Jackson, E. A., American Heart Association Prevention Science Committee of the Council on Epidemiology and Prevention and Council on Cardiovascular and Stroke Nursing, Council on Clinical Cardiology, Council on Lifestyle and Cardiometabolic Health, Council on Peripheral Vascular Disease, Council on Quality of Care and Outcomes Research, ; & Stroke Council. (2023). Implementation of prevention science to eliminate health care inequities in achieving cardiovascular health: A scientific statement from the American Heart Association, *Circulation, 148*(15), 1183–1193. Retrieved from https://www.ahajournals.org/doi/10.1161/CIR.0000000000001171

American College of Cardiology. (2017). New ACC/AHA high blood pressure guidelines: Lower definition of hypertension. Retrieved from https://www.acc.org/latest-in-cardiology/articles/2017/11/08/11/47/mon-5pm-bp-guideline-aha-2017

Centers for Disease Control and Prevention. (2023). Heart disease. Retrieved from https://www.cdc.gov/heartdisease/index.htm

Harvard Health Publishing. (last accessed 2023, October 15). Coronary artery disease. Retrieved from https://www.health.harvard.edu/topics/coronary-artery-disease

Harvard Health Publishing. (last accessed 2023, October 15). Heart disease. Retrieved from https://www.health.harvard.edu/topics/coronary-artery-disease

Journal of the American College of Cardiology. (2018). JACC instructions for authors. Retrieved from http://www.onlinejacc.org/content/71/19

Mayo Clinic. (2021). Nutrition and healthy eating. Retrieved from https://www.mayoclinic.org/healthy-lifestyle/nutrition-and-healthy-eating/basics/nutrition-basics/hlv-20049477

Mayo Clinic. (2022). What is thirdhand smoke, and why is it a concern? Retrieved from https://www.mayoclinic.org/healthy-lifestyle/adult-health/expert-answers/third-hand-smoke/faq-20057791

National Heart, Lung, and Blood Institute. (2021). Know the difference fact sheet. Retrieved from https://www.nhlbi.nih.gov/resources/know-differences-cardiovascular-disease-heart-disease-coronary-heart-disease

National Heart, Lung, and Blood Institute. (2022a). Coronary heart disease. Retrieved from https://www.nhlbi.nih.gov/health-topics/ischemic-heart-disease

National Heart, Lung, and Blood Institute. (2022b). *Smoking and your heart.* Retrieved from https://www.nhlbi.nih.gov/health/heart/smoking

National Heart, Lung, and Blood Institute. (2022c). *Heart healthy living.* Retrieved from https://www.nhlbi.nih.gov/health/heart-healthy-living/risks

National Institute of Diabetes and Digestive and Kidney Diseases. (2021). Diabetes, heart disease, and stroke. Retrieved from https://www.niddk.nih.gov/health-information/diabetes/overview/preventing-problems/heart-disease-stroke

Whelton, P. K., Carey, R. M., Aronow, W. S., Casey, D. E., Jr, Collins, K. J., Dennison Himmelfarb, C., DePalma, S. M., Gidding, S., Jamerson, K. A., Jones, D. W., MacLaughlin, E. J., Muntner, P., Ovbiagele, B., Smith, S. C. Jr, Spencer, C. C., Stafford, R. S., Taler, S. J., Thomas, R. J., Williams, K. A. Sr, Williamson, J. D., & Wright, J. T. Jr. (2018). 2017 ACC/AHA/AAPA/ABC/ACPM/AGS/APhA/ASH/ASPC/NMA/PCNA guideline for the prevention, detection, evaluation, and management of high blood pressure in adults: A report of the American College of Cardiology/American heart association Task Force on clinical practice guidelines. *Journal of the American College of Cardiology, 71*(19), e127–e248. https://doi.org/10.1016/j.jacc.2017.11.006

Chapter 4

Diagnostic tests and procedures

Just the facts

In this chapter, you'll learn:

◆ normal and abnormal laboratory findings

◆ tests for diagnosing cardiovascular disorders

◆ procedures used in cardiovascular care

◆ monitoring techniques for patients with cardiovascular disorders.

A look at diagnostic tests and procedures

Advances in diagnostic testing allow for earlier and easier diagnosis and treatment of cardiovascular disorders. For example, in some patients, transthoracic echocardiography—a noninvasive and risk-free test—can provide as much diagnostic information about valvular heart disease as can cardiac catheterization—an invasive and high-risk test. Monitoring and testing also help guide diagnosis, evaluate treatment, as well as identify complications. Before the patient undergoes testing, explain the procedure in terms they can easily understand. Make sure an informed consent form is signed, if necessary. These tests may cause anxiety, so be sure to provide emotional support.

Cardiac tests range from the relatively simple (analyzing the patient's blood for cardiac enzymes, proteins, and clotting time) to the very sophisticated (imaging and radiographic tests, which reveal a detailed image of the heart). Other cardiac tests include various forms of electrocardiography and hemodynamic monitoring.

Cardiac enzymes and proteins

Analyzing cardiac enzymes and proteins (markers) is an important step in diagnosing acute myocardial infarction (MI) and in evaluating other cardiac disorders. After an MI, damaged cardiac tissue releases significant amounts of enzymes and proteins into the blood. CK-MB levels do NOT usually rise with transient chest pain caused

General Nursing Considerations

Be sure to follow hospital policy for all lab draws. Confirm the following:
• Type of collection tube (and volume of sample)
• Required additives
• How quickly sample must be sent to the lab
• Whether the sample can be room temperature or sent on ice

by angina, pulmonary embolism, or acute congestive heart failure. Specific blood tests help reveal the extent of cardiac damage and help monitor healing progress. (See *Cardiac enzyme and protein patterns*, page 59.)

Cardiac markers to monitor include the following:

- troponin I and troponin T
- creatine kinase (CK-MB)
- myoglobin
- homocysteine
- C-reactive protein (CRP)
- B-type natriuretic peptide (BNP)
- N-terminal pro-BNP (NT-proBNP).

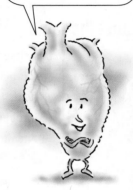

Levels of cardiac enzymes and proteins typically rise when I'm damaged.

Troponin

Troponin is a protein found in skeletal and cardiac muscles. Troponin I, troponin T, and high sensitivity cardiac troponin (hs-cTn) are isotypes found in the myocardium. Troponin T may also be found in skeletal muscle. Troponin I, however, is found only in the myocardium and is more specific to myocardial damage than CK, CK-MB isoenzymes, and myoglobin. However, the use of hs-cTn in the diagnosis of acute coronary syndrome is recommended as it is the most specific marker for cardiac injury (Gulati et al., 2021; Rajarao et al., 2018; Sandoval et al., 2022).

Normal hs-cTn is less than 14 ng/L. It raises within 1 hour of cardiac injury and can remain elevated for 7 to 14 days post MI (Rajarao, et al., 2018). Troponin I levels are less than 0.04 ng/mL; normal troponin T levels are less than 0.1 ng/mL. Troponin I and T levels elevate in 4 to 6 hours after MI and remain elevated for 5 to 7 days. Because troponin levels stay elevated for a prolonged time, they can detect an infarction that occurred several days earlier.

Nursing considerations

- Inform the patient that they need not restrict food or fluids before the test.
- Tell the patient that multiple blood samples may be drawn.
- Sustained vigorous exercise, cardiotoxic drugs renal disease, and certain surgical procedures can cause elevated troponin T levels.

Creatine kinase

CK is present in heart muscle, skeletal muscle, and brain tissue. Its isoenzyme CK-MB is found specifically in the heart muscle.

Cardiac enzyme and protein patterns

Because they're released by damaged tissue, serum proteins and isoenzymes (catalytic proteins that vary in concentration in specific organs) can help identify the compromised organ and assess the extent of damage. After acute myocardial infarction, cardiac enzymes, and proteins rise and fall in a characteristic pattern, as shown in the graph below.

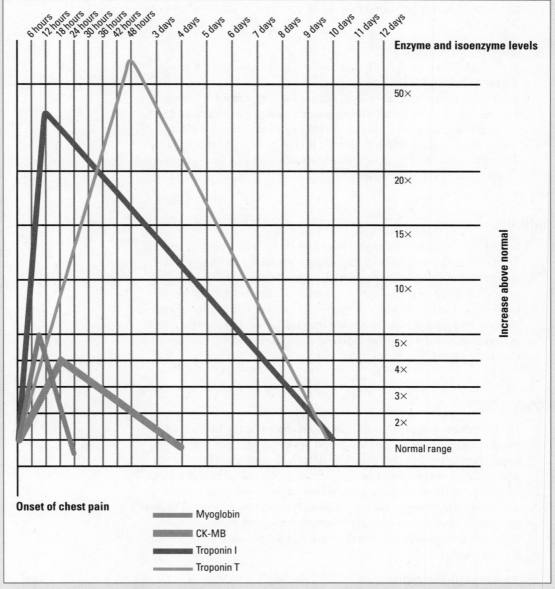

High Sensitivity Cardiac Troponin. Elevates within 1 hour of cardiac injury and remains increased for 7 to 14 days post MI (Gulati et al., 2021; Rajarao et al., 2018; Sandoval et al., 2022).

Creatine kinase (CK–MB)

Generally, CK-MB levels rise about 4 to 6 hours after the onset of acute MI, peak after about 12 to 24 hours, and may remain elevated for up to 72 hours. Normal CK levels are 55 to 170 U/L for males and 30 to 135 U/L for females. Remember, CK normal values are always laboratory specific so there can be a slight deviation of the normal values provided here from the normal values of your laboratory.

Nursing considerations
- Explain to the patient that the test will help confirm or rule out MI.
- Inform the patient that blood samples will be drawn at timed intervals. Be aware that muscle trauma caused by intramuscular injections can raise CK levels. Other causes may include electrical injuries, defibrillation, heart injury (e.g., from a car accident), inflammation of the heart muscle usually due to a virus (myocarditis), or open-heart surgery.

Myoglobin

Myoglobin, which is normally found in skeletal and cardiac muscle, functions as an oxygen-bonding muscle protein providing extra oxygen for muscles to stay at a high level of activity for longer periods of time. It's released into the bloodstream when ischemia, trauma, and inflammation of the muscle occur. The kidneys help remove myoglobin from the body into the urine. In large amounts, myoglobin can damage the kidneys. Normal myoglobin values are 0 to 0.09 μg/mL.

Homocysteine

Homocysteine is an amino acid that's produced by the body. High homocysteine levels can irritate blood vessels, leading to atherosclerosis. High levels can also raise low-density lipoprotein (LDL) levels and make blood clot more easily, increasing the risk of blood vessel blockages. Patients with elevated homocysteine levels may benefit from folic acid, vitamin B_6, and vitamin B_{12} to reduce elevated homocysteine levels. Determining the homocysteine level is an optimal approach in high-risk patients. Normal homocysteine levels are from 4 to 14 μmol/L.

Nursing considerations
- Inform the patient that they must be fasting.

C-reactive protein

CRP is a substance produced by the liver. A high CRP level indicates that inflammation exists at some location in the body. Other diagnostic tests are needed to determine the location of the inflammation and its cause. Elevated CRP levels can indicate such conditions as MI, angina, systemic lupus erythematosus, postoperative infection, trauma, and heatstroke. A more sensitive CRP test, called a high-sensitivity CRP (hs-CRP) assay, is available to determine a person's risk for heart disease. CRP level may be a strong predictor of future cardiovascular events.

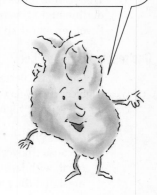

An elevated CRP level indicates that inflammation exists somewhere in the body.

B-type natriuretic peptide

BNP and NT-proBNP are both polypeptide hormones secreted by ventricular tissues in the heart. The substance is secreted as a response to the increased ventricular volume and pressure that occur when a patient is in heart failure.

A grade for heart failure

A BNP or NT-proBNP test helps accurately diagnose and grade the severity of heart failure. A quick diagnosis of heart failure in patients who present with dyspnea is important in order to begin appropriate treatment early.

A BNP result greater than 100 pg/mL and an NT-proBNP greater than 300 pg/mL is abnormal. The higher the number, the more likely heart failure is present and the more severe it is. Patients in renal failure, on dialysis, or waiting for dialysis may have elevated levels whether or not heart failure is present. As a result, the BNP and NT-proBNP assay is not useful in renal failure patients. Patients with right-sided heart failure (due to pulmonary hypertension, cor pulmonale, or pulmonary emboli) also have elevated levels (usually 300 to 400 pg/mL).

Lipid studies

Lipid studies include triglycerides, total cholesterol, and lipoprotein fractionation. They measure lipid levels in the body and help evaluate the risk of coronary artery disease (CAD).

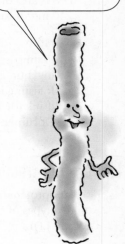

Lipid studies can tell you if arteries are becoming clogged, putting you at risk for coronary artery disease or stroke.

Triglycerides

Triglycerides, or neutral fats, are the main storage form of lipids and constitute about 90% of fatty tissue. Monitoring triglyceride levels in the blood helps with the early identification of hyperlipidemia and identification of patients at risk for CAD.

What's normal?

Triglyceride values less than 150 mg/dL are widely accepted as normal.

What's abnormal?

Triglyceride levels between 150 and 199 mg/dL are considered borderline high. Levels between 200 and 499 mg/dL are considered high. Levels greater than 500 mg/dL are very high.

One test leads to another

Measuring cholesterol may also be necessary because cholesterol and triglyceride levels vary independently. If both triglyceride and cholesterol levels are high, the patient is at risk for CAD.

Nursing considerations

- Because triglycerides are highly affected by a fat-containing meal, with levels rising and peaking 4 hours after ingesting a meal, tell the patient that they should abstain from food for 9 to 12 hours before the test and from alcohol for 24 hours before the test. The patient may drink water.

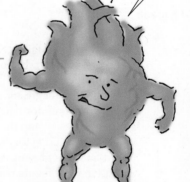

A desirable total cholesterol level is less than 200 mg/dl.

Total cholesterol

The total serum cholesterol test measures the circulating levels of the two forms in which cholesterol appears in the body—free cholesterol and cholesterol esters.

What's your level?

For adults, a desirable cholesterol level is less than 200 mg/dL. Levels are considered borderline high if they're between 200 and 240 mg/dL and high if they're greater than 240 mg/dL.

Nursing considerations

- Fasting isn't needed for isolated total cholesterol checks or screening, but fasting is required if cholesterol is part of a lipid profile. If fasting is required, instruct the patient to abstain from food and drink for 12 hours before the test.
- Document any drugs the patient is taking.

Lipoprotein fractionation

Lipoprotein fractionation tests are used to isolate and measure the two types of cholesterol in blood: high-density lipoproteins (HDLs) and LDLs.

This is good

HDL level is inversely related to the risk of CAD—that is, the higher the HDL level, the lower the incidence of CAD. For males, normal HDL values are greater than 55 mg/dL; in females, normal values are greater than 45 mg/dL.

This is bad

Conversely, the higher the LDL level, the higher the incidence of CAD. For individuals who don't have CAD, desirable LDL levels are less than 130 mg/dL, borderline high levels are in the range of 130 to 159 mg/dL, and high levels are more than 160 mg/dL. For individuals who have CAD, optimal levels are less than 100 mg/dL, and higher than optimal levels are more than 100 mg/dL.

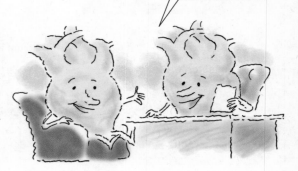

A high HDL level means a lower incidence of CAD, but a high LDL level means a higher incidence of CAD.

Nursing considerations

- Tell the patient to maintain a normal diet for 2 weeks before the test.
- Tell the patient to abstain from alcohol for 24 hours before the test.
- As ordered, tell the patient to discontinue use of thyroid hormone, hormonal contraceptives, and antilipemic agents until after the test because the medications alter results.

Evaluating lipid test results

Use this chart to determine an adult patient's risk of CAD.

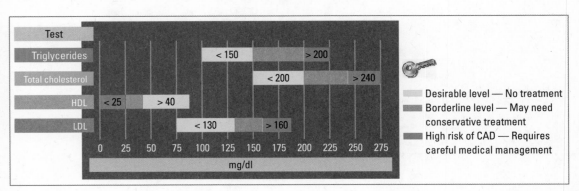

Coagulation tests

Partial thromboplastin time (PTT), prothrombin time (PT), and activated clotting time are tests that measure clotting time. They're used to measure response to treatment as well as to screen for clotting disorders.

Understanding clotting

Clotting is initiated through two different pathways.

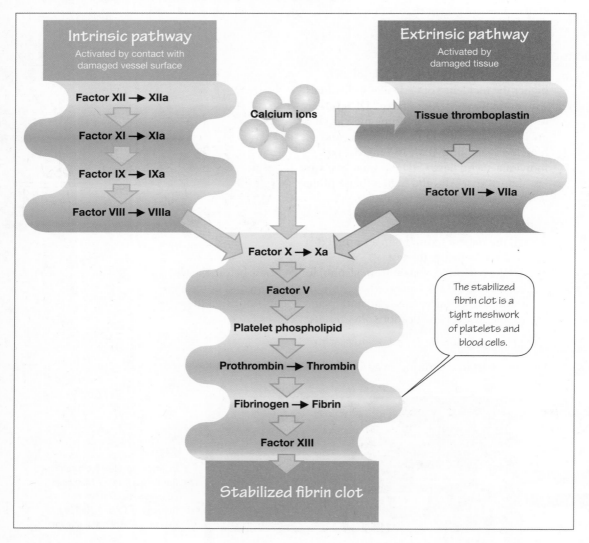

Intrinsic pathway
Activated by contact with damaged vessel surface

Factor XII → XIIa

Factor XI → XIa

Factor IX → IXa

Factor VIII → VIIIa

Extrinsic pathway
Activated by damaged tissue

Calcium ions

Tissue thromboplastin

Factor VII → VIIa

Factor X → Xa

Factor V

Platelet phospholipid

Prothrombin → Thrombin

Fibrinogen → Fibrin

Factor XIII

The stabilized fibrin clot is a tight meshwork of platelets and blood cells.

Stabilized fibrin clot

Partial thromboplastin time

The PTT test evaluates all the clotting factors of the intrinsic pathway, except platelets. It's done by measuring the time it takes a clot to form after adding calcium and phospholipid emulsion to a plasma sample. Normally, a clot forms 25 to 35 seconds after the reagents are added.

The PTT test also helps monitor a patient's response to heparin therapy. For a patient on anticoagulant therapy, check with the attending healthcare provider to find out what PTT test results to expect.

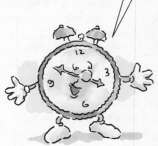

A clot should form 25 to 35 seconds after beginning the PTT test.

Nursing considerations

- Tell the patient receiving heparin therapy that this test may be repeated at regular intervals to assess response to treatment.
- For a patient on anticoagulant therapy, additional pressure may be needed at the venipuncture site to control bleeding.

Prothrombin time

Prothrombin, or factor II, is a plasma protein produced by the liver. The PT test (also known as *pro time*) measures the time required for a clot to form in a citrated plasma sample after the addition of calcium ions and tissue thromboplastin (factor III).

Excellent choice!

The PT test is an excellent screening procedure for the overall evaluation of extrinsic coagulation factors V, VII, and X and of prothrombin and fibrinogen. It's also the test of choice for monitoring oral anticoagulant therapy.

Count to 10 (or more)

Normally, PT ranges from 11 to 13 seconds. In a patient receiving warfarin (Coumadin) therapy, the goal of treatment is to attain a PT level 1.5 to 2 times the normal control value—for example, a level of 16 to 26 seconds. (See *Understanding the INR.*)

Foods rich in vitamin K can decrease clotting time. Some of these foods include beef liver, broccoli, Brussels sprouts, cabbage, collard greens, endive, kale, lettuce, mustard greens, parsley, soybeans, spinach, Swiss chard, turnip greens, watercress, and other green leafy vegetables. Moderate to high levels of vitamin K are also found in other foods such as asparagus, avocados, dill pickles, green peas, green tea, canola oil, margarine, mayonnaise, olive oil, and soybean oil. *The diet in general should remain consistent* because other foods containing little or no vitamin K such as mangos and soy milk have been reported to interact with warfarin. Patients should also consider avoiding or limiting the consumption of cranberry juice, pomegranate juice, black currant juice, and black currant seed oil.

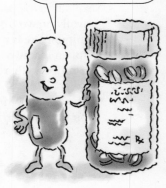

Be on the lookout for food and drugs that may affect PT test results, including vitamin K, vitamin E, and antibiotics.

Understanding the INR

The international normalized ratio (INR) system is generally viewed as the best means of standardizing measurement of prothrombin time to monitor oral anticoagulant therapy.

Guidelines for patients receiving warfarin (Coumadin) therapy recommend an INR result of 2.0 to 3.0. For patients with mechanical prosthetic heart valves, an INR result of 2.5 to 3.5 is recommended.

What's the problem?

Increased INR values may indicate disseminated intravascular coagulation, cirrhosis, hepatitis, vitamin K deficiency, salicylate intoxication, uncontrolled oral anticoagulation caused by dietary indiscretions, or massive blood transfusion.

Nursing considerations

- Check the patient's history for use of medications that may affect test results, such as vitamin K or antibiotics.

Activated clotting time

Activated clotting time, or automated coagulation time, measures the time it takes whole blood to clot. This test is commonly performed during procedures that require extracorporeal (occurring outside the body) circulation, such as cardiopulmonary bypass, ultrafiltration, hemodialysis, and extracorporeal membrane oxygenation. It is also commonly used in cardiac and radiological invasive procedures such as stent angioplasty or ablations.

Nursing considerations

- Explain to the patient that the test requires a blood sample that's usually drawn from an existing vascular access site; therefore, no venipuncture is necessary.
- Explain that two samples will be drawn. The first one will be discarded so that heparin in the tubing doesn't interfere with the results.
- If the sample is drawn from a line with a continuous infusion, stop the infusion before drawing the sample.

Electrocardiography

The heart's electrical conduction system can be recorded numerous ways, but the most common methods are a 12-lead electrocardiogram (ECG), continuous cardiac monitoring, an exercise ECG, Holter monitoring, and electrophysiology studies (EPS).

12-Lead electrocardiogram

The 12-lead ECG measures the heart's electrical activity and records it as waveforms. The ECG does not provide information about the mechanical response of the heart muscle.

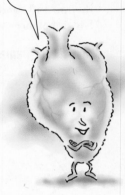

ECG is a valuable and commonly used tool, so take a systematic approach and look for changes compared to the patient's previous ECG results.

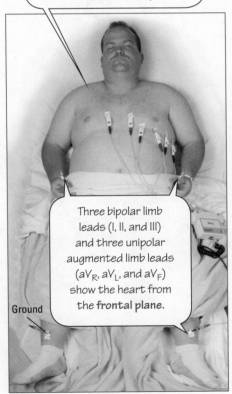

Six unipolar precordial leads (V$_1$ to V$_6$) show the heart from the horizontal plane.

Three bipolar limb leads (I, II, and III) and three unipolar augmented limb leads (aV$_R$, aV$_L$, and aV$_F$) show the heart from the frontal plane.

Ground

A test with 12 views

The standard 12-lead ECG uses a series of electrodes placed on the patient's extremities and chest wall to assess the heart from 12 different views (leads). The 12 leads include three bipolar limb leads (I, II, and III), three unipolar augmented limb leads (aV_R, aV_L, and aV_F), and six unipolar precordial limb leads (V_1 to V_6). The limb leads and augmented leads show the heart from the frontal plane. The precordial leads show the heart from the horizontal plane.

ECG can be used to identify myocardial ischemia and infarction, rhythm and conduction disturbances, chamber enlargement, electrolyte imbalances, and drug toxicity.

Locating myocardial damage with a 12–lead ECG

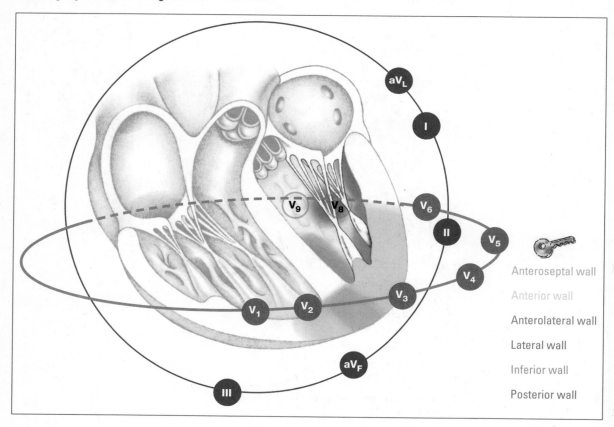

Anteroseptal wall

Anterior wall

Anterolateral wall

Lateral wall

Inferior wall

Posterior wall

Wall affected	Leads	Artery involved	Reciprocal changes
Anteroseptal	V_1, V_2, V_3, V_4	Left anterior descending (LAD)	None
Anterior	V_2, V_3, V_4	Left coronary artery (LCA) and LAD	II, III, aV_F
Anterolateral	I, aV_L, V_3, V_4, V_5, V_6	LAD and diagonal branches, circum-flex and marginal branches	II, III, aV_F
Lateral	I, aV_L, V_5, V_6	Circumflex branch of LCA	II, III, aV_F
Inferior	II, III, aV_F	Right coronary artery (RCA)	I, aV_L
Posterior	V_8, V_9	RCA or circumflex	V_1, V_2, V_3, V_4 (R greater than S in V_1 and V_2, ST-segment depression, elevated T wave)

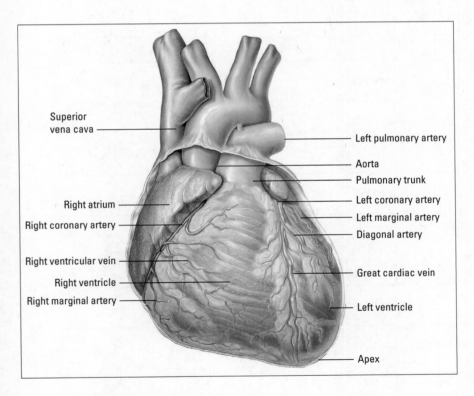

Nursing considerations

- Use a systematic approach to interpret the ECG recording. (See *Normal ECG waveforms*, page 70.) Compare the patient's previous ECG with the current one, if available. Doing so will help you identify changes.

Normal ECG waveforms

Each of the 12 standard leads of an electrocardiogram (ECG) takes a different view of heart activity, and each generates its own characteristic tracing. The tracings shown here represent a normal heart rhythm viewed from each of the 12 leads. Keep in mind the following:
• An upward (positive) deflection indicates that the wave of depolarization flows toward the positive electrode.
• A downward (negative) deflection indicates that the wave of depolarization flows away from the positive electrode.

• An equally positive and negative (biphasic) deflection indicates that the wave of depolarization flows perpendicularly to the positive electrode.

Each lead represents a picture of a different anatomic area; when you find abnormal tracings, compare information from the different leads to pinpoint areas of cardiac damage.

Lead I

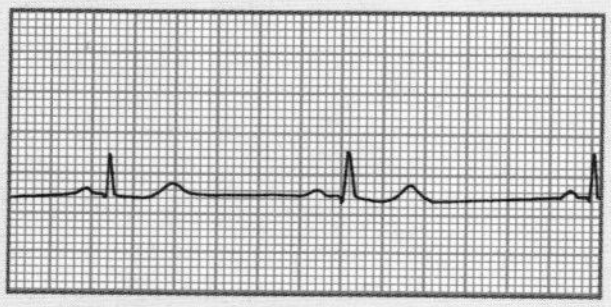

Lead aV$_L$

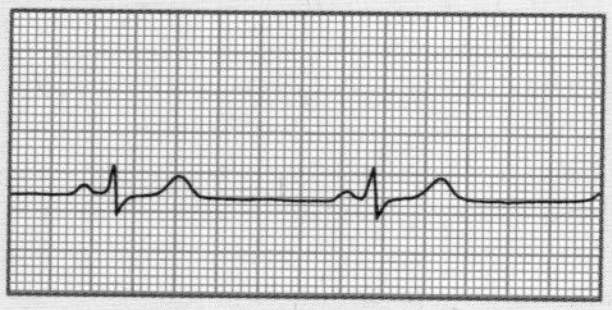

Lead V$_3$

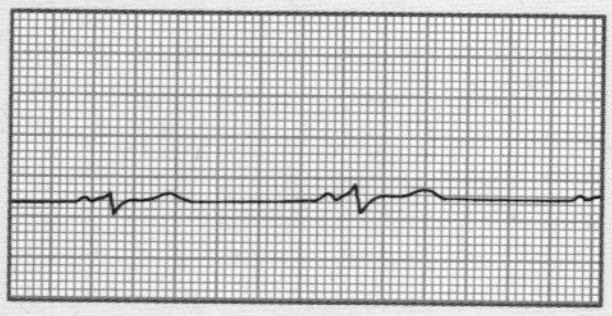

Lead II

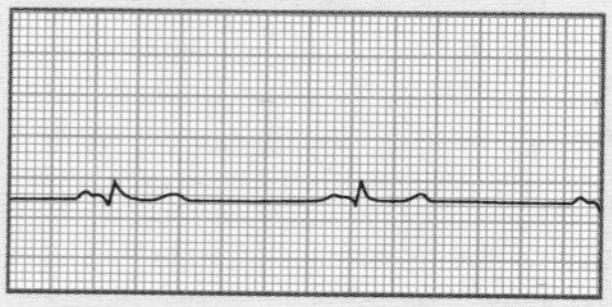

Lead aV$_F$

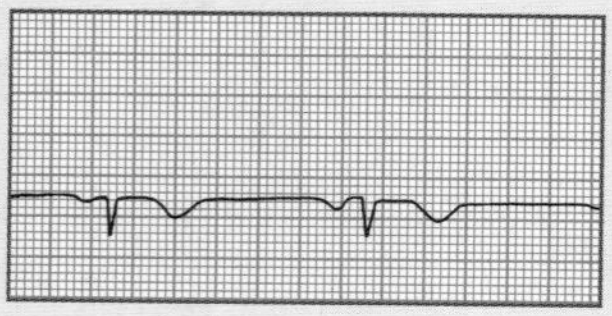

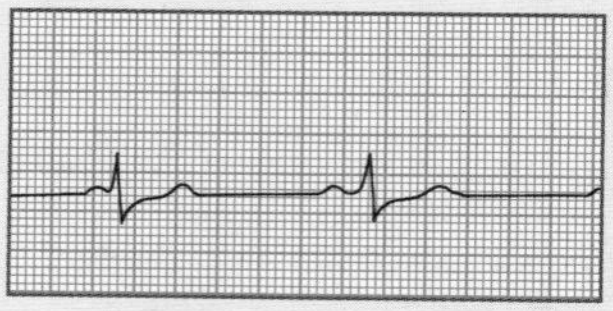

Lead V$_4$

Lead III

Lead V$_1$

Lead V$_5$

Lead aV$_R$

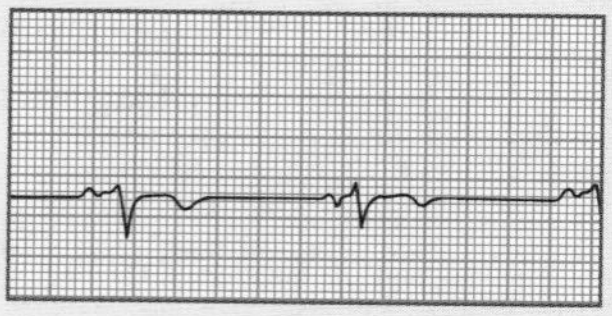

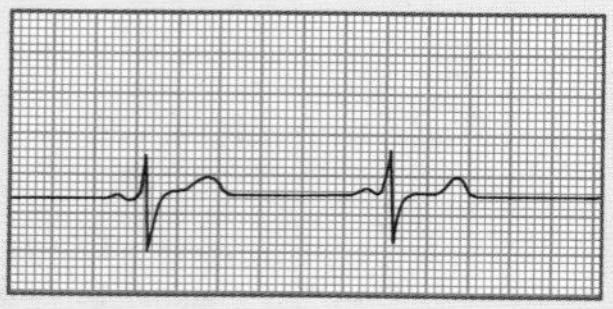

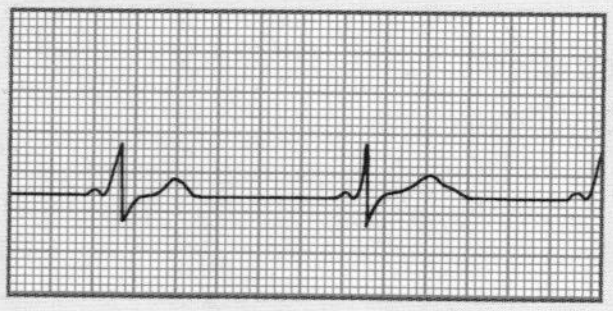

Lead V$_2$

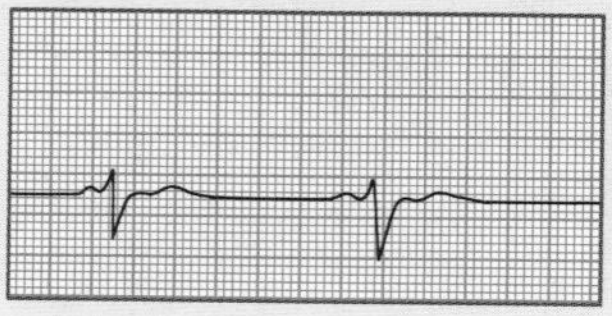

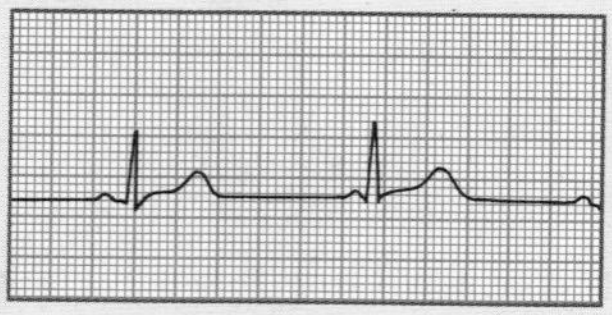

Lead V$_6$

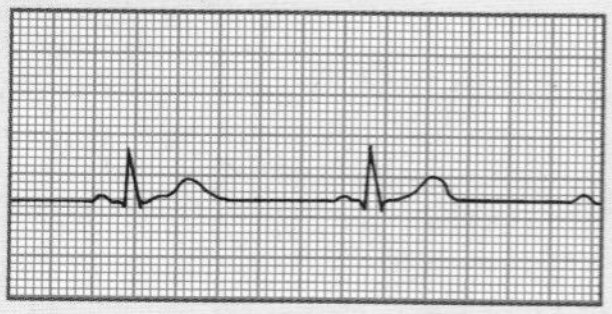

Waves of waves

- P waves should be upright; however, they may be inverted in lead aV_R or biphasic or inverted in leads III, aV_L, and V_1.
- PR intervals should always be constant, like QRS-complex durations.
- QRS-complex deflections vary in different leads. Observe for pathologic Q waves, which are defined as one-third the height of the R wave, greater than 0.04 seconds in width, and must be present in contiguous or groups of leads representing the different walls of the heart.
- ST segments should be isoelectric or have minimal deviation.
- ST-segment elevation greater than 1 mm above the baseline and ST-segment depression greater than 0.5 mm below the baseline are considered abnormal and must be present in contiguous leads. Leads facing toward an injured area have ST-segment elevations, and leads facing away show ST-segment depressions.

Don't sound the alarm—yet

- The T wave normally deflects upward in leads I, II, and V_3 to V_6. It's inverted in lead aV_R and variable in the other leads. T-wave changes have many causes and aren't always a reason for alarm. Excessively tall, flat, or inverted T waves occurring with such symptoms as chest pain may indicate myocardial ischemia.
- A normal Q wave generally has a duration less than 0.04 second. An abnormal Q wave has a duration of 0.04 second or more, a depth greater than 4 mm, or a height one-fourth of the R wave. Abnormal Q waves indicate myocardial necrosis, developing when depolarization can't follow its normal path because of damaged tissue in the area.
- Remember that aV_R normally has a large Q wave, so disregard this lead when searching for abnormal Q waves.

Continuous cardiac monitoring

Because it allows continuous observation of the heart's electrical activity, cardiac monitoring is used in patients at risk for life-threatening arrhythmias. Like other forms of electrocardiography, cardiac monitoring uses electrodes placed on the patient's chest to transmit electrical signals that are converted into a cardiac rhythm tracing on an oscilloscope. (See *Positioning monitor leads*, page 72.)

Hardwire versus wireless

Two types of monitoring may be performed: hardwire or telemetry. In *hardwire monitoring*, the patient is connected to a monitor at the bedside. The rhythm display appears at the bedside, or it may be transmitted to a console at a remote location. *Telemetry* uses a small transmitter connected to leads on the ambulatory patient to send electrical signals to another location, where they're displayed on a monitor screen.

Peak technique

Positioning monitor leads

These illustrations show correct electrode positions for some of the monitoring leads you'll use most often. The abbreviations used are RA, right arm; LA, left arm; RL, right leg; LL, left leg; C, chest; and G, ground. For each lead, you'll see electrode placement for a five-lead system and a three-lead telemetry system.

One for one

In the five-lead system, the electrode position for one lead may be identical to the electrode position for another lead. In this case, simply change the lead selector switch to the setting that corresponds to the lead you want. In some cases, you'll need to reposition the electrodes.

Two for three

In the three-lead telemetry system, you can create the same lead with two electrodes that you do with three simply by eliminating the ground electrode.

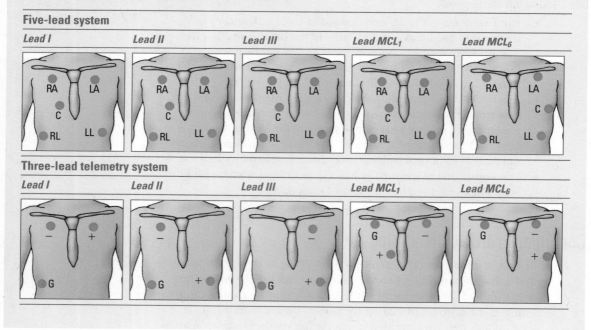

Five-lead system

| Lead I | Lead II | Lead III | Lead MCL₁ | Lead MCL₆ |

Three-lead telemetry system

| Lead I | Lead II | Lead III | Lead MCL₁ | Lead MCL₆ |

Job description

Regardless of the type, cardiac monitors can display the patient's heart rate and rhythm, produce a printed record of cardiac rhythm, and sound an alarm if the heart rate exceeds or falls below specified limits. Monitors also recognize and count abnormal heartbeats as well as changes. (See *Identifying cardiac monitor problems*, page 73.)

Identifying cardiac monitor problems

Problem	Possible causes	Solutions
False–high-rate alarm	Monitor interpreting large T waves as QRS complexes, which doubles the rate	• Reposition electrodes to a lead where QRS complexes are taller than T waves.
	Skeletal muscle activity	• Place electrodes away from major muscle masses.
False–low-rate alarm	Shift in electrical axis from patient's movement, making QRS complexes too small to register	• Reapply electrodes. Set gain so height of complex is greater than 1 mV.
	Low amplitude of QRS	• Increase gain.
	Poor contact between electrode and skin	• Reapply new electrodes.
Artifact (waveform interference)	Patient having seizures, chills, or anxiety	• Notify the healthcare provider and treat the patient as ordered. • Keep the patient warm and reassure them.
	Patient movement	• Help the patient relax.
	Electrodes applied improperly	• Check electrodes and reapply, if necessary.
	Dry electrodes or too little gel	• Make sure cables don't have exposed connectors.
	Static electricity	• Change static-causing bedclothes.
	Electrical short circuit in leads or cable	• Replace broken equipment. Use stress loops when applying leads.
	Interference from decreased room humidity	• Regulate humidity to 40%.

Nursing considerations
- Make sure all electrical equipment and outlets are grounded to avoid electric shock and interference (artifacts). Also ensure that the patient is clean and dry to prevent electric shock.
- If the patient's skin is very oily, scaly, or diaphoretic, rub the electrode site with a dry 4 × 4″ gauze pad before applying the electrode to help reduce interference in the tracing.
- Assess skin integrity and change the electrodes every 24 hours or as necessary.
- Document a rhythm strip at least every 8 hours and with any change in the patient's condition (or as stated by your facility's policy).

Exercise electrocardiography

Exercise electrocardiography is a noninvasive test that helps assess cardiovascular response to an increased workload. Commonly known as a *stress test*, it provides diagnostic information that can't be obtained from a resting ECG. This test may also assess response to treatment. You will usually be asked to avoid caffeine for 24 hours before the test. This includes the following:

- tea and coffee
- all sodas, even ones that are labeled caffeine-free
- chocolates
- certain pain relievers that contain caffeine.

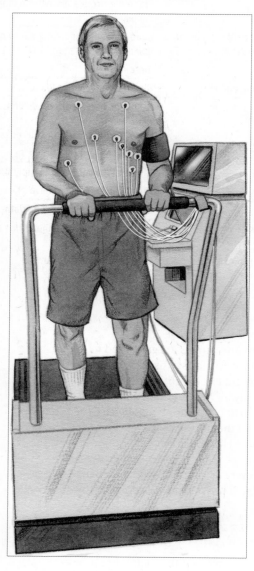

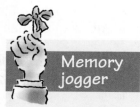

Memory jogger

To help you remember where to place electrodes in a five-electrode configuration, think of the phrase "white to the upper right." Then think of snow over grass (white electrode over green electrode) and smoke over fire (black electrode above red electrode). And of course, chocolate (brown electrode) lies close to the heart.

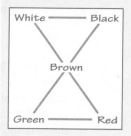

Drug-induced stress tests

If a patient can't tolerate physical activity, a drug (dipyridamole, adenosine, or dobutamine) can be administered to cause the heart to react as if the person were exercising. The drug is given IV along with a radioactive substance known as a *tracer*. Those areas of the heart muscle that lack adequate blood supply pick up the tracer very slowly, if at all.

A nuclear scanner records a set of images; a second set of images is taken 30 minutes to 3 hours later. A cardiologist uses these images to determine the areas of heart muscle with diminished blood supply or permanent damage from an MI.

Stop in a hurry

Stop the test if the patient experiences chest pain, fatigue, or other signs and symptoms that reflect exercise intolerance. These findings may include severe dyspnea, claudication, weakness or dizziness, hypotension, pallor or vasoconstriction, disorientation, ataxia, ischemic ECG changes (with or without pain), rhythm disturbances or heart block, and ventricular conduction abnormalities.

Drugs do it, too

If the patient can't perform physical exercise, a stress test can be performed by intravenous (IV) injection of a coronary vasodilator, such as dipyridamole (Persantine) or adenosine. Other methods of stressing the heart include dobutamine administration and pacing (for patient with a pacemaker or an implantable cardioverter-defibrillator [ICD]). During the stress test, nuclear scanning or echocardiography may also be performed. (See *Drug-induced stress tests*, page 76.)

Nursing considerations

- Tell the patient not to eat, drink caffeinated beverages, or smoke cigarettes for 4 hours before the test.
- Explain that they should wear loose, lightweight clothing, and sneakers and emphasize that they should immediately report any chest pain, leg discomfort, breathlessness, or fatigue.
- Check the healthcare provider's orders to determine which cardiac drugs should be administered or withheld before the test. Beta-adrenergic blockers, for example, can limit the patient's ability to raise their heart rate and are generally withheld the day of the test. Obtain an informed written consent prior to the procedure.

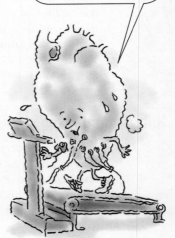

Stop electrocardiography if the patient experiences chest pain, fatigue, or other signs and symptoms that reflect exercise intolerance.

Drug-induced stress tests

If a patient can't tolerate or perform physical activity, a drug-induced stress test can be used so that the healthcare provider can measure the reaction of the heart to exertion.

Exercise without the effort

A drug such as dipyridamole (Persantine) or dobutamine is administered to the patient, which causes the heart to react as if the person were exercising, although the patient is actually at rest.

No blood, no tracer

The drug will either dilate the coronary arteries (dipyridamole [Persantine]) or increase the heart rate (dobutamine). The medication is given through an IV access,

along with thallium or sestamibi (a radioactive substance known as a tracer). These substances travel through the bloodstream to the heart, where they're picked up by the heart muscle cells. Those areas of the heart muscle that lack an adequate blood supply pick up the tracer very slowly or not at all.

A baseline set of images is recorded, with a second set of images taken 3 to 4 hours later. A cardiologist reads the scan to determine areas of the heart muscle that have diminished blood supply or have suffered permanent damage from a heart attack. If an area reveals ischemia, further cardiac testing or medications may be prescribed.

- Inform the patient that they may receive an injection of thallium during the test so that the healthcare provider can evaluate coronary blood flow. Reassure the patient that the injection involves negligible radiation exposure.
- Tell the patient that during and after the test, blood pressure, heart rate, and ECG will be monitored for a period of time.

Holter monitoring

Also called *ambulatory electrocardiography,* Holter monitoring allows recording of heart activity as the patient follows their normal routine. Like exercise electrocardiography, Holter monitoring can provide considerably more diagnostic information than a standard resting ECG. In addition, Holter monitoring can record intermittent arrhythmias.

This test can last from 24 hours up to 14 days. The monitor is connected to electrodes on the chest and is worn at all times. The patient keeps a diary of activities. Patients use this diary to record their daily activities. This is used to compare symptoms the patient may be having to recorded rhythms.

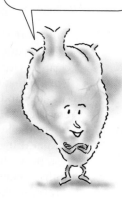

Holter monitoring records the heart's activity for 24 hours while the patient follows a normal routine.

A look at a Holter monitor

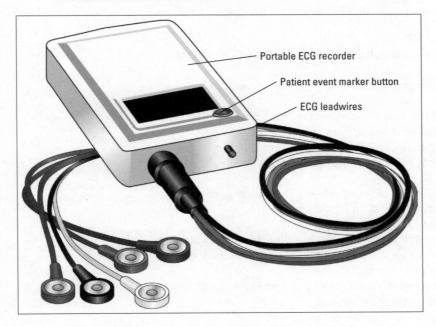

Portable ECG recorder

Patient event marker button

ECG leadwires

Nursing considerations

- Urge the patient not to tamper with the monitor or disconnect leads or electrodes. Demonstrate how to check the recorder for proper function.
- Tell the patient that they can't bathe or shower while wearing the monitor. They also need to avoid electrical appliances, which can interfere with the monitor's recording.
- Emphasize to the patient the importance of keeping track of their activities, regardless of symptoms.
- Evaluation of the recordings will guide further treatment.

Electrophysiology studies

EPS are used to diagnose abnormal heart rhythms. The procedure involves passing two to three temporary electrode catheters into the right-sided heart chambers. The electrodes are usually positioned in the high right atrium, bundle of His region, apex of the right ventricle, and right ventricle outflow area (beneath the pulmonary valve). The electrodes stimulate (pace) the heart and record the heart's electrical conduction and reaction to the pacing stimulus.

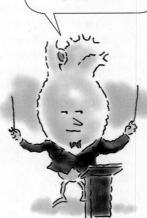

EPS evaluates my conduction system. The results may determine if I need a permanent pacemaker or an ICD or possibly an ablation to stop arrhythmias such as SVT or Afib.

Normal conduction intervals in adults are as follows: HV interval, 35 to 55 ms; AH interval, 55 to 130 ms; and PA interval, 20 to 50 ms.

Nursing considerations

- Explain to the patient that EPS evaluates the heart's conduction system.
- Instruct them to restrict food and fluids for at least 6 to 8 hours before the test.
- Inform the patient that the studies take 1 to 3 hours.
- Have the patient void before the test.
- Monitor the patient's vital signs, as ordered. If they're unstable, check them every 15 minutes and alert the healthcare provider.
- Observe for shortness of breath; chest pain; pallor; or changes in pulse rate, cardiac rhythm, or blood pressure.
- Enforce bed rest for 4 to 6 hours.
- Check the catheter insertion site for bleeding; first, apply manual pressure to the site until hemostasis is achieved and then apply a bandage to the puncture site(s).
- Pressure bandages aren't used for all patients. Remember these are venous access as opposed to arterial.

Cardiac catheterization

Cardiac catheterization involves passing catheters into the right, left, or both sides of the heart.

A multipurpose procedure

This procedure permits measurement of blood pressure and blood flow in the chambers of the heart. It's used to determine valve competence and cardiac wall contractility and to detect intracardiac shunts. The procedure is also used for blood sample collection and can be used to obtain diagnostic images of the ventricles (ventriculography) and arteries (coronary arteriography or angiography). It is the preferred method for restoring blood flow through an obstructed coronary artery.

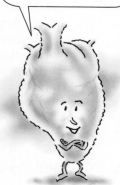

Cardiac catheterization can confirm the presence of CAD, myocardial incompetence, valvular heart disease, and septal defects. Pretty thorough!

Right-sided heart catheterization

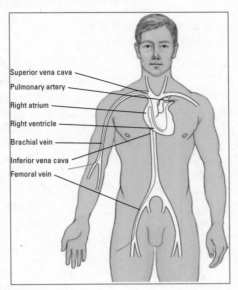

Superior vena cava
Pulmonary artery
Right atrium
Right ventricle
Brachial vein
Inferior vena cava
Femoral vein

Upper limits of normal pressure curves

Chambers of the right side of the heart

Two pressure complexes are represented for each chamber. Complexes at the far right in this diagram represent simultaneous recordings of pressures from the right atrium, right ventricle, and pulmonary artery.

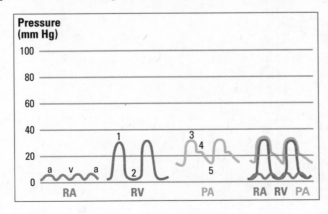

RA = Right atrium
RV = Right ventricle
PA = Pulmonary artery
a wave = Contraction
v wave = Passive filling
1 = RV peak systolic pressure
2 = RV end-diastolic pressure
3 = PA peak systolic pressure
4 = PA dicrotic notch
5 = PA diastolic pressure

Chambers of the left side of the heart

Overall pressure configurations in the left side of the heart are similar to those of the right side of the heart, but pressures are significantly higher because systemic flow resistance is much greater than pulmonary resistance.

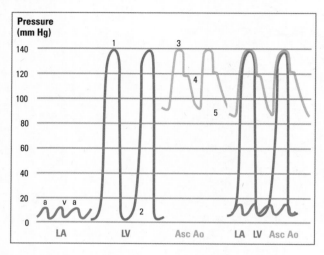

Left-sided heart catheterization

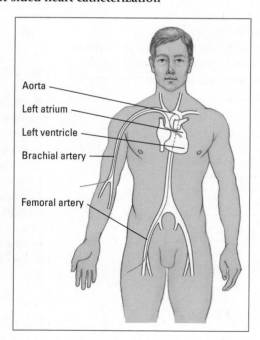

LA = Left atrium
LV = Left ventricle
Asc Ao = Ascending aorta
a wave = Contraction
v wave = Passive filling
1 = LV peak systolic pressure
2 = LV end-diastolic pressure
3 = PA peak systolic pressure
4 = PA dicrotic notch
5 = PA diastolic pressure

Bumpy road ahead

Watch your patient for bradycardia, hypotension, and nausea during femoral catheter removal.

Confirming common problems

Common abnormalities and defects that can be confirmed by cardiac catheterization include CAD, myocardial wall motion abnormalities, valvular heart disease, and septal defects.

Nursing considerations

When caring for a patient undergoing a cardiac catheterization, describe the procedure and events after it and take steps to prevent postoperative complications.

Before the procedure

- Explain that this test is used to evaluate the function of the heart and its vessels. Instruct the patient to restrict food and fluids for at least 6 hours before the test. Tell the patient that the procedure takes 1 to 2 hours and that they may receive a mild sedative during the procedure.
- Tell the patient that the catheters are inserted into an artery or vein in the arm or leg. Tell them that they will experience a transient stinging sensation when a local anesthetic is injected to numb the catheter insertion site.
- Inform the patient that injection of the contrast medium through the catheter may produce a hot, flushing sensation or nausea that quickly passes; instruct the patient to follow directions to cough or breathe deeply. Explain that they may be given medication if they experience chest pain during the procedure. Explain that nitroglycerin may be given periodically to dilate coronary vessels and aid visualization. If the patient develops a headache, inform the staff. Reassure the patient that complications, such as MI and thromboembolism, are rare.
- Make sure that the patient or a responsible family member has signed an informed consent form.
- Check for and tell the healthcare provider about hypersensitivity to shellfish, iodine, or contrast media used in other diagnostic tests. The patient may then require prophylactic medication such as diphenhydramine (Benadryl) and steroids.
- Discontinue anticoagulant therapy, as ordered, to reduce the risk of complications from bleeding.
- Review activity restrictions and position requirements that may be necessary for the patient after the procedure, such as lying flat with the limb extended for 4 to 6 hours and using sandbags as a reminder not to move the affected leg.
- Document the presence of peripheral pulses, noting their intensity. Mark the pulses, so they may be easily located after the procedure and used as a consistent reference spot.

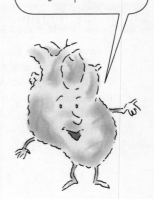

Be sure to discuss postprocedure instructions with your patient.

After the procedure

- Determine if a hemostatic device, such as a collagen plug or suture closure system, was used to close the vessel puncture site. If either method was used, inspect the site for bleeding or oozing, redness, swelling, or hematoma formation. Maintain the patient on bed rest for 1 to 2 hours.
- Enforce bed rest for 4 to 8 hours if no hemostatic device was used. If the femoral route was used for catheter insertion, keep the patient's leg extended for 4 to 8 hours; if the antecubital fossa route was used, keep the arm extended for at least 3 hours; and if the radial artery was used, wrist movement should be limited for 24 hours.
- Monitor vital signs every 15 minutes for 2 hours, then every 30 minutes for the next 2 hours, and then every hour for 2 hours. If no hematoma or other problems arise, check every 4 hours. If signs are unstable, check every 5 minutes and notify the healthcare provider.
- Continually assess the insertion site for a hematoma or blood loss and reinforce the pressure dressing as needed. If the radial artery was used, a radial artery compression band should be placed for at least 2 to 4 hours.
- Check the patient's color, skin temperature, and peripheral pulse below the puncture site.
- Administer IV fluids as ordered (usually 100 mL/hour) to promote excretion of the contrast medium. Monitor for signs of fluid overload.
- Watch for signs of chest pain, shortness of breath, abnormal heart rate, dizziness, diaphoresis, nausea or vomiting, or extreme fatigue. Notify the healthcare provider immediately if these complications occur.

Imaging and radiographic tests

Imaging and radiographic testing produces detailed images of the heart and its ability to function. These tests include echocardiography, coronary computed tomography (CT) angiography, cardiac magnetic resonance imaging (MRI), cardiac positron-emission tomography (PET) scanning, cardiac blood pool imaging, technetium-99m (^{99m}Tc) pyrophosphate scanning, thallium scanning, duplex ultrasonography, and venography.

Echocardiography

An echocardiograph uses ultra-high-frequency sound waves to help examine the size, shape, and motion of the heart's structures. Here's how it works.

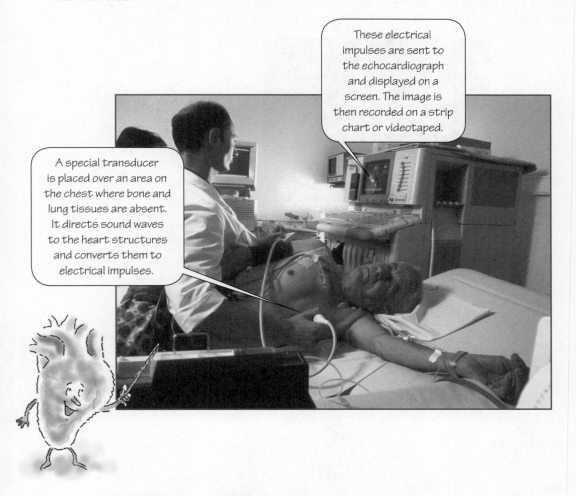

These electrical impulses are sent to the echocardiograph and displayed on a screen. The image is then recorded on a strip chart or videotaped.

A special transducer is placed over an area on the chest where bone and lung tissues are absent. It directs sound waves to the heart structures and converts them to electrical impulses.

Comparing two types of echocardiography

The most commonly used echocardiographic techniques are M-mode (motion mode) and two-dimensional. In many cases, the techniques are performed together to complement each other. Echocardiography may be used to detect mitral stenosis, mitral valve prolapse, aortic insufficiency, wall motion abnormalities, and pericardial effusion. The shaded areas beneath the transducer identify cardiac structures that intercept and reflect the transducer's ultrasonic waves.

Picture this!

This computer graphic depicts an image of the heart's chambers and valves that's more detailed than an x-ray. The ultrasound waves that rebound (or echo) off the heart can show the size, shape, and movement of cardiac structures as well as the flow of blood through the heart, which helps analyze valvular function and heart pressures.

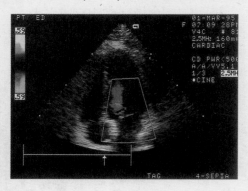

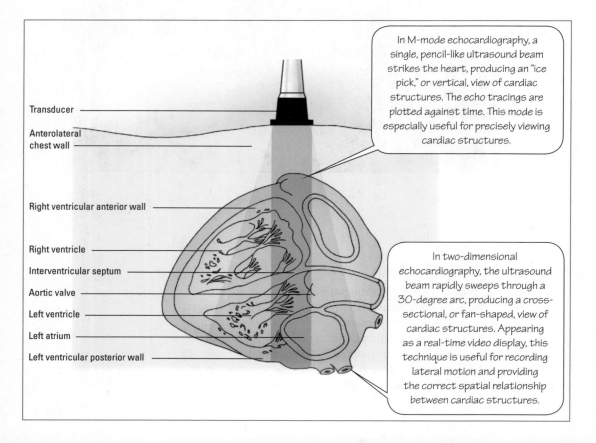

Transducer

Anterolateral chest wall

Right ventricular anterior wall

Right ventricle

Interventricular septum

Aortic valve

Left ventricle

Left atrium

Left ventricular posterior wall

In M-mode echocardiography, a single, pencil-like ultrasound beam strikes the heart, producing an "ice pick," or vertical, view of cardiac structures. The echo tracings are plotted against time. This mode is especially useful for precisely viewing cardiac structures.

In two-dimensional echocardiography, the ultrasound beam rapidly sweeps through a 30-degree arc, producing a cross-sectional, or fan-shaped, view of cardiac structures. Appearing as a real-time video display, this technique is useful for recording lateral motion and providing the correct spatial relationship between cardiac structures.

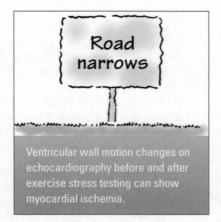

Ventricular wall motion changes on echocardiography before and after exercise stress testing can show myocardial ischemia.

TEE

In transesophageal echocardiography, ultrasonography is combined with endoscopy to provide a better view of the heart's structures. (See *A closer look at TEE*.)

In exercise echocardiography and dobutamine stress echocardiography, a two-dimensional echocardiogram records cardiac wall motion during exercise or while dobutamine is being infused. (See *Teaching about cardiac stress testing*.)

A closer look at TEE

In transesophageal echocardiography (TEE), ultrasonography is combined with endoscopy to provide a better view of the heart's structures.

How it's done
A small transducer attached to the end of a gastroscope is inserted into the esophagus so that images of the heart's structure can be taken from the posterior of the heart. This test has less tissue penetration and interference from chest wall structures and produces high-quality images of the thoracic aorta (except for the superior ascending aorta, which is shadowed by the trachea). The patient is usually given medications to numb the gag reflex and intravenous (IV) sedatives because of the size of the probe.

And why
TEE is used to evaluate valvular disease or repairs. It's also used to diagnose the following:
- thoracic and aortic disorders
- endocarditis
- congenital heart disease
- intracardiac thrombi (commonly done precardioversion)
- tumors.

Teaching about cardiac stress testing

Exercise echocardiography and dobutamine stress echocardiography are the types of cardiac stress testing that detect changes in heart wall motion through the use of two-dimensional echocardiography during exercise or a dobutamine infusion. Imaging is done before and after either exercise or dobutamine administration. Usually, these tests are performed to do the following:

- identify the cause of chest pain
- detect heart abnormalities, obstructions, or damage
- determine the heart's functional capacity after myocardial infarction or cardiac surgery
- evaluate myocardial perfusion
- measure the heart chambers
- set limits for an exercise program.

Preparing your patient

When preparing your patient for these tests, cover the following points:

- Explain that this test will evaluate how their heart performs under stress and how specific heart structures work under stress.
- Instruct the patient not to eat, smoke, or drink alcohol or caffeinated beverages for at least 4 hours before the test.
- Advise the patient to ask their healthcare provider whether they should withhold current medications before the test.
- Tell the patient to wear a two-piece outfit because they will be removing all clothing above the waist and will wear a hospital gown.
- Explain that electrodes will be placed on their chest and arms to obtain an initial electrocardiogram (ECG). Mention that the areas where electrodes are placed will be cleaned with alcohol and that the skin will be rubbed for optimal electrode contact.
- Tell the patient that an initial echocardiogram will be performed while they're lying down. Conductive gel, which feels warm, will be placed on their chest. Then, a special transducer will be placed at various angles

on their chest to visualize different parts of their heart. Emphasize that they must remain still to prevent distorting the images.

- Inform the patient that the entire procedure should take 60 to 90 minutes. Explain that the healthcare provider will compare these echocardiograms to diagnose abnormal their heart conditions.

Explaining exercise echocardiography

If the patient will have an exercise stress test after the initial echocardiogram, cover these teaching points:

- Tell the patient that they will walk on the treadmill at a prescribed rate for a predetermined time to raise their heart rate. After they reach the prescribed heart rate, they will lie down and a second echocardiogram will be done.
- Explain that they may feel tired, sweaty, and slightly short of breath during the test. If their symptoms are severe or chest pain develops, the test will be stopped.
- Reassure the patient that their blood pressure will be monitored during the test. After the test is complete, their ECG and blood pressure will be monitored for a minimum of 10 minutes.

Describing the dobutamine stress test

If the patient will undergo a dobutamine stress test after the initial echocardiogram, cover these teaching points:

- Explain that an intravenous (IV) line will be inserted into their vein for the dobutamine infusion. Tell the patient that this drug will increase their heart rate without exercise. Tell them to expect initial discomfort when the IV line is inserted. Mention that, during the infusion, they may feel palpitations, shortness of breath, and fatigue.
- Inform the patient that a second echocardiogram will be done during the dobutamine infusion. After the drug is infused and their heart rate reaches the desired level, a third echocardiogram will be obtained.
- Reassure the patient that their blood pressure will be monitored during the test.

Echo abnormalities

The echocardiogram may detect congenital heart disease, mitral stenosis, mitral valve prolapse, aortic insufficiency, wall motion abnormalities, and pericardial effusion (excess pericardial fluid), endocarditis, intracardiac thrombi, and tumors.

Nursing considerations

- Explain the procedure to the patient and advise them to remain still during the test because movement can distort results. Tell the patient that conductive gel is applied to the chest and a transducer head is placed directly over the gel. Because pressure is exerted to keep the transducer in contact with the skin, warn the patient that they may feel minor discomfort.
- After the procedure, remove the conductive gel from the skin.

Coronary CT angiography

Also known as coronary calcium score, CT uses an injection of iodine-containing contrast material to examine the arteries that supply blood to the heart and determine whether they have narrowing of arteries. The plaque formation can be quantified (calcium score) by a low-dose x-ray detector.

Nursing considerations

- Assess for iodine or shellfish allergy.
- Instruct the patient not to eat or drink anything for 4 hours before the test.
- Encourage the patient to verbalize concerns of claustrophobia.
- Explain to the patient that they may experience a salty taste, flushing, and warmth from the dye injection.
- After the procedure, encourage the patient to increase fluid intake to flush dye from the kidneys.

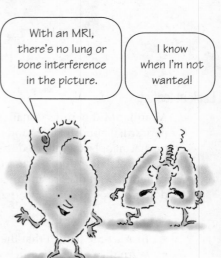

With an MRI, there's no lung or bone interference in the picture.

I know when I'm not wanted!

Cardiac magnetic resonance imaging

Also known as *nuclear magnetic resonance*, MRI yields high-resolution, tomographic, three-dimensional images of body structures. It takes advantage of certain magnetically aligned body nuclei that fall out of alignment after radiofrequency transmission. The MRI scanner records the signals the nuclei emit as they realign in a process called *precession* and then translates the signals into detailed pictures of body structures. The resulting images show tissue characteristics without lung or bone interference.

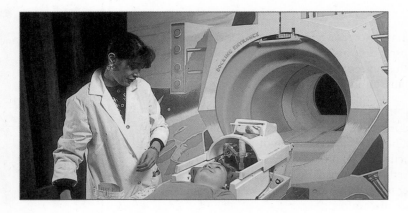

The MRI scanner records the electromagnetic signals the nuclei emit. The scanner then translates the signals into detailed pictures. The resulting images show tissue characteristics without lung or bone interference, as shown here.

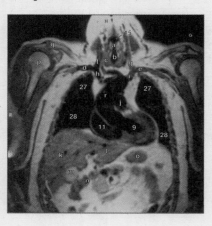

Dangerous intersection

Don't let your patients with pacemakers, implantable cardioverter defibrillators, or transdermal drug patches in here; metal attracts!

Look at leaflets

A cardiac MRI permits visualization of valve leaflets and structures, pericardial abnormalities and processes, ventricular hypertrophy, cardiac neoplasm, infarcted tissue, anatomic malformations, and structural deformities. It can be used to monitor the progression of ischemic heart disease and the effectiveness of treatment because it does not look at coronary arteries.

Nursing considerations

- Instruct the patient that they will need to lie still during the test.
- Warn the patient that they will hear a thumping noise.

- Encourage the patient to verbalize concerns of claustrophobia.
- Tell the patient that they will be given a signal button to notify staff of any problems.

Lose the jewels

- Have the patient remove all jewelry and other metallic objects before testing. A patient with an internal surgical clip, scalp vein needle, pacemaker or ICD, gold fillings, heart valve prosthesis, or other metal object in their body can't undergo an MRI.
- Permit the patient to resume activities as ordered.

Cardiac positron-emission tomography

Cardiac PET scanning combines elements of CT scanning and conventional radionuclide imaging. Here's how it works: Radioisotopes are administered to the patient. These isotopes emit particles called *positrons*, which the PET scanner detects and reconstructs to form an image. One distinct advantage of PET scans is that positron emitters can be chemically "tagged" to biologically active molecules, such as glucose, enabling study of their uptake and distribution in tissue.

Cardiac PET scanning is used to detect CAD, evaluate myocardial metabolism and contractility, and distinguish viable cardiac tissue from infarcted tissue, especially during the early stages of MI. Reduced blood flow with increased glucose use indicates ischemia. Reduced blood flow with decreased glucose use indicates necrotic, scarred tissue. Normally, no areas of ischemic tissue are present on the scan.

How it works

Radioisotopes are administered to the patient by injection, inhalation, or IV infusion. One isotope targets blood; one targets glucose.

1.
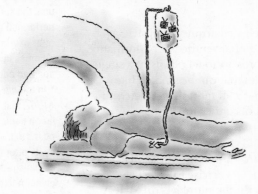

These isotopes emit particles called *positrons*.

2.

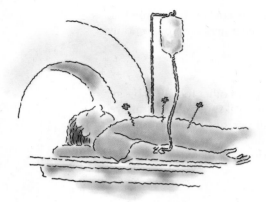

3. The PET scanner detects and reconstructs the positrons to form an image.

Nursing considerations

*   Warn the patient that cigarette smoking is restricted, and medication use may be restricted before the test.
*   Make sure the patient has signed an informed consent form.
*   Document and report all allergies.
*   Advise the patient that they may be connected to a cardiac monitor.
*   Instruct the patient that they will need to lie still during the test.
*   Explain to the patient that they will be given a radioactive substance, either by injection, by inhalation, or by IV infusion.
*   Tell the patient that the test is usually painless. If an IV infusion is planned, the patient may experience slight discomfort from the needle puncture and tourniquet. If the radioisotope will be inhaled, explain to the patient that this procedure is painless.

Cardiac blood pool imaging

Cardiac blood pool imaging (multiple-gated acquisition [MUGA] scan) is used to evaluate regional and global ventricular performance. During a MUGA scan, the camera records 14 to 64 points of a single cardiac cycle, yielding sequential images that can be studied like a motion picture film to evaluate regional wall motion and determine the ejection fraction and other indices of cardiac function.

Various variations

There are many variations of the MUGA scan. In the stress MUGA test, the same test is performed at rest and after exercise to detect changes in ejection fraction and cardiac output. In the nitroglycerin MUGA test, the scintillation camera records points in the cardiac cycle after the sublingual administration of nitroglycerin to assess the drug's effect on ventricular function.

What it shows

*   Normal blood flow and glucose metabolism indicates good coronary perfusion.
*   Decreased blood flow with increased glucose metabolism indicates ischemia.
*   Decreased blood flow with decreased glucose metabolism shows necrotic or scarred heart tissue.

Varieties are the spice of life

Many variations of the MUGA scan are available:
*   In the *stress MUGA* test, the same test is performed at rest and after exercise to detect changes in ejection fraction and cardiac output.
*   In the *nitroglycerin MUGA* test, the scintillation camera records points in the cardiac cycle after the sublingual administration of nitroglycerin to assess the drug's effect on ventricular function.

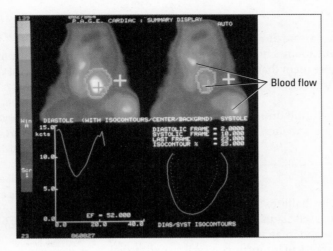

Blood flow

Nursing considerations

- An ECG is required to signal the computer and the camera to take images for each cardiac cycle.
- If arrhythmias interfere with a reliable ECG, the test may need to be postponed.

---

^{99m}Tc pyrophosphate scanning

^{99m}Tc pyrophosphate scanning, also known as *hot spot imaging* or PYP scanning, helps diagnose acute myocardial injury by showing the location and size of newly damaged myocardial tissue. Especially useful for diagnosing transmural infarction, this test works best when performed 12 hours to 6 days after symptom onset. It also helps diagnose right ventricular infarctions; locate true posterior infarctions; assess trauma, ventricular aneurysm, and heart tumors; and detect myocardial damage from a recent electric shock such as defibrillation.

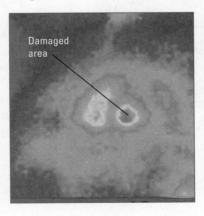

Damaged area

How it works

- ^{99m}Tc pyrophosphate is injected into the patient.
- Isotopes are absorbed by damaged cells.
- Damaged areas show as orange to bright red spots on the image.
- The scan reveals transmural, right ventricular, and posterior infarctions.
- Ventricular aneurysms and tumors are also visible.

Nursing considerations
- Tell the patient that the healthcare provider will inject ^{99m}Tc pyrophosphate into an arm vein about 3 hours before the start of this 45-minute test. Reassure them that the injection causes only transient discomfort and that it involves only negligible radiation exposure.
- Instruct the patient to remain still during the test.
- Permit the patient to resume activities, as ordered.

Test tip

Tell your patient to expect to lie on their back with the arms above the head during and up to 30 minutes after the test. This allows the scanner to move 360° around the body.

Thallium scanning

Also known as *cold spot imaging*, thallium scanning evaluates myocardial blood flow and myocardial cell status. This test helps determine areas of ischemic myocardium and infarcted tissue. It can also help evaluate coronary artery and ventricular function as well as pericardial effusion. Thallium imaging can also detect an MI in its first few hours. (See *How it works*.)

Cold-hearted

The test uses thallium-201, a radioactive isotope that emits gamma rays and closely resembles potassium. When injected IV, the isotope enters healthy myocardial tissue rapidly but enters areas with poor blood flow and damaged cells slowly. A camera counts the gamma rays and displays an image. Areas with heavy isotope uptake appear light, whereas areas with poor uptake, known as "cold spots," look dark. Cold spots represent areas of reduced myocardial perfusion.

How it works

- Tl^{201} is injected into the patient.
- Isotopes are rapidly absorbed by healthy heart tissue and emit gamma rays. Unhealthy tissue slowly absorbs isotopes.
- Damaged areas show as **dark** spots on the image.
- The scan reveals ischemic and infarcted areas.
- The test is also used to evaluate ventricular function and the presence of pericardial effusion.

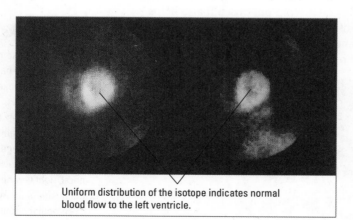

Uniform distribution of the isotope indicates normal blood flow to the left ventricle.

Test tip

If your patient can't raise the arms, one-dimensional Tl^{201} scanning can still be done. Pictures are taken from three different views (called *planar imaging*).

Nursing considerations
- Tell the patient to avoid heavy meals, cigarette smoking, and strenuous activity for 24 hours before the test.
- If the patient is scheduled for an exercise thallium scan, advise them to wear comfortable clothes such as sweatpants or pajamas and sneakers.
- After the procedure, permit the patient to resume activities, as ordered.

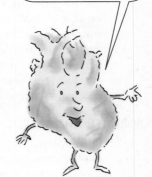

With duplex ultrasonography, a handheld transducer directs high-frequency sound waves that help to evaluate blood flow.

Duplex ultrasonography

Duplex ultrasonography is a noninvasive method used to evaluate blood flow in the major arteries and veins of the arms, legs, abdomen, and extracranial cerebrovascular system. The procedure involves using a handheld transducer to direct high-frequency sound waves into an artery or vein and its surrounding tissues.

Two-step process

In the first part of the test, the sound waves reflect off the blood vessel and surrounding tissues, creating images that are displayed on a monitor. Then additional sound waves are directed specifically into the vessel to be studied. These sound waves strike moving red blood cells within the vessel at one frequency and are reflected back to the

Duplex scan of popliteal artery

Color flow duplex image of popliteal artery with normal triphasic spectral waveform.

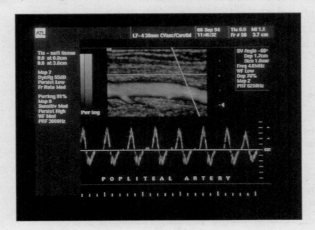

transducer at another frequency. This change in frequency produces an audible Doppler signal that corresponds to blood flow velocity within the vessel. The speed, direction, and pattern of the blood flow are displayed on the monitor as a spectral waveform. The size and shape of the imaged blood vessel can also be measured.

Diagnosing duplex

Duplex ultrasonography can be used to diagnose diseases of the arteries and the veins, such as atherosclerotic blockages, arterial thrombosis or emboli, aneurysms, pseudoaneurysm, arterial dissections, congenital abnormalities, arteriovenous fistulae, thrombophlebitis, and venous insufficiency. It can also be used to create maps of a patient's arteries and veins prior to transplant or bypass surgery. It is also used to assess and detect complications after invasive procedures involving femoral vascular access.

Additional arterial analysis

Pulse volume recorder testing may be performed along with arterial duplex ultrasonography. This test yields quantitative recordings of the differences in arterial blood flow between various segments of the arms or legs. Several blood pressure cuffs are placed on the extremity, and a handheld Doppler is used to record segmental systolic pressures and spectral waveforms from each cuff. By comparing the difference between each segment, the presence, location, and extent of arterial blockage can be determined.

Nursing considerations

- Explain the test to the patient. Emphasize that the test is noninvasive and that they won't feel the sound waves.
- Inform the patient that water-soluble conductive gel will be applied to their skin to conduct the sound waves into their tissues.
- Check with the vascular laboratory to determine whether special instructions or preparation is necessary. Note that some tests may require the patient to fast.

Suggested references

Adams, M. P., & Urban, C. Q. (2019). Pharmacotherapy of hyperlipidemia. In Adams, M. P. & Urban, C. Q. (Eds.), *Pharmacology: Connections to nursing practice* (4th ed., pp. 488–509). Pearson.

American Association of Critical Care Nurses. (2009). *AACN practice alert: Pulmonary artery/central venous pressure measurement.* Retrieved from http://www.aacn.org/wd/practice/docs/pap-measurement.pdf

Barohn, R. J. (2007). Muscle diseases. In Goldman, L. & Ausiello, D. (Eds.), *Cecil medicine* (23rd ed., pp. 2817–2833). Saunders Elsevier.

Bridges, E. J. (2006). Pulmonary artery pressure monitoring: When, how, and what else to use. *AACN Advanced Critical Care, 17*(3), 286–303.

Darovic, G. O. (2004). *Handbook of hemodynamic monitoring* (2nd ed.). Saunders Elsevier.

Doering, L. V. (1993). The effect of positioning on hemodynamics and gas exchange in the critically ill: A review. *American Journal of Critical Care, 2*(3), 208–216.

Ellis, K. M. (2017). *EKG plain and simple* (4th ed.). Pearson.

Gulati, M., Levy, P. D., Mukherjee, D., Amsterdam, E., Bhatt, D. L., Birtcher, K. K., Blankstein, R, Boyd, J., Bullock-Palmer, R. P., Conejo, T., Diercks, D. B., Gentile, F., Greenwood, J. P., Hess, E. P., Hollenberg, S. M., Jaber, W. A., Jneid, H., Joglar, J. A., Morrow, D. A., … Shaw, L. J. (2021). *144, .* 2021 AHA/ACC/ASE/CHEST/SAEM/SCCT/SCMR guideline for the evaluation and diagnosis of chest pain: A report of the American College of Cardiology/American Heart Association Joint Committee on Clinical Practice Guidelines. *Circulation,* 2021(22) e368–e454. https://doi.org/10.1161/CIR.0000000000001029

Lewis, S. M., Heitkemper, M. M., & Dirksen, S. R. (2017). *Medical-surgical nursing: Assessment and management of clinical problems* (10th ed.). Mosby.

Pagana, K. D., & Pagana, T. J. (2018). *Mosby's manual of diagnostics and laboratory tests* (6th ed.). Elsevier.

Rajarao, M.P., Al Kharoosi, A. M., Panduranga, P. (2018). *19,* Clinical significance of elevated high-sensitivity troponin T in low likelihood acute coronary syndrome patients. *Heart View, 2018*(2), 54–57.

Sandoval, Y., Apple, F. S, Mahler, S. A., Body, R. Collinson, P. O., Jaffe, A. S., International Federation of Clinical Chemistry and Laboratory Medicine Committee on the Clinical Application of Cardiac Biomarkers. (2022). High-sensitivity cardiac troponin and the 2021 AHA/ACC/ASE/CHEST/SAEM/SCCT/SCMR guidelines for the evaluation and diagnosis of acute chest pain. *Circulation, 146*(7) 569–581. https://doi.org/10.1161/CIRCULATIONAHA.122.059678

Smith, L. W. (2015). Cardiac and vascular assessment. In Smith, L. W. (Ed.), *Cardiac-vascular nursing review and resource manual* (4th ed., pp. 181–223). American Nurses Association.

Virani, S. S., Newby, L. K., Arnold, S. V., Bittner, V., Brewer, L. C., Demeter, S. H., , Dixon, DL, Fearon, WF, Hess, B, Johnson, HM, Kazi, DS, Kolte, D, Kumbhani, DJ, LoFaso, J, Mahtta, D, Mark, DB, Minissian, M, Navar, AM, Patel, AR, … Williams, MS. (2023). 2023 AHA/ACC/ACCP/ASPC/NLA/PCNA Guideline for the Management of patients with chronic coronary disease: A report of the American Heart Association/American College of Cardiology Joint Committee on Clinical Practice Guidelines. *Circulation, 148*(9) e9–e119. https://doi.org/10.1161/CIR.0000000000001168

Chapter 5

Arrhythmias

Just the facts

In this chapter, you'll learn:

- ◆ ways to identify various arrhythmias
- ◆ causes of each type of arrhythmia
- ◆ significance of, treatment for, and nursing implications of each type of arrhythmia
- ◆ assessment findings for each type of arrhythmia.

A look at arrhythmias

Cardiac arrhythmias are variations in the normal pattern of electrical stimulation of the heart. Arrhythmias vary in severity—from those that are mild, cause no symptoms, and require no treatment (such as sinus arrhythmia) to those that require emergency intervention (such as ventricular fibrillation). Arrhythmias are generally classified according to their origin (ventricular or supraventricular).

The most common types of arrhythmias include sinus node arrhythmias, atrial arrhythmias, junctional arrhythmias, ventricular arrhythmias, and atrioventricular (AV) blocks.

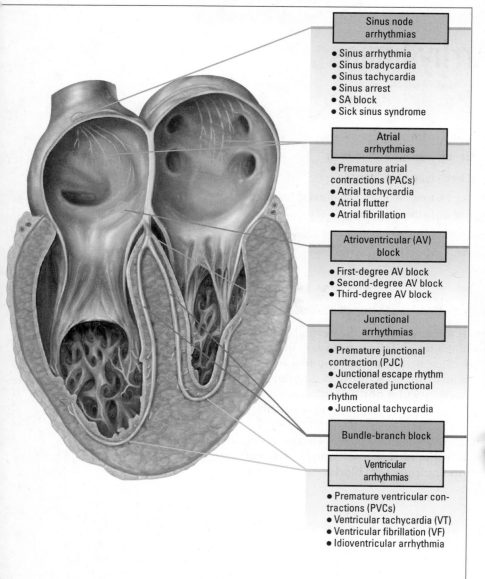

Sinus node arrhythmias

- Sinus arrhythmia
- Sinus bradycardia
- Sinus tachycardia
- Sinus arrest
- SA block
- Sick sinus syndrome

Atrial arrhythmias

- Premature atrial contractions (PACs)
- Atrial tachycardia
- Atrial flutter
- Atrial fibrillation

Atrioventricular (AV) block

- First-degree AV block
- Second-degree AV block
- Third-degree AV block

Junctional arrhythmias

- Premature junctional contraction (PJC)
- Junctional escape rhythm
- Accelerated junctional rhythm
- Junctional tachycardia

Bundle-branch block

Ventricular arrhythmias

- Premature ventricular contractions (PVCs)
- Ventricular tachycardia (VT)
- Ventricular fibrillation (VF)
- Idioventricular arrhythmia

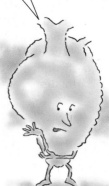

Arrhythmias are variations in my normal pattern of electrical stimulation. Bummer!

Sinus node arrhythmias

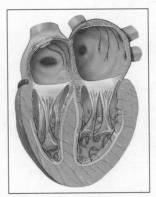

When a heart is functioning normally, the sinoatrial (SA) node, also called the *sinus node*, acts as the primary pacemaker. The sinus node assumes this role because its automatic firing rate exceeds that of the heart's other pacemakers. In an adult at rest, the sinus node has an inherent firing rate of 60 to 100 times/min.

What nerve!

The SA node's blood supply comes from the right coronary artery and left circumflex artery. The autonomic nervous system richly innervates the sinus node through the vagus nerve, a parasympathetic nerve, and several sympathetic nerves. Stimulation of the vagus nerve decreases the node's firing rate, and stimulation of the sympathetic system increases it.

Types of sinus node arrhythmias include sinus arrhythmia, sinus bradycardia, sinus tachycardia, sinus arrest, and sick sinus syndrome.

Sinus arrhythmia

In sinus arrhythmia, the pacemaker cells of the SA node fire irregularly. The cardiac rate stays within normal limits, but the rhythm is irregular and corresponds to the respiratory cycle. Sinus arrhythmias commonly occur in athletes, children, and older people but rarely occur in infants. Conditions unrelated to respiration may also produce sinus arrhythmia, including inferior-wall myocardial infarction (MI), advanced age, use of digoxin (Lanoxin) or morphine, and increased intracranial pressure.

How it happens

During inspiration, blood flow to the heart increases. This increase reduces vagal tone, which in turn increases heart rate. During expiration, venous return decreases. This increases vagal tone, slowing the heart rate. (See *Breathing and sinus arrhythmia.*)

Breathing and sinus arrhythmia

When sinus arrhythmia is related to respirations, you'll see an increase in heart rate with inspiration and a decrease with expiration, as shown here.

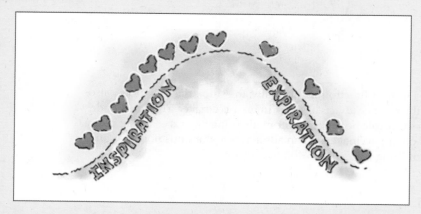

Rhythm
- Irregular
- Corresponds to the respiratory cycle
- P-P interval and R-R interval shorter during respiratory inspiration; longer during expiration
- Difference between longest and shortest P-P interval exceeds 0.12 second

Rate
- Usually within normal limits (60 to 100 beats/min)
- Varies with respiration (increases during inspiration; decreases during expiration due to the effect on the vagus nerve)

P wave
- Normal size
- Normal configuration
- P wave before each QRS complex

PR interval
- May vary slightly
- Within normal limits

QRS complex
- Preceded by **P wave**

T wave
- Normal size
- Normal configuration

QT interval
- May vary slightly
- Usually within normal limits

Other
- Phasic slowing and quickening

What to look for

To identify sinus arrhythmia, observe the patient's heart rhythm during respiration. The atrial and ventricular rates should be within normal limits (60 to 100 beats/min) but increase during inspiration and slow with expiration. Electrocardiogram (ECG) complexes fall closer together during inspiration, shortening the P-P interval (the time elapsed between two consecutive P waves). During expiration, the P-P interval lengthens. The difference between the shortest and longest P-P intervals exceeds 0.12 second. (See *Recognizing sinus arrhythmia*.)

Breathing easy

Check the patient's peripheral pulse rate. It, too, should increase during inspiration and decrease during expiration. If the arrhythmia is caused by an underlying condition, you may note signs and symptoms of that condition as well.

When evaluating sinus arrhythmia, be sure to check the monitor carefully. A marked variation in P-P intervals in an older patient may indicate sick sinus syndrome, a related but more serious phenomenon. (See *A longer look at sinus arrhythmia*.)

Recognizing sinus arrhythmia

Take a look at this example of how sinus arrhythmia appears on a rhythm strip. Notice its distinguishing characteristics.

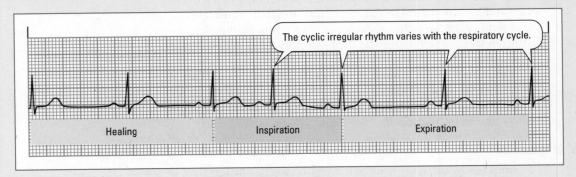

The cyclic irregular rhythm varies with the respiratory cycle.

Healing | Inspiration | Expiration

- *Rhythm:* Irregular
- *Rate:* 60 beats/min
- *P wave:* Normal
- *PR interval:* 0.16 second
- *QRS complex:* 0.06 second and preceded by a P wave
- *T wave:* Normal
- *QT interval:* 0.36 second
- *Other:* Phasic slowing and quickening

How you intervene

Unless the patient is symptomatic, treatment usually isn't necessary. If sinus arrhythmia is unrelated to respiration, the underlying cause may require treatment.

On the alert

If sinus arrhythmia is caused by drugs, such as morphine or other sedatives, the healthcare provider may decide to continue those medications. If a patient taking digoxin suddenly develops sinus arrhythmia, notify the healthcare provider immediately. The patient may be experiencing digoxin toxicity. Illicit drugs, such as cocaine, can also cause arrhythmias.

Sinus bradycardia

Sinus bradycardia is a heart rate less than 60 beats/min. This may be a normal cardiac rhythm for some individuals, such as very fit athletes. The clinical significance of sinus bradycardia depends on the rate and whether the patient is symptomatic. Most adults can tolerate a sinus bradycardia of 45 to 59 beats/min. If the heart rate decreases abnormally, to rates below 45 beats/min in individuals who are not athletes, they may exhibit signs and symptoms of decreased cardiac output and hypotension, such as dizziness, confusion, and, possibly, syncope.

How it happens

Sinus bradycardia usually occurs as a normal response to a reduced demand for blood flow. In this case, vagal stimulation increases and sympathetic stimulation decreases. As a result, automaticity (the tendency of cells to initiate their own impulses) in the SA node diminishes.

Sinus bradycardia commonly occurs after an inferior-wall MI involving the right coronary artery, which supplies blood to the SA node. Numerous other conditions and the use of certain drugs may also cause sinus bradycardia. (See *Causes of sinus bradycardia*.)

What to look for

In sinus bradycardia, the heartbeat is regular with a rate less than 60 beats/min. All other ECG findings are normal: A P wave precedes each QRS complex and the PR interval, QRS complex, T wave, and QT interval are all normal. (See *Recognizing sinus bradycardia*.)

Symptoms? Problem!

If the rate falls below 45 beats/min, patients usually have signs and symptoms of decreased cardiac output, such as hypotension, dizziness, confusion, or syncope (Stokes-Adams attack). Keep in mind,

Causes of sinus bradycardia

Sinus bradycardia may be caused by the following:

- noncardiac disorders, such as hyperkalemia, increased intracranial pressure, hypothyroidism, hypothermia, sleep apnea, and glaucoma
- conditions producing excess vagal stimulation or decreased sympathetic stimulation, such as sleep, deep relaxation, Valsalva maneuver, carotid sinus massage, and vomiting
- cardiac diseases, such as sinoatrial node disease, cardiomyopathy, myocarditis, myocardial ischemia, and heart block; sinus bradycardia can also occur immediately following an inferior-wall myocardial infarction
- certain drugs, especially beta-adrenergic blockers; digoxin (Lanoxin); calcium channel blockers; lithium (Eskalith); and antiarrhythmics, such as sotalol (Betapace), amiodarone (Cordarone), propafenone (Rythmol), and quinidine.

too, that patients with underlying cardiac disease may be less tolerant of a decreased heart rate.

Bradycardia may trigger more serious arrhythmias as well. Ectopic beats, such as premature atrial, junctional, or ventricular contractions, may also occur, causing palpitations and an irregular pulse.

Recognizing sinus bradycardia

Take a look at this example of how sinus bradycardia appears on a rhythm strip. Notice its distinguishing characteristics.

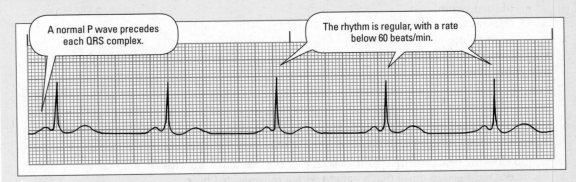

- *Rhythm:* Regular
- *Rate:* 48 beats/min
- *P wave:* Normal
- *PR interval:* 0.16 second
- *QRS complex:* 0.08 second
- *T wave:* Normal
- *QT interval:* 0.50 second
- *Other:* None

In a patient with acute inferior-wall MI, sinus bradycardia is considered a favorable prognostic sign, unless it's accompanied by hypotension. That's because with a slower heart rate, the heart uses less oxygen and avoids ischemia. Sinus bradycardia rarely affects children.

How you intervene

If the patient is asymptomatic and their vital signs are stable, treatment isn't necessary. Continue to observe their heart rhythm, monitoring the progression and duration of bradycardia. Evaluate their tolerance of the rhythm at rest and with activity. Also, review the drugs they are taking. Check with the healthcare provider about stopping medications that may be depressing the SA node, such as digoxin, beta-adrenergic blockers, and calcium channel blockers. Before giving those drugs, make sure the heart rate is within a safe range.

If the patient is symptomatic, treatment aims to identify and correct the underlying cause. Meanwhile, drugs such as atropine, epinephrine, and dopamine, or a temporary pacemaker can help to maintain an adequate heart rate. Patients with chronic, symptom-producing sinus bradycardia may require insertion of a permanent pacemaker. (See *Treating symptom-producing bradycardia*, page 104.)

Check the ABCs

If the patient abruptly develops a significant sinus bradycardia, assess their airway, breathing, and circulation (ABC). If these are adequate, determine whether the patient has an effective cardiac output. If not, they may develop these signs and symptoms:
- hypotension
- cool, clammy skin
- altered mental status
- dizziness
- blurred vision
- crackles, dyspnea, and a third heart sound (S_3), which indicate heart failure
- chest pain
- syncope.

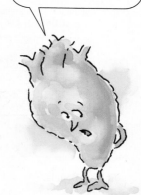

Sinus bradycardia in a child is an ominous sign.

Treatment sequence

If the patient has poor perfusion, atropine 1 mg IV should be administered as a first-line treatment and may be repeated to a total dose of 3 mg. Atropine doses lower than 0.5 mg may have a paradoxical effect and slow the heart rate even further, so it is important to double check the dosage. Keep in mind that a patient with a transplanted heart won't respond to atropine and may require pacing for emergency treatment.

Peak technique

Treating symptom-producing bradycardia

This algorithm shows the steps for treating bradycardia in a patient not in cardiac arrest.

Perform initial assessment and early interventions:

- Assess airway, breathing, and circulation.
- Secure the patient's airway noninvasively.
- Assess whether invasive airway management is needed.
- Make sure a monitor defibrillator is available.
- Assess vital signs, and apply a pulse oximeter and an automatic sphygmomanometer.

- Perform a physical examination.
- Review the patient's history.
- Develop a differential diagnosis.
- Obtain and review a 12-lead electrocardiogram.
- Obtain and review a portable chest X-ray.

---

1   Bradycardia
Heart rate <60 beats/min and inadequate for clinical condition

---

2
- Maintain patent airway; assist breathing as needed.
- Give oxygen.
- Monitor electrocardiogram (ECG) (identify rhythm), blood pressure, oximetry.
- Establish IV access.

---

3   Signs or symptoms of poor perfusion caused by the bradycardia? (for example, acute altered mental status, acute heart failure, ongoing chest pain, hypotension, or other signs of shock)

Adequate perfusion ← | → **Inadequate perfusion**

4A   Observe/monitor

If pulseless arrest develops, go to the American Heart Association's adult cardiac arrest algorithm, Asystole/PEA. Search for and treat possible contributing factors, such as:
- hydrogen ion (acidosis)
- hypokalemia or hyperkalemia
- hypothermia
- hypovolemia
- hypoxia
- tamponade, cardiac
- tension pneumothorax
- thrombosis (coronary or pulmonary)
- toxins

4
- Give atropine. Atropine IV dose: First dose: 1 mg bolus. Repeat every 3–5 minutes. Maximum: 3 mg.
- If atropine ineffective: (1) Transcutaneous pacing and/or (2) Dopamine infusion or (3) Epinephrine infusion
- Dopamine IV infusion: Usual infusion rate is 5–20 µg/kg/min. Titrate to patient response; taper slowly.
- Epinephrine IV infusion: 2–10 µg/min infusion. Titrate to patient response.

5
- Prepare for transvenous pacing.
- Treat contributing causes.
- Consider expert consultation.

See also:
2020 Handbook of Emergency Cardiovascular Care for Healthcare Providers. © 2020, American Heart Association
Advanced Cardiovascular Life Support Provider Manual. © 2020, American Heart Association.
Source: American Heart Association, Inc.

Sinus tachycardia

If sinus bradycardia is the tortoise of the sinus arrhythmias, sinus tachycardia is the hare. Sinus tachycardia in an adult is characterized by a sinus rate greater than 100 beats/min. The rate rarely exceeds 180 beats/min except during strenuous exercise; the maximum rate achievable with exercise decreases with age.

How it happens

The clinical significance of sinus tachycardia depends on the underlying cause. (See *Causes of sinus tachycardia.*)

Sinus tachycardia in a patient who has had an acute MI suggests massive heart damage and is a poor prognostic sign. Persistent tachycardia may also signal impending heart failure or cardiogenic shock.

What to look for

In sinus tachycardia, atrial and ventricular rhythms are regular. Both rates are equal, generally 100 to 160 beats/min. As in sinus bradycardia, the P wave is of normal size and shape and precedes each QRS, but it may increase in amplitude. As the heart rate increases, the P wave may be superimposed on the preceding T wave and difficult to identify. The PR interval, QRS complex, and T wave are normal. The QT interval normally shortens with tachycardia. (See *Recognizing sinus tachycardia*, page 107.)

Symptoms

If cardiac output falls and compensatory mechanisms fail, the patient may experience hypotension, syncope, and blurred vision. They may report chest pain and palpitations, commonly described as a pounding chest or a sensation of skipped heartbeats. They may also report a sense of nervousness or anxiety. If heart failure develops, they may exhibit lung crackles, an extra heart sound (S_3), and jugular vein distention. (See *What happens in tachycardia*, page 108.) Because the heart demands more oxygen at higher rates, tachycardia can trigger chest pain in patients with coronary artery disease (CAD). An increase in heart rate can also be detrimental for patients with obstructive types of heart conditions, such as aortic stenosis and hypertrophic cardiomyopathy.

How to intervene

No treatment for sinus tachycardia is necessary if the patient is asymptomatic or if the rhythm is the result of physical exertion. In other cases, the underlying cause may be treated, which usually resolves the arrhythmia.

Causes of sinus tachycardia

Sinus tachycardia may be a normal response to exercise; pain; stress; fever; or strong emotions, such as fear and anxiety. It can also occur:
- with certain cardiac conditions, such as heart failure, cardiogenic shock, and pericarditis
- as a compensatory mechanism in shock, anemia, respiratory distress, pulmonary embolism, sepsis, electrolyte imbalances, and hyperthyroidism
- when taking such drugs as atropine, isoproterenol (Isuprel), aminophylline, dopamine, dobutamine, epinephrine, and amphetamines
- with use of alcohol, caffeine, and nicotine.

Recognizing sinus tachycardia

Take a look at this example of how sinus tachycardia appears on a rhythm strip. Notice its distinguishing characteristics.

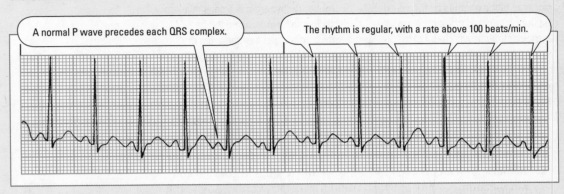

A normal P wave precedes each QRS complex.

The rhythm is regular, with a rate above 100 beats/min.

- *Rhythm:* Regular
- *Rate:* 120 beats/min
- *P wave:* Normal

- *PR interval:* 0.14 second
- *QRS complex:* 0.06 second
- *T wave:* Normal

- *QT interval:* 0.34 second
- *Other:* None

Slow it down

If sinus tachycardia leads to cardiac ischemia, treatment may include medications to slow the heart rate. For rates less than 150 beats/min, the most commonly used drugs include beta-adrenergic blockers, such as metoprolol (Lopressor) and atenolol (Tenormin), or calcium channel blockers, such as verapamil (Isoptin) and diltiazem (Cardizem). For sinus tachycardia with a narrow QRS complex and rate greater than 150 beats/min, vagal maneuvers and adenosine may be used. Adenosine is given by rapid injection and followed with a normal saline flush.

The goal of an intervention for the patient with sinus tachycardia is to maintain adequate cardiac output and tissue perfusion and to identify and correct the underlying cause.

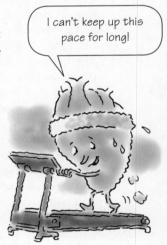

I can't keep up this pace for long!

Getting at the history

Check the patient's medication history. Over-the-counter sympathomimetic agents, which mimic the effects of the sympathetic nervous system, may contribute to sinus tachycardia. These agents may be contained in nose drops and cold formulas.

What happens in tachycardia

Tachycardia can lower cardiac output by reducing ventricular filling time and the amount of blood pumped by the ventricles during each contraction. Normally, ventricular volume reaches 120 to 130 mL during diastole. In tachycardia, decreased ventricular volume leads to hypotension and decreased peripheral perfusion.

As cardiac output plummets, arterial pressure, and peripheral perfusion decrease. Tachycardia worsens myocardial ischemia by increasing the heart's demand for oxygen and reducing the duration of diastole—the period of greatest coronary flow.

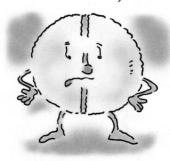

Over-the-counter cold medicines may contribute to sinus tachycardia.

You should also ask about the patient's use of caffeine, nicotine, herbal supplements, alcohol, and such illicit drugs as cocaine and amphetamines—any of which could trigger tachycardia. Advise them to avoid these substances.

Part of the plan

Here are other steps you should take for the patient with sinus tachycardia:

- Because sinus tachycardia can lead to injury of the heart muscle, check for chest pain or angina. Also assess for signs and symptoms of heart failure, including crackles, an S_3 heart sound, and jugular vein distention.
- Monitor intake and output as well as daily weight.
- Check the patient's level of consciousness (LOC) to assess cerebral perfusion.
- Provide the patient with a calm environment. Help reduce fear and anxiety, which can fuel the arrhythmia.
- Teach about procedures and treatments. Include relaxation techniques in the information you provide.
- Be aware that a sudden onset of sinus tachycardia after an MI may signal extension of the infarction. Prompt recognition is vital so treatment can be started.

Sinus arrest

A disorder of impulse formation, sinus arrest results from a lack of electrical activity in the atrium (atrial standstill). During atrial standstill, the atria aren't stimulated and an entire PQRST complex is missing from the ECG strip.

Except for this missing complex, or pause, the ECG usually remains normal. Atrial standstill is called *sinus pause* when one or two beats aren't formed and *sinus arrest* when three or more beats aren't formed.

Sinus arrest closely resembles third-degree SA block, also called *exit block*, on the ECG strip.

How it happens

Sinus arrest occurs when the SA node fails to generate an impulse. Such failure may result from several conditions, including acute infection, heart disease, and vagal stimulation. Pauses of 2 to 3 seconds normally occur in healthy adults during sleep and occasionally in patients with increased vagal tone or hypersensitive carotid sinus disease. Sinus arrest may be associated with sick sinus syndrome, a collection of sinus arrhythmias that includes sinus bradycardia and other abnormalities of the sinus conduction system. (See *Causes of sinus arrest*, page 110.)

What to look for

When assessing for sinus pause, you'll find on the ECG that atrial and ventricular rhythms are regular except for a missing complex at the onset of atrial standstill. Atrial and ventricular rates are equal and are usually within normal limits. The rate may vary, however, as a result of the pauses. (See *Recognizing sinus arrest*, page 110.)

Failing to make an appearance

A P wave that's of normal size and shape precedes each QRS complex but is absent during a pause. The PR interval is normal and constant when the P wave is present and not measurable when it's absent. The QRS complex, the T wave, and the QT interval are normal when present and are absent during a pause.

Junctional escape beats, including premature atrial, junctional, or ventricular contractions, may also be present. With sinus arrest, the length of the pause isn't a multiple of the previous R-R intervals.

Memory board

When your patient experiences sinus arrest, use this acronym to remember the characteristics and ways to **ARREST** the situation:

Absence of three or more PQRST complexes is involved.

Rate is slowed.

Rhythm is irregular.

Excess digoxin (Lanoxin), procainamide (Pronestyl), or other antiarrhythmics may be the cause.

Syncope, dizziness, confusion, angina, or heart failure may occur.

Treat with atropine and a pacemaker if the patient is unstable.

Causes of sinus arrest

Sinus arrest can be caused by the following:

• sinus node disease, such as fibrosis and idiopathic degeneration

• increased vagal tone, as occurring in Valsalva maneuver, carotid sinus massage, and vomiting

• digoxin (Lanoxin), quinidine, procainamide (Pronestyl), and salicylates, especially if given at toxic levels

• excessive doses of beta-adrenergic blockers, such as metoprolol (Lopressor) and propranolol (Inderal)

• cardiac disorders, such as chronic coronary artery disease, acute myocarditis, cardiomyopathy, and hypertensive heart disease

• Lyme disease

• acute inferior-wall myocardial infarction.

Recognizing sinus arrest

Take a look at this example of how sinus arrest appears on a rhythm strip. Notice its distinguishing characteristics.

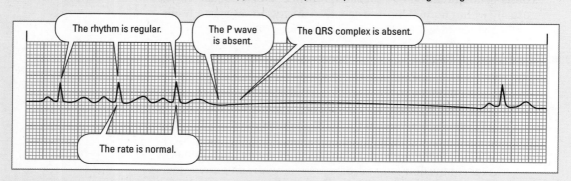

• *Rhythm:* Regular, except for the missing PQRST complexes

• *Rate:* 88 beats/min except during pause

• *P wave:* Normal; missing during pause

• *PR interval:* 0.20 second

• *QRS complex:* 0.08 second; absent during pause

• *T wave:* Normal; absent during pause

• *QT interval:* 0.40 second; absent during pause

• *Other:* None

Taking a break

You won't be able to detect a pulse or heart sounds when sinus arrest occurs. If the pauses are short and infrequent, the patient will most likely be asymptomatic and won't require treatment. They may have a normal sinus rhythm for days or weeks between episodes of sinus arrest, and they may not be able to feel the arrhythmias at all.

Too many for too long

Recurrent and prolonged pauses may cause signs of decreased cardiac output, such as low blood pressure; altered mental status; and cool, clammy skin. The patient may also complain of dizziness or blurred vision. The arrhythmias can produce syncope or near-syncopal episodes within 7 seconds of asystole.

How you intervene

An asymptomatic patient needs no treatment. For a patient displaying mild symptoms, treatment focuses on maintaining cardiac output and identifying the cause of the sinus arrest. That may involve stopping medications that contribute to SA node suppression, such as digoxin, beta-adrenergic blockers, and calcium channel blockers.

Don't let sleeping pauses lie

Examine the circumstances under which sinus pauses occur. A sinus pause may be insignificant if detected while the patient is sleeping. If the pauses are recurrent, assess the patient for evidence of decreased cardiac output, such as altered mental status; low blood pressure; and cool, clammy skin.

Ask them whether they are dizzy or light-headed or has blurred vision. Do they feel as if they have passed out? If so, they may be experiencing syncope from a prolonged sinus arrest.

Document the patient's vital signs and how they feel during pauses as well as what activities they were involved in when they occurred. Activities that increase vagal stimulation, such as Valsalva maneuver or vomiting, increase the likelihood of sinus pauses.

When matters get even worse

Assess for a progression of the arrhythmia. Notify the healthcare provider immediately if the patient becomes unstable. Withhold medications that may contribute to sinus pauses and check with the healthcare provider about whether those drugs should be continued.

If appropriate, be alert for signs of digoxin (Lanoxin), quinidine, or procainamide (Pronestyl) toxicity. Obtain a serum digoxin level and a serum electrolyte level.

Arresting the arrest

A patient who develops signs of circulatory collapse needs immediate treatment. As with sinus bradycardia, emergency treatment includes administration of atropine or epinephrine and the use of a temporary pacemaker. A permanent pacemaker may be implanted for long-term management.

The goal for the patient with sinus arrest is to maintain adequate cardiac output and perfusion. Be sure to record and document the frequency and duration of pauses. Determine whether a pause is the result of sinus arrest or SA block. If a pacemaker is implanted, give the patient discharge instructions about pacemaker care.

Sick sinus syndrome

Also called *sinus nodal dysfunction*, sick sinus syndrome refers to a wide spectrum of SA node abnormalities. The syndrome is caused by disturbances in the way impulses are generated or the inability to conduct impulses to the atrium.

Sick sinus syndrome usually shows up as bradycardia, with episodes of sinus arrest and SA block interspersed with sudden, brief periods of rapid atrial fibrillation. Patients are also prone to paroxysms of other atrial tachyarrhythmias, such as atrial flutter and ectopic atrial tachycardia, a condition sometimes referred to as *bradycardia-tachycardia (or tachy-brady) syndrome.*

Most patients with sick sinus syndrome are older than age 60, but anyone can develop the arrhythmia. It's rare in children except after open-heart surgery that results in SA node damage. The arrhythmia affects males and females equally. The onset is progressive, insidious, and chronic.

How it happens

Sick sinus syndrome results either from a dysfunction of the sinus node's automaticity or from abnormal conduction or blockages of impulses coming out of the nodal region. These conditions, in turn, stem from a degeneration of the area's autonomic nervous system and partial destruction of the sinus node, as may occur with an interrupted blood supply after an inferior-wall MI. (See *Causes of sick sinus syndrome.*)

Blocked exits

In addition, certain conditions can affect the atrial wall surrounding the SA node and cause exit blocks. Conditions that cause inflammation or degeneration of atrial tissue can also lead to sick sinus syndrome. In many patients, though, the exact cause of sick sinus syndrome is never identified.

Causes of sick sinus syndrome

Sick sinus syndrome may result from the following:
• conditions leading to fibrosis of the sinoatrial (SA) node, such as increased age, atherosclerotic heart disease, hypertension, and cardiomyopathy
• trauma to the SA node caused by open-heart surgery (especially valvular surgery), pericarditis, or rheumatic heart disease
• autonomic disturbances affecting autonomic innervation, such as hypervagotonia and degeneration of the autonomic system
• cardioactive medications, such as digoxin (Lanoxin), beta-adrenergic blockers, and calcium channel blockers.

What to look for

Sick sinus syndrome encompasses several potential rhythm disturbances that may be intermittent or chronic. (See *Recognizing sick sinus
syndrome.*) Those rhythm disturbances include one or a combination
of the following conditions:

- sinus bradycardia
- SA block
- sinus arrest
- sinus bradycardia alternating with sinus tachycardia
- episodes of atrial tachyarrhythmias, such as atrial fibrillation and
  atrial flutter
- failure of the sinus node to increase heart rate with exercise.

Check for speed bumps

Look for an irregular rhythm with sinus pauses and abrupt rate
changes. Atrial and ventricular rates may be fast, slow, or alternating
periods of fast rates and slow rates interrupted by pauses.

The P wave varies with the rhythm and usually precedes each QRS
complex. The PR interval is usually within normal limits but varies
with changes in the rhythm. The QRS complex and T wave are usually
normal, as is the QT interval, which may vary with rhythm changes.

Recognizing sick sinus syndrome

Take a look at this example of how sick sinus syndrome appears on a rhythm strip. Notice its distinguishing
characteristics.

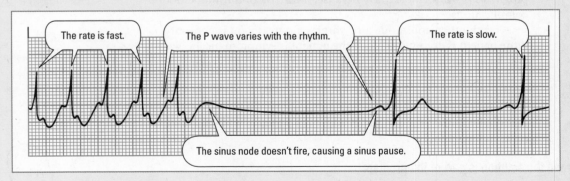

- *Rhythm:* Irregular
- *Rate:* Atrial—60 beats/min; ven-
  tricular—70 beats/min
- *P wave:* Configuration varies
- *PR interval:* Varies with rhythm
- *QRS complex:* 0.10 second
- *T wave:* Configuration varies
- *QT interval:* Varies with rhythm
  changes
- *Other:* None

Make up your mind!

The patient's pulse rate may be fast, slow, or normal, and the rhythm may be regular or irregular. You can usually detect an irregularity on the monitor or when palpating the pulse, which may feel inappropriately slow and then becomes rapid.

If you monitor the patient's heart rate during exercise or exertion, you may observe an inappropriate response to exercise, such as a failure of the heart rate to increase. You may also detect episodes of tachy-brady syndrome, atrial flutter, atrial fibrillation, SA block, or sinus arrest on the monitor.

That sinking feeling

The patient may show signs and symptoms of decreased cardiac output, such as hypotension, blurred vision, and syncope, a common experience with this arrhythmia. The length of a pause significant enough to cause syncope varies with the patient's age, posture at the time, and cerebrovascular status. Consider any pause that lasts 2 to 3 seconds significant.

Other assessment findings depend on the patient's condition. For instance, they may have crackles in the lungs, an S_3 heart sound, or a dilated and displaced left ventricular (LV) apical impulse if they have underlying cardiomyopathy.

How you intervene

The significance of sick sinus syndrome depends on the patient's age, the presence of other diseases, and the type and duration of the specific arrhythmias that occur. If atrial fibrillation is involved, the prognosis is worse, most likely because of the risk of thromboembolic complications.

As with other sinus node arrhythmias, no treatment is necessary if the patient is asymptomatic. If the patient is symptomatic, however, treatment aims to alleviate signs and symptoms and correct the underlying cause of the arrhythmia.

Atropine or epinephrine may be given initially for an acute attack. A pacemaker may be used until the underlying disorder resolves. Tachyarrhythmias may be treated with beta-adrenergic blockers or calcium channel blockers.

When the solution is part of the problem

Unfortunately, medications used to suppress tachyarrhythmias may worsen underlying SA node disease and bradyarrhythmias. The patient may need anticoagulants if they develop sudden bursts, or paroxysms, of atrial fibrillation. The anticoagulants help prevent thromboembolism and stroke, a complication of the condition. Because the syndrome is progressive and chronic, a symptomatic patient needs lifelong treatment.

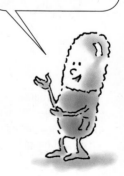

Drugs that suppress tachyarrhythmias may worsen underlying SA node disease.

Keep a running total

When caring for a patient with sick sinus syndrome, monitor and document all arrhythmias they experience and signs or symptoms they develop. Assess how their rhythm responds to activity and pain and look for changes in the rhythm.

Watch the patient carefully after starting calcium channel blockers, beta-adrenergic blockers, or other antiarrhythmic medications. If treatment includes anticoagulant therapy and/or the insertion of a pacemaker, make sure the patient and family receive appropriate instruction.

Atrial arrhythmias

The most common cardiac rhythm disturbances, atrial arrhythmias, result from impulses originating in areas outside the SA node. They can affect ventricular filling time and diminish the strength of the atrial kick (the contraction that normally provides the ventricles with about 30% of their blood), resulting in decreased cardiac output.

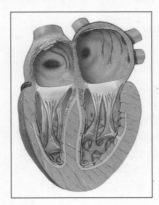

Triple play

Atrial arrhythmias are thought to result from three mechanisms: altered automaticity, circuit reentry, and afterdepolarization. Let's take a look at each cause and review specific atrial arrhythmias:

Mechanism	Characteristics	Possible Causes
Altered automaticity	• Ability of atrial cardiac cells to initiate impulses on their own increases, triggering abnormal impulses.	• Hypoxia • Hypocalcemia • Digoxin (Lanoxin) toxicity • Conditions that diminish sinoatrial node function

Mechanism	Characteristics	Possible Causes
Reentry	• The impulse remains active enough to produce another impulse during myocardial repolarization. • The impulse does not stop or die out, as it normally would. This creates a loop of repeated depolarizations until it is interrupted.	• Coronary artery disease • Cardiomyopathy • Myocardial infarction
Afterdepolarization	• An injured cell only partly repolarizes. • Partial repolarization can lead to a repetitive ectopic firing called *triggered activity*. • Triggered activity produces depolarization and can lead to atrial or ventricular tachycardia.	• Cell injury • Digoxin (Lanoxin) toxicity

Premature atrial contractions

Premature atrial contractions, usually referred to as PACs, originate from an irritable spot, or *focus*, in the atria that takes over as pacemaker for one or more beats. In a patient with heart disease, PACs may lead to more serious arrhythmias, such as atrial fibrillation and atrial flutter. In a patient who has had an acute MI, PACs can serve as an early sign of heart failure or an electrolyte imbalance.

How it happens

PACs commonly occur in a normal heart and are rarely dangerous in a patient who doesn't have heart disease. In fact, they usually cause no symptoms and can go unrecognized for years. (See *Causes of PACs*.)

A sign of things to come

However, in patients with heart disease, PACs may lead to more serious arrhythmias, such as atrial fibrillation and atrial flutter. In a patient who has had an acute MI, PACs can serve as an early sign of heart failure or an electrolyte imbalance. PACs can also result from the release of the neurohormone catecholamine during episodes of pain or anxiety.

What to look for

With PACs, atrial and ventricular rates are irregular, but the underlying rhythm may be regular. When the PAC is conducted through the

Causes of PACs

Premature atrial contractions (PACs) may be triggered by the following:
• alcohol and nicotine use
• anxiety
• fatigue
• fever
• infection
• coronary or valvular heart disease
• acute respiratory failure or hypoxia
• pulmonary disease
• digoxin toxicity
• electrolyte imbalances.

ventricles, the QRS complex appears normal on the patient's ECG. (See *Recognizing PACs*, page 117.)

A hallmark moment

The hallmark ECG characteristic of a PAC is a premature P wave with an abnormal configuration (when compared with a sinus P wave). It may be lost in the previous T wave, distorting that wave's configuration. (The T wave might be bigger or have an extra bump.) Varying configurations of the P wave indicate more than one ectopic site. (See *Nonconducted PACs and second-degree AV block*.)

The PR interval is usually normal but may be shortened or slightly prolonged, depending on the origin of the ectopic focus. If no QRS complex follows the premature P wave, a nonconducted PAC has occurred.

PACs may occur in bigeminy (every other beat is a PAC), trigeminy (every third beat is a PAC), or couplets (two PACs at a time). The patient may have an irregular peripheral or apical pulse rhythm when the PACs occur. They may complain of palpitations, skipped beats, or a fluttering sensation. In a patient with heart disease, signs and symptoms of decreased cardiac output—such as hypotension and syncope—may occur.

Recognizing PACs

Take a look at this example of how premature atrial contractions (PACs) appear on a rhythm strip. Notice the distinguishing characteristics.

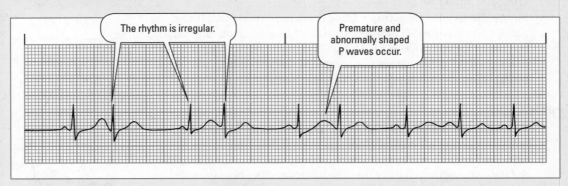

The rhythm is irregular.

Premature and abnormally shaped P waves occur.

- *Rhythm:* Irregular
- *Rate:* 90 beats/min
- *P wave:* Abnormal with PAC; some lost in previous T wave
- *PR interval:* 0.12 second
- *QRS complex:* 0.08 second
- *T wave:* Abnormal with some embedded P waves
- *QT interval:* 0.32 second
- *Other:* Noncompensatory pause

Nonconducted PACs and second-degree AV block

Don't confuse nonconducted premature atrial contractions (PACs) with type II second-degree atrioventricular (AV) block. In type II second-degree AV block, the P-P interval is regular. A nonconducted PAC, however, is an atrial impulse that arrives early to the AV node, when the node isn't yet repolarized.

As a result, the premature P wave fails to be conducted to the ventricle. The rhythm strip below shows a P wave embedded in the preceding T wave.

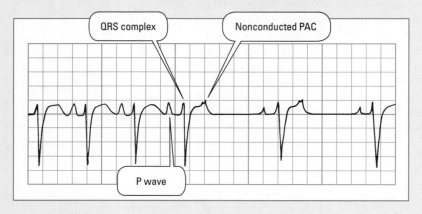

QRS complex

Nonconducted PAC

P wave

How you intervene

Most patients who are asymptomatic don't need treatment. If the patient is symptomatic, however, treatment may focus on eliminating the cause, such as caffeine or alcohol, and ruling out any serious heart conditions. Medications are not commonly used, but beta-adrenergic blockers or calcium channel blockers may be helpful.

The patient's part

When caring for a patient with PACs, assess them to help determine what's triggering the ectopic beats. Tailor your patient teaching to help the patient correct or avoid the underlying cause. For example, the patient might need to avoid caffeine or smoking or learn stress reduction techniques to lessen their anxiety.

If the patient has ischemic or valvular heart disease, monitor them for signs and symptoms of heart failure, electrolyte imbalances, and the development of more severe atrial arrhythmias.

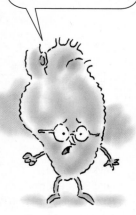

Too much caffeine and stress can cause PACs.

Atrial flutter

Atrial flutter, a supraventricular tachycardia (a rapid rhythm in which the impulse comes from above the ventricle), is characterized by an atrial rate of 250 to 400 beats/min, although it's generally around 300 beats/min. Originating in a single atrial focus, this rhythm results from circuit reentry and possibly increased automaticity.

How it happens

Atrial flutter is commonly associated with second-degree block. In that instance, the AV node fails to allow conduction of all the impulses to the ventricles. As a result, the ventricular rate is slower. Atrial flutter rarely occurs in a healthy person. When it does, it may indicate intrinsic cardiac disease. (See *Causes of atrial flutter*.)

What to look for

Atrial flutter is characterized by abnormal P waves that lose their distinction because of the rapid atrial rate. The waves blend together, creating a saw-toothed or shark fin appearance and are called *flutter waves*, or *F waves*. Varying degrees of AV block produce ventricular rates one-half to one-fourth of the atrial rate. The QRS complex is usually normal but may be widened if flutter waves are buried in the complex. You won't be able to identify a T wave or will you be able to measure the QT interval. (See *Recognizing atrial flutter*.)

Causes of atrial flutter

Atrial flutter may be caused by the following:
• conditions that enlarge atrial tissue and elevate atrial pressures, such as severe mitral valve disease, hyperthyroidism, pericardial disease, and primary myocardial disease
• cardiac surgery
• acute myocardial infarction
• chronic obstructive pulmonary disease
• systemic arterial hypoxia.

Recognizing atrial flutter

Take a look at this example of how atrial flutter appears on a rhythm strip. Notice its distinguishing characteristics.

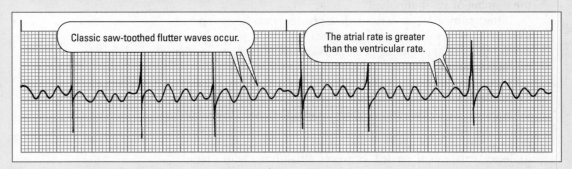

Classic saw-toothed flutter waves occur.

The atrial rate is greater than the ventricular rate.

• *Rhythm:* Atrial—regular; ventricular—irregular
• *Rate:* Atrial—280 beats/min; ventricular—60 beats/min
• *P wave:* Classic saw-toothed appearance
• *PR interval:* Unmeasurable
• *QRS complex:* 0.08 second
• *T wave:* Unidentifiable
• *QT interval:* Unidentifiable
• *Other:* None

A flitter, a flutter

The atrial rhythm may vary between fibrillatory waves and flutter waves, an arrhythmia commonly referred to as *atrial fibrillation* and *flutter*. Fibrillatory waves are uneven baseline fibrillation waves caused by the initiation of chaotic impulses from multiple ectopic sites in the atria. Depolarization can't spread in an organized manner because the atria quiver instead of contract.

Rating the ratio

The clinical significance of atrial flutter is determined by the number of impulses conducted through the node—expressed as a conduction ratio, for example, 2:1 or 4:1 (meaning that for every 2 atrial impulses, 1 is conducted; or for every 4, 1 is conducted)—and the resulting ventricular rate. If the ventricular rate is too slow (less than 40 beats/min) or too fast (greater than 150 beats/min), cardiac output may be seriously compromised.

Usually, the faster the ventricular rate, the more dangerous the arrhythmia. The rapid rate reduces ventricular filling time and coronary perfusion, which can cause angina, heart failure, pulmonary edema, hypotension, and syncope.

One of the most common rates is 150 beats/min. With an atrial rate of 300, that rhythm is referred to as a 2:1 block. (See *Atrial flutter and sinus tachycardia*.)

Misleading pulses

When caring for a patient with atrial flutter, you may note that their peripheral or apical pulse is normal in rate and rhythm. That's because the pulse reflects the number of ventricular contractions, not the number of atrial impulses.

If the ventricular rate is normal, the patient may be asymptomatic. However, if the ventricular rate is rapid, the patient may exhibit signs and symptoms of reduced cardiac output and cardiac decompensation.

How you intervene

If the patient is asymptomatic and with no other acute underlying or associated conditions, monitor them. They may be prescribed with medications, such as a beta-blocker or a calcium channel blocker, to decrease the rate if needed. However, atrial flutter with a rapid ventricular response and reduced cardiac output requires immediate intervention. Therapy aims to control the ventricular rate and convert the atrial ectopic rhythm to a normal sinus rhythm. Although stimulation of the vagus nerve may temporarily increase the block ratio and slow the ventricular rate, the effects won't last. For that reason, cardioversion remains the treatment of choice for a symptomatic patient exhibiting atrial flutter.

Advice from the experts

Atrial flutter and sinus tachycardia

Whenever you see sinus tachycardia with a rate of 150 beats/min, take another look. That rate is a common one for atrial flutter with 2:1 conduction. Look closely for flutter waves, which may be difficult to see if they're hidden in the QRS complex. You may need to check another lead to clearly see them.

A shocking solution

Synchronized cardioversion delivers an electrical stimulus during depolarization. The stimulus makes part of the myocardium refractory to ectopic impulses and terminates circuit reentry movements.

Become a convert

Drug therapy includes beta-adrenergic blockers and calcium channel blockers, such as diltiazem and verapamil, which may be used to control the heart rate. For patients who remain symptomatic and have not responded to cardioversion, dofetilide, or ibutilide may be used to control heart rhythm. If possible, the underlying cause of the atrial flutter should be treated. However, it should only be used if the atrial flutter or fibrillation has been going on for less than 48 hours and there is a high risk for arrhythmias in patients who show LV dysfunction. If treatment is to be administered, synchronized cardioversion is still the best option, especially for the unstable patient.

Keeping watch

Because atrial flutter may be an indication of intrinsic cardiac disease, monitor the patient closely for signs and symptoms of low cardiac output. If cardioversion is indicated, prepare the patient for intravenous (IV) administration of a sedative or anesthetic as ordered. The American Heart Association recommends caution with the use of sedation and/or analgesia if the patient is hypotensive (systolic blood pressure is greater than 90) or has any neurologic compromise; however, it should be remembered that this is an extremely uncomfortable and even painful procedure for most patients. Keep resuscitative equipment at the bedside. Be alert to the effects of digoxin, which depresses the SA node. Also, be alert for bradycardia because cardioversion can decrease the heart rate.

Atrial fibrillation

Atrial fibrillation, sometimes called *A-fib*, is defined as chaotic, asynchronous, electrical activity in atrial tissue. The ectopic impulses may fire at a rate of 400 to 600 times/min, causing the atria to quiver instead of contract. The previously described atrial kick no longer exists.

The ventricles respond only to those impulses that make it through the AV node. On an ECG, atrial activity is no longer represented by P waves but by erratic baseline waves called *fibrillatory waves*, or *F waves*. This rhythm may either be sustained or paroxysmal (occurring in bursts). It can be preceded by, or result from, PACs. Atrial fibrillation is one of the leading causes of ischemic strokes and the risk increases with age.

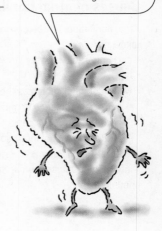

Sometimes my atria get so wired I just can't beat straight.

How it happens

Atrial fibrillation occurs more commonly than atrial flutter or atrial tachycardia. It stems from the firing of several impulses in circuit reentry pathways. (See *Causes of atrial fibrillation.*)

What to look for

In atrial fibrillation, small sections of the atria are activated individually. This situation causes the atrial muscle to quiver, or *fibrillate*, instead of contract. On an ECG, you'll see uneven baseline F waves rather than clearly distinguishable P waves. Also, when several ectopic sites in the atria fire impulses, depolarization can't spread in an organized manner, which causes an irregular ventricular response. (See *Recognizing atrial fibrillation*, page 123.)

That fabulous filter

The AV node protects the ventricles from the 400 to 600 erratic atrial impulses that occur each minute by acting as a filter and blocking some of the impulses. The AV node itself doesn't receive all the impulses, however. If muscle tissue around the AV node is in a refractory state, impulses from other areas of the atria can't reach the AV node, which further reduces the number of atrial impulses conducted through to the ventricles. These two factors help explain the characteristic-wide variation in R-R intervals in atrial fibrillation.

Fast and furious

The atrial rate is almost indiscernible (unable to distinguish) but is usually greater than 400 beats/min. The ventricular rate usually varies from 100 to 150 beats/min but can be lower. Atrial fibrillation is

---

Causes of atrial fibrillation

Atrial fibrillation may be caused by the following:
- cardiothoracic surgery
- heart failure
- Heart conditions such as the following:
  - mitral insufficiency or mitral stenosis
  - coronary artery disease
  - acute myocardial infarction
  - atrial septal defects
- infections, such as pericarditis and pneumonia

- hypertension,
- sleep apnea
- pulmonary embolisms
- hyperthyroidism
- inflammatory diseases
- coffee, alcohol, or nicotine use
- obesity and diabetes

Recognizing atrial fibrillation

Take a look at this example of how atrial fibrillation appears on a rhythm strip. Notice its distinguishing characteristics.

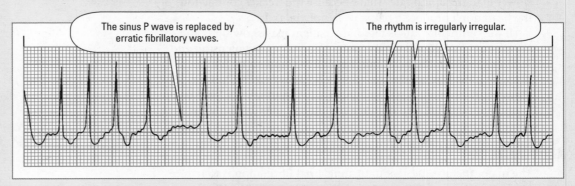

The sinus P wave is replaced by erratic fibrillatory waves.

The rhythm is irregularly irregular.

- *Rhythm:* Irregularly irregular
- *Rate:* Atrial—indiscernible; ventricular—130 beats/min
- *P wave:* Absent; replaced by fine fibrillatory waves
- *PR interval:* unable to distinguish
- *QRS complex:* 0.08 second
- *T wave:* unable to distinguish
- *QT interval:* Unmeasurable
- *Other:* None

called *coarse* if the F waves are pronounced; the fibrillation is called *fine* if they aren't. Atrial fibrillation and flutter may also occur simultaneously.

As with other atrial arrhythmias, atrial fibrillation eliminates atrial systole (also known as *atrial kick*). That loss, combined with the decreased filling times associated with rapid rates, can lead to clinically significant problems. If the ventricular rate is greater than 100 beats/min—a condition called *uncontrolled atrial fibrillation* or *rapid ventricular response*—the patient may develop heart failure, angina, or syncope.

Pre-existing problems

Patients with pre-existing cardiac disease, such as hypertrophic obstructive cardiomyopathy, mitral stenosis, rheumatic heart disease, and mitral prosthetic valves, tend to tolerate atrial fibrillation poorly and may develop shock and severe heart failure. Left untreated, atrial fibrillation can lead to cardiovascular collapse, thrombus formation, and systemic arterial or pulmonary embolism.

Atrial fibrillation greatly increases the risk of strokes, heart failure, and dementia. The stroke risk is particularly high for individuals who have atrial fibrillation and mitral stenosis.

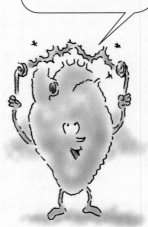

The AV node blocks erratic atrial impulses to protect the ventricles.

How you intervene

When assessing a patient with atrial fibrillation, assess both the peripheral and apical pulses. You may find that the radial pulse rate is slower than the apical rate. That's because the weaker contractions of the heart don't produce a palpable peripheral pulse.

If the ventricular rate is rapid, the patient may show signs and symptoms of decreased cardiac output, including hypotension and light-headedness. The heart may be able to compensate for the decrease if the fibrillation lasts long enough to become chronic. However, the patient is still at a greater-than-normal risk for developing pulmonary, cerebral, or other emboli and may exhibit signs of those conditions.

Goal: Reduce the rate

The major therapeutic goal in treating atrial fibrillation is to reduce the ventricular response rate to less than 100 beats/min. When the onset of atrial fibrillation is acute and the patient is stable, vagal maneuvers or carotid sinus massage may slow the ventricular response but won't convert the arrhythmia.

The ventricular rate may be controlled with calcium channel blockers, such as diltiazem (Cardizem) and verapamil (Isoptin) and beta-adrenergic blockers. Amiodarone can be used to control ventricular rate. Flecainide, dofetilide, propafenone, or other antiarrhythmics can be used to convert atrial fibrillation to normal sinus rhythm, usually after anticoagulation. Digoxin may also be used, but it is not a first-line agent.

A jolting recovery

If the patient is symptomatic, immediate synchronized cardioversion is necessary. Cardioversion is most successful if used within the first 3 days of treatment and less successful if the rhythm has existed for a long time. Due to the likelihood of blood pooling in the atria secondary to the loss of atrial kick (and resulting passive flow of blood into the ventricle), clot formation is a dangerous risk that must be considered if cardioversion is to be implemented.

If possible, anticoagulants should be administered first because conversion to normal sinus rhythm causes forceful atrial contractions to resume abruptly. A transesophageal echocardiogram may be performed prior to cardioversion to check for a thrombus. If a thrombus has formed in the atria, the resumption of contractions can result in systemic emboli.

Resuming a commanding role

If cardioversion is not an option or is unsuccessful, antiarrhythmics can be used to attempt pharmacologic conversion in patients who are symptomatic. Some of these drugs prolong the atrial refractory period, giving the SA node an opportunity to re-establish its role as the heart's pacemaker, whereas others primarily slow AV node conduction, controlling the ventricular rate.

If drug therapy is used, monitor serum drug levels, and observe the patient for evidence of toxicity. Tell the patient to report pulse rate changes; syncope or dizziness; chest pain; or signs of heart failure, such as increasing dyspnea and peripheral edema.

Patients who remain in atrial fibrillation, or at a high risk for recurrence, may require long-term treatment to prevent thromboembolisms. Antithrombotic therapy decisions should be made after assessing both stroke and bleeding risks. In the past, warfarin was the anticoagulant of choice, but there are several newer medications that can also be used for reducing the risk of stroke from atrial fibrillation.

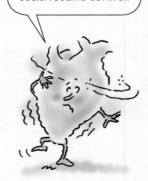

If all those other impulses would calm down, my SA node could resume control.

Radio blackout

Symptom-producing atrial fibrillation that doesn't respond to routine treatment may be treated with *radiofrequency ablation therapy*. In this invasive procedure, a transvenous catheter is used to locate the area within the heart that participates in initiating or perpetuating certain tachyarrhythmias. Radiofrequency energy is then delivered to the myocardium through this catheter to produce a small area of necrosis. The damaged tissue can no longer cause or participate in the tachyarrhythmia. If the energy is delivered close to the AV node, bundle of His, or bundle branches, a block can occur.

Atrial tachycardia

Atrial tachycardia is a supraventricular tachycardia, which means the impulses driving the rapid rhythm originate above the ventricles. Atrial tachycardia is characterized by an atrial rate of 150 to 250 beats/ min. The rapid rate shortens diastole, resulting in a loss of atrial kick, reduced cardiac output, reduced coronary perfusion, and ischemic myocardial changes.

Three types of atrial tachycardia exist: atrial tachycardia with block, multifocal atrial tachycardia (MAT) (or chaotic atrial rhythm), and paroxysmal atrial tachycardia (PAT).

How it happens

In a healthy person, atrial tachycardia is usually benign. However, this rhythm may be a forerunner of a more serious ventricular arrhythmia, especially if it occurs in a patient with an underlying heart condition. (See *Causes of atrial tachycardia.*)

The increased ventricular rate of atrial tachycardia decreases the time allowed for the ventricles to fill, increases myocardial oxygen consumption, and decreases oxygen supply. Angina, heart failure, ischemic myocardial changes, and even MI can result.

What to look for

Atrial tachycardia is characterized by three or more successive ectopic atrial beats at a rate of 140 to 250 beats/min. The P wave is usually upright, if visible, and followed by a QRS complex.

Keep in mind that atrial beats may be conducted on a 1:1 basis into the ventricles (meaning that each P wave has a QRS complex); if this is the case, atrial and ventricular rates will be equal. In other cases, atrial beats may be conducted only periodically, meaning there's a block in the AV conduction system. The block keeps the ventricles from receiving every impulse.

Hold it right there!

Think of the AV node as a gatekeeper or doorman. Sometimes it lets atrial impulses through to the ventricles regularly (every other impulse, for instance), and sometimes it lets them in irregularly (two impulses might get through, for instance, and then three, and then one).

Fast but regular

When assessing a rhythm strip for atrial tachycardia, you'll see that atrial rhythm is always regular, and ventricular rhythm is regular when the block is constant and irregular when it isn't. The rate consists of three or more successive ectopic atrial beats at a rate of 140 to 250 beats/min. The ventricular rate varies according to the AV conduction ratio. (See *Recognizing atrial tachycardia*.)

The P wave has a 1:1 ratio with the QRS complex unless a block is present. The P wave may not be discernible because of the rapid rate and may be hidden in the previous ST segment or T wave. You may not be able to measure the PR interval if the P wave can't be distinguished from the preceding T wave.

The QRS complex is usually normal, unless the impulses are being conducted abnormally through the ventricles. The T wave may be normal or inverted if ischemia is present. The QT interval is usually within normal limits but may be shorter because of the rapid rate. ST-segment and T-wave changes may appear if ischemia occurs with a prolonged arrhythmia. (See *Identifying types of atrial tachycardia*.)

Feel the rhythm

Atrial tachycardia is characterized by a rapid apical or peripheral pulse rate. The rhythm may be regular or irregular, depending on the type of atrial tachycardia. A patient with PAT may complain of suddenly feeling rapid heartbeats or palpitations. Persistent tachycardia and rapid ventricular rate cause decreased cardiac output, which can lead to blurred vision, syncope, and hypotension.

Causes of atrial tachycardia

Atrial tachycardia can occur in patients with normal heart. In those cases, the condition is commonly related to excessive use of caffeine or other stimulants, marijuana use, electrolyte imbalances, hypoxia, and physical or psychological stress. Atrial tachycardia may also be a component of sick sinus syndrome.

Other causes may include the following:
- digoxin toxicity (most common cause)
- myocardial infarction, cardiomyopathy, congenital anomalies, Wolff-Parkinson-White syndrome, and valvular disease
- cor pulmonale
- hyperthyroidism
- systemic hypertension.

Recognizing atrial tachycardia

Take a look at this example of how atrial tachycardia appears on a rhythm strip. Notice its distinguishing characteristics.

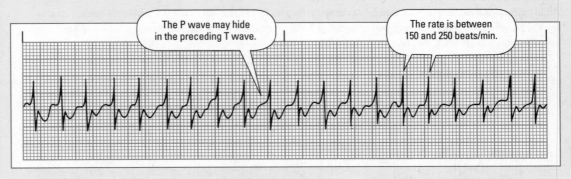

The P wave may hide in the preceding T wave.

The rate is between 150 and 250 beats/min.

- *Rhythm:* Regular
- *Rate:* 200 beats/min
- *P wave:* Abnormal

- *PR interval:* 0.12 second
- *QRS complex:* 0.10 second
- *T wave:* Distorted by P wave

- *QT interval:* 0.20 second
- *Other:* None

How you intervene

Treatment depends on the type of tachycardia and the severity of the patient's symptoms. Because one of the most common causes of atrial tachycardia is digoxin toxicity, monitor levels of the drug. (See *Signs of digoxin toxicity*, page 129.)

Vagal stimulation, such as Valsalva maneuver and carotid sinus massage, may be used to treat PAT. Vagal maneuvers are particularly effective when the tachycardia is caused by circuit re-entry, which is signaled by frequent PACs. There are no contraindications to Valsalva maneuvers in hemodynamically stable patients (See *Understanding carotid sinus massage*, page 130.)

Making a bigger block

Other treatment options include drugs that increase the degree of AV block, which in turn decreases the ventricular response and slows the rate. Such drugs include digoxin, beta-adrenergic blockers, and calcium channel blockers.

In addition, adenosine (Adenocard) may be used to stop atrial tachycardia. If the patient is stable, beta-adrenergic blockers or calcium channel blockers, such as diltiazem or verapamil, may be given. When other treatments fail, synchronized cardioversion may be used.

Identifying types of atrial tachycardia

Atrial tachycardia comes in three varieties. Here's a quick rundown of each.

Atrial tachycardia with block

Atrial tachycardia with block is caused by increased automaticity of the atrial tissue. As atrial rate speeds up and the atrioventricular conduction becomes impaired, a 2:1 block typically occurs. Occasionally, a type 1 (Wenckebach) second-degree heart block may be seen.

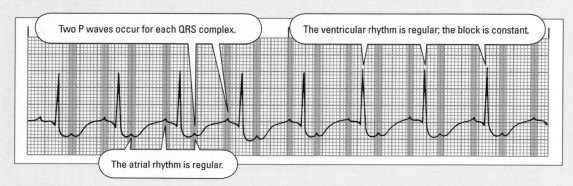

Two P waves occur for each QRS complex.

The ventricular rhythm is regular; the block is constant.

The atrial rhythm is regular.

Interpretation

- *Rhythm:* Atrial—regular; ventricular—regular if block is constant, irregular if block is variable
- *Rate:* Atrial—140 to 250 beats/min, multiple of ventricular rate; ventricular—varies with block
- *P wave:* Slightly abnormal
- *PR interval:* Usually normal; may be hidden
- *QRS complex:* Usually normal
- *Other:* More than one P wave for each QRS

Multifocal atrial tachycardia

In multifocal atrial tachycardia (MAT), atrial tachycardia occurs with numerous atrial foci firing intermittently. MAT produces varying P waves on the strip and occurs most commonly in patients with chronic pulmonary disease. The irregular baseline in this strip is caused by movement of the chest wall.

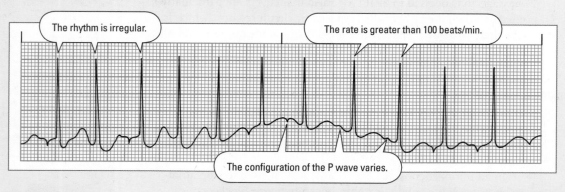

The rhythm is irregular.

The rate is greater than 100 beats/min.

The configuration of the P wave varies.

Interpretation

- *Rhythm:* Both irregular
- *Rate:* Atrial—100 to 250 beats/min (usually under 160); ventricular—100 to 250 beats/min
- *P wave:* Configuration varies; must see at least three different P wave shapes
- *PR interval:* Varies
- *Other:* None

Identifying types of atrial tachycardia *(continued)*

Paroxysmal atrial tachycardia

A type of paroxysmal supraventricular tachycardia, paroxysmal atrial tachycardia (PAT) features brief periods of tachycardia that alternate with periods of normal sinus rhythm. PAT starts and stops suddenly as a result of rapid firing of an ectopic focus. It commonly follows frequent premature atrial contractions (PACs), one of which initiates the tachycardia.

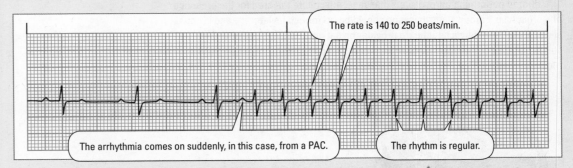

The rate is 140 to 250 beats/min.

The arrhythmia comes on suddenly, in this case, from a PAC.

The rhythm is regular.

Interpretation
- *Rhythm:* Regular
- *Rate:* 140 to 250 beats/min

- *P wave:* Abnormal; possibly hidden in previous T wave
- *PR interval:* Identical for each cycle

- *QRS complex:* Possibly aberrantly conducted
- *Other:* One P wave for each QRS complex

Signs of digoxin toxicity

With digoxin toxicity, atrial tachycardia isn't the only change you might see in your patient. Be alert for the following signs and symptoms, especially if the patient is taking digoxin (Lanoxin) and his potassium level is low or if he's also taking amiodarone (Cordarone). Both combinations can increase the risk of digoxin toxicity.

Central nervous system
- Fatigue and general muscle weakness
- Agitation
- Hallucinations

Eyes, ears, nose, and throat
- Yellow-green halos around visual images
- Blurred vision

Gastrointestinal
- Anorexia
- Nausea and vomiting

Cardiovascular
- Arrhythmias (most commonly, conduction disturbances with or without atrioventricular block, premature ventricular contractions, and supraventricular arrhythmias)
- Increased severity of heart failure
- Hypotension
   Digoxin's toxic effects on the heart may be life threatening, and they always require immediate attention.

Understanding carotid sinus massage

Carotid sinus massage (shown below) may be used to stop paroxysmal atrial tachycardia. Massaging the carotid sinus stimulates the vagus nerve, which then inhibits firing of the sinoatrial (SA) node and slows atrioventricular node conduction. As a result, the SA node can resume its job as primary pacemaker. Carotid massage should be avoided in individuals who have a carotid bruit or a history of a stroke or TIA. Prior to performing carotid sinus massage, auscultate the area for the presence of a bruit. Also, carotid sinus massage should be performed unilaterally and is generally only performed by a healthcare provider on patients who are hemodynamically stable because of the risks. Risks include decreased heart rate, vasodilation, ventricular arrhythmias, stroke, and cardiac standstill.

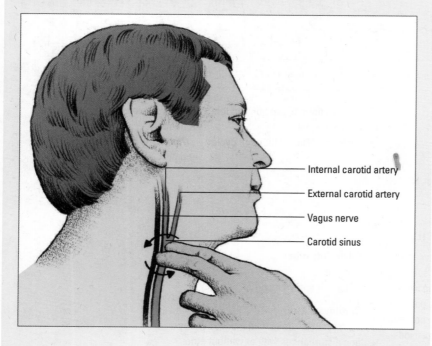

— Internal carotid artery

— External carotid artery

— Vagus nerve

— Carotid sinus

Going into overdrive

Atrial overdrive pacing (also called *burst pacing* or *rapid atrial pacing*) may be used to stop the arrhythmia. In this procedure, the patient's atrial rate is electronically paced slightly higher than the intrinsic rate. With some patients, the atria are paced using much faster bursts or are paced prematurely at a critical time in the conduction cycle. Whichever variation is used, the result is the same. The pacing interferes with the conduction circuit and renders part of it unresponsive to the reentrant impulse. Atrial tachycardia stops, and the SA node resumes its normal role as pacemaker. Overdrive pacing is a feature in many permanent pacemakers. Although it can be effective, permanent pacemakers should not be implanted in individuals with atrial fibrillation who do not have other indications for having one.

If the arrhythmia is associated with Wolff-Parkinson-White syndrome, or WPW (the occurrence of an abnormal extra conductive pathway in the heart can result in intermittent bursts of tachycardia accompanied by a "delta" wave on ECG), radiofrequency ablation therapy may be used to control recurrent episodes of PAT. Because MAT commonly occurs in patients with chronic obstructive pulmonary disease, the rhythm may not respond to treatment. Treatment efforts are focused on correct the hypoxia.

Keeping tabs on troublemakers

When caring for a patient with atrial tachycardia, carefully monitor the patient's rhythm strips. Doing so may provide information about the cause of atrial tachycardia, which in turn can facilitate treatment. Also monitor the patient for chest pain, indications of decreased cardiac output, and signs and symptoms of heart failure or myocardial ischemia.

Junctional arrhythmias

Junctional arrhythmias originate in the AV junction—the area around the AV node and the bundle of His. These arrhythmias occur when the SA node is suppressed and fails to conduct impulses, or when a block occurs in conduction. Electrical impulses may then be initiated by pacemaker cells in the AV junction.

In normal impulse conduction, the AV node slows transmission of the impulse from the atria to the ventricles, which allows the atria to pump as much blood as they can into the ventricles before the ventricles contract. However, impulses aren't always conducted normally. (See *Conduction in Wolff-Parkinson-White syndrome*, page 132.)

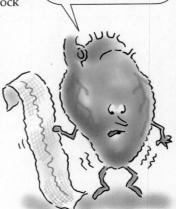

Don't mistake an atrial arrhythmia for a junctional arrhythmia. Check the PR interval.

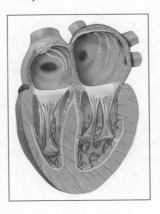

Conduction in Wolff-Parkinson-White syndrome

Conduction doesn't always take place in a normal way. In Wolff-Parkinson-White syndrome, a conduction bypass develops outside the atrioventricular (AV) junction and connects the atria with the ventricles, as shown at right. Wolff-Parkinson-White syndrome (commonly called *WPW*) is typically a congenital rhythm disorder that occurs mainly in young children and in adults ages 20 to 35.

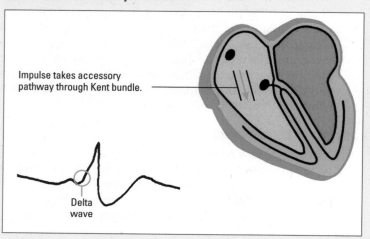

Impulse takes accessory pathway through Kent bundle.

Delta wave

Rapidly conducted

The bypass formed in Wolff-Parkinson-White syndrome, known as *Kent bundle*, conducts impulses to the atria or the ventricles. Impulses aren't delayed at the AV node, so conduction is abnormally fast. Retrograde conduction, re-entry, and re-entrant tachycardia can result.

Checking the ECG

Wolff-Parkinson-White syndrome causes a shortened PR interval (less than 0.10 second) and a widened QRS complex (greater than 0.10 second).

The beginning or upstroke of the QRS complex may look slurred because of altered ventricular depolarization. The hallmark sign of this syndrome is called a *delta wave*, shown in the inset above.

Because the AV junction is located in the middle of the heart, impulses generated in this area cause the heart to be depolarized in an abnormal way. The impulse moves upward and causes backward, or retrograde, depolarization of the atria. This results in inverted (rather than upright) P waves in leads II, III, and aV$_F$, leads in which you would usually see upright P waves. (See *Finding the P wave*, page 133.)

Which way did the impulse go?

The impulse also moves down toward the ventricles, causing forward, or antegrade, depolarization of the ventricles and an upright QRS complex. Arrhythmias that cause inverted P waves on an ECG may be atrial or junctional in origin.

Finding the P wave

When the pacemaker fires in the AV junction, the impulse may reach the atria or the ventricles first. Therefore, the inverted P wave and the following QRS complex won't have a consistent relationship. These rhythm strips show the various positions the P wave can take in junctional rhythms.

Atria first
If the atria are depolarized first, the P wave will occur before the QRS complex.

Ventricles first
If the ventricles are depolarized first, the QRS complex will come before the P wave.

Simultaneous
If the ventricles and atria are depolarized simultaneously, the P wave will be hidden in the QRS complex.

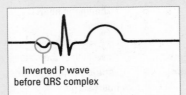

Inverted P wave before QRS complex

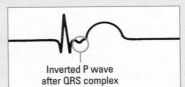

Inverted P wave after QRS complex

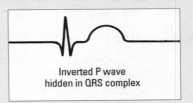

Inverted P wave hidden in QRS complex

Junctional mimic

Atrial arrhythmias are sometimes mistaken for junctional arrhythmias because impulses are generated so low in the atria that they cause retrograde depolarization and inverted P waves. Looking at the PR interval helps you determine whether an arrhythmia is atrial or junctional.

Bad PR

An arrhythmia with an inverted P wave before the QRS complex and a normal PR interval (0.12 to 0.20 second) originated in the atria. An arrhythmia with a PR interval less than 0.12 second originated in the AV junction.

Junctional arrhythmias include premature junctional contractions (PJCs), junctional escape rhythm, accelerated junctional rhythm, and junctional tachycardia.

Premature junctional contraction

A PJC is a beat that occurs before a normal beat and causes an irregular rhythm. This ectopic beat occurs when an irritable location within the AV junction acts as a pacemaker and fires either prematurely or out of sequence.

As with all beats produced by the AV junction, the atria depolarize in retrograde fashion, causing an inverted P wave on the ECG. The ventricles depolarize normally.

How it happens

PJCs commonly occur in a normal heart and are rarely dangerous. In fact, they usually cause no symptoms and can go unrecognized for years. (See *Causes of PJCs.*)

What to look for

A PJC appears on a rhythm strip as an early beat causing an irregularity. The rest of the strip may show regular atrial and ventricular rhythms, depending on the patient's underlying rhythm.

When upside down your feeling

Look for an inverted P wave in leads II, III, and aV$_F$. Depending on when the impulse occurs, the P wave may fall before, during, or after the QRS complex. If it falls during the QRS complex, it's hidden. If it comes before the QRS complex, the PR interval is less than 0.12 second. (See *Recognizing a PJC*, page 135.)

Because the ventricles usually depolarize normally, the QRS complex has a normal configuration and a normal duration of less than 0.12 second. The T wave and the QT interval are usually normal.

That quickening feeling

The patient may be asymptomatic, or they may complain of palpitations or a feeling of quickening in the chest. Palpation may reveal an irregular pulse. If the PJCs are frequent, the patient may have hypotension from a transient decrease in cardiac output.

How you intervene

Although PJCs themselves usually aren't dangerous, you'll need to monitor the patient carefully and assess them for other signs of intrinsic pacemaker failure. If digoxin toxicity is the culprit, check with the patient's healthcare provider about discontinuing the medication and monitoring serum drug levels.

You should also monitor the patient for hemodynamic instability. If ectopic beats are frequent, the patient should decrease or eliminate his caffeine intake.

Causes of PJCs

Premature junctional contractions (PJCs) may be caused by the following:

- toxic levels of digoxin (Lanoxin) (level greater than 2.5 ng/mL)
- excessive caffeine intake
- inferior-wall myocardial infarction
- rheumatic heart disease
- valvular disease
- swelling of the atrioventricular junction after heart surgery.

Recognizing a PJC

Take a look at this example of how a premature junctional contraction (PJC)—a junctional beat that occurs before a normal sinus beat—appears on a rhythm strip. Notice its distinguishing characteristics.

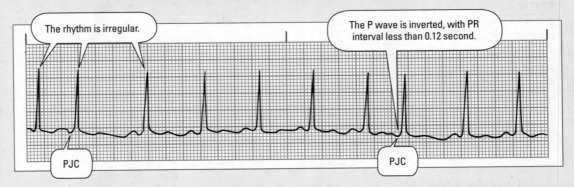

The rhythm is irregular.

The P wave is inverted, with PR interval less than 0.12 second.

PJC

PJC

- *Rhythm:* Atrial and ventricular—irregular
- *Rate:* 100 beats/min
- *P wave:* Inverted and precedes the QRS complex

- *PR interval:* 0.14 second for the underlying rhythm and 0.06 second for the PJC
- *QRS complex:* 0.06 second

- *T wave:* Normal configuration
- *QT interval:* 0.36 second
- *Other:* Pause after PJC

Junctional escape rhythm

A junctional escape rhythm is a string of beats that occurs after a conduction delay from the atria. The normal intrinsic firing rate for cells in the AV junction is 40 to 60 beats/min.

Remember that the AV junction can take over as the heart's pacemaker if higher pacemaker sites slow down or fail to fire or conduct. The junctional escape beat is an example of this compensatory mechanism. Because junctional escape beats prevent ventricular standstill, they should never be suppressed.

Backward and upside down

In a junctional escape rhythm, as in all junctional arrhythmias, the atria are depolarized by means of retrograde conduction. The P waves are inverted, and impulse conduction through the ventricles is normal.

How it happens

A junctional escape rhythm can be caused by any condition that disturbs SA node function or enhances AV junction automaticity. (See *Causes of junctional escape rhythm.*)

Causes of junctional escape rhythm

Junctional escape rhythm can be caused by any condition that disturbs sinoatrial node function or enhances atrioventricular junction automaticity, including the following:

- sick sinus syndrome
- vagal stimulation
- digoxin toxicity
- inferior-wall myocardial infarction
- rheumatic heart disease
- Lyme disease
- medications such as beta-adrenergic blockers and calcium channel blockers
- postcardiac surgery, particularly in children.

What to look for

A junctional escape rhythm shows a regular rhythm of 40 to 60 beats/min on an ECG strip. Look for inverted P waves in leads II, III, and aV$_F$.

The P waves will occur before, after, or hidden within the QRS complex. The PR interval is less than 0.12 second and is measurable only if the P wave comes before the QRS complex. (See *Recognizing junctional escape rhythm*, page 137.)

The rest of the ECG waveform—including the QRS complex, T wave, and QT interval—should appear normal because impulses through the ventricles are usually conducted normally.

I may be slow, but at least I'm regular

A patient with a junctional escape rhythm has a slow, regular pulse rate of 40 to 60 beats/min. The patient may be asymptomatic. Whether or not a junctional escape rhythm harms the patient depends on how well the patient's heart tolerates a decreased heart rate and decreased cardiac output. Typically, pulse rates less than 60 beats/min may lead to inadequate cardiac output, causing hypotension, syncope, or blurred vision.

How you intervene

Treatment of a junctional escape rhythm involves correcting the underlying cause. Atropine may be given to increase the heart rate, or a temporary or permanent pacemaker may be inserted.

Nursing care includes monitoring the patient's serum digoxin and electrolyte levels and watching for signs of decreased cardiac output, such as hypotension, syncope, or blurred vision. If the patient is hypotensive, lower the head of their bed as far as they can tolerate and keep atropine at the bedside.

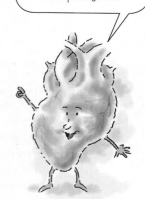

If I can tolerate a low heart rate and cardiac output, I can handle a junctional escape rhythm.

Recognizing junctional escape rhythm

Take a look at this example of how junctional escape rhythm appears on a rhythm strip. Note the inverted P wave.

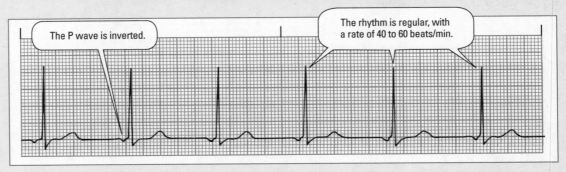

The P wave is inverted.

The rhythm is regular, with a rate of 40 to 60 beats/min.

- *Rhythm:* Regular
- *Rate:* 60 beats/min
- *P wave:* Inverted and preceding each QRS complex

- *PR interval:* 0.10 second
- *QRS complex:* 0.10 second
- *T wave:* Normal

- *QT interval:* 0.44 second
- *Other:* None

Accelerated junctional rhythm

An accelerated junctional rhythm results when an irritable focus in the AV junction speeds up and takes over as the heart's pacemaker. The atria depolarize by retrograde conduction, whereas the ventricles depolarize normally. The accelerated rate is usually between 60 and 100 beats/min.

How it happens

Conditions that affect SA node or AV node automaticity can cause accelerated junctional rhythm. (See *Causes of accelerated junctional rhythm.*)

What to look for

With an accelerated junctional rhythm, look for a regular rhythm and a rate of 60 to 100 beats/min. If a P wave is present, it's inverted in leads II, III, and aV$_F$ and occurs before or after the QRS complex or may be hidden in it. If the P wave comes before the QRS complex, the PR interval is less than 0.12 second. The QRS complex, T wave, and QT interval all appear normal. (See *Recognizing accelerated junctional rhythm.*)

Low-down, dizzy, and confused

The patient may be asymptomatic because accelerated junctional rhythm has the same rate as sinus rhythm. This arrhythmia is

Causes of accelerated junctional rhythm

Accelerated junctional rhythm can be caused by conditions that affect sinoatrial node or atrioventricular node automaticity, including the following:
- digoxin toxicity
- hypokalemia
- inferior- or posterior-wall myocardial infarction
- rheumatic heart disease
- valvular heart disease
- hypoxemia.

Recognizing accelerated junctional rhythm

Take a look at this example of how an accelerated junctional rhythm appears on a rhythm strip. Notice its distinguishing characteristics.

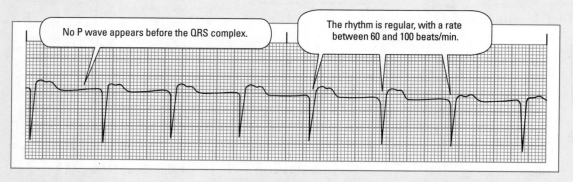

> No P wave appears before the QRS complex.

> The rhythm is regular, with a rate between 60 and 100 beats/min.

- *Rhythm:* Regular
- *Rate:* 80 beats/min
- *P wave:* Absent

- *PR interval:* Unmeasurable
- *QRS complex:* 0.10 second
- *T wave:* Normal

- *QT interval:* 0.32 second
- *Other:* None

significant if the patient has symptoms of decreased cardiac output—hypotension, syncope, and blurred vision. These can occur if the atria are depolarized after the QRS complex, which prevents blood ejection from the atria into the ventricles, or atrial kick.

How you intervene

Treatment of accelerated junctional arrhythmia involves correcting the underlying cause. Nursing interventions include observing the patient for signs of decreased cardiac output and monitoring their vital signs for hemodynamic instability. You should also assess the levels of potassium and other electrolytes and administer supplements as ordered. Finally, monitor the patient's digoxin level and withhold their digoxin dose if indicated.

Junctional tachycardia

In junctional tachycardia, three or more PJCs occur in a row. The rate is usually 100 to 200 beats/min.

How it happens

This supraventricular tachycardia occurs when an irritable focus from the AV junction has enhanced automaticity, overriding the SA node's ability to function as the heart's pacemaker. In this arrhythmia, the atria are depolarized by retrograde conduction; however, conduction through the ventricles remains normal. (See *Causes of junctional tachycardia.*)

What to look for

When assessing a rhythm strip for junctional tachycardia, look for a rate of 100 to 200 beats/min. The P wave is inverted in leads II, III, and aV$_F$ and can occur before, during (hidden P wave), or after the QRS complex. If it comes before the QRS complex, the only time the PR interval can be measured, it's always less than 0.12 second. (See *Recognizing junctional tachycardia.*)

The QRS complexes look normal, as does the T wave, unless a P wave occurs in it, or the rate is so fast that the T wave can't be detected. (See *Junctional and supraventricular tachycardia.*)

Compromisin' rhythm

The significance of junctional tachycardia depends on the rate, underlying cause, and severity of the accompanying cardiac disease. At higher ventricular rates, junctional tachycardia may compromise cardiac output by decreasing the amount of blood filling the ventricles with each beat. Higher rates also result in the loss of atrial kick. As a

Causes of junctional tachycardia

The most common cause of junctional tachycardia is digoxin toxicity, which can be enhanced by hypokalemia.

Other possible causes include the following:
- inferior- or posterior-wall myocardial infarction or ischemia
- congenital heart disease in children
- swelling of the atrioventricular junction after heart surgery.

Recognizing junctional tachycardia

Take a look at this example of how junctional tachycardia appears on a rhythm strip. Notice its distinguishing characteristics.

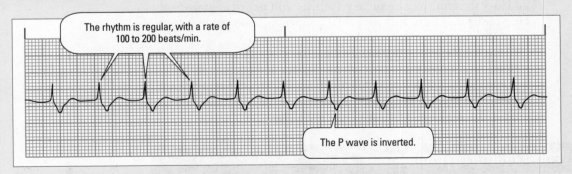

The rhythm is regular, with a rate of 100 to 200 beats/min.

The P wave is inverted.

- *Rhythm:* Regular
- *Rate:* Atrial and ventricular rates—115 beats/min
- *P wave:* Inverted; follows QRS complex
- *PR interval:* Unmeasurable
- *QRS complex:* 0.08 second
- *T wave:* Normal
- *QT interval:* 0.36 second
- *Other:* None

Junctional and supraventricular tachycardia

If a tachycardia has a narrow QRS complex, you may have trouble deciding whether its source is junctional or atrial. When the rate approaches 150 beats/min, a formerly visible P wave is hidden in the previous T wave, so you won't be able to use the P wave to figure out where the rhythm originated.

In these cases, call the rhythm *supraventricular tachycardia*, a general term that refers to the origin as being above the ventricles. Examples of supraventricular tachycardia include atrial flutter, multifocal atrial tachycardia, and junctional tachycardia.

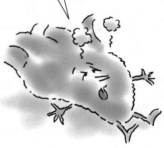

A higher ventricular rate means more problems for me!

result, the patient may exhibit signs and symptoms of decreased cardiac output, such as a rapid pulse, low blood pressure, and dizziness.

How you intervene

The underlying cause of junctional tachycardia should be treated. If the cause is digoxin toxicity, digoxin should be discontinued. Vagal maneuvers and medications, such as verapamil, may slow the heart rate for the symptomatic patient.

Setting the pace

If the patient recently had an MI or heart surgery, they may need a temporary pacemaker to reset the heart's rhythm. Children with permanent arrhythmias may be resistant to drug therapy and may therefore require surgery. Patients with recurrent junctional tachycardia may be treated with ablation therapy, followed by permanent pacemaker insertion.

Monitor patients with junctional tachycardia for signs of decreased cardiac output. You should also check digoxin and potassium levels and administer potassium supplements, as ordered. If symptoms are severe and digoxin is the culprit, the healthcare provider may order digoxin immune fab (Digibind), a digoxin-binding drug.

Ventricular arrhythmias

Ventricular arrhythmias originate in the ventricles below the bundle of His. They occur when electrical impulses depolarize the myocardium using a different pathway from normal impulses.

Ventricular arrhythmias appear on an ECG in characteristic ways. The QRS complex is wider than normal because of the prolonged conduction time through the ventricles. The T wave and the QRS complex deflect in opposite directions because of the difference in the action potential during ventricular depolarization and repolarization. Also, the P wave is absent because atrial depolarization doesn't occur. The QT interval is often prolonged.

You've lost your kick

When electrical impulses originate in the ventricles instead of the atria, atrial kick is lost and cardiac output decreases by as much as 30%. As a result, patients with ventricular arrhythmias may show signs and symptoms of cardiac decompensation, including hypotension, angina, syncope, and respiratory distress.

Potential to kill

Although ventricular arrhythmias may be benign, they're potentially deadly because the ventricles are ultimately responsible for cardiac output. Rapid recognition and treatment of ventricular arrhythmias increases the chance for successful resuscitation.

Ventricular arrhythmias include premature ventricular contractions (PVCs), ventricular tachycardia, ventricular fibrillation, and idioventricular rhythms. This section also discusses asystole, which is the lack of ventricular movement.

Premature ventricular contraction

A PVC is an ectopic beat originating low in the ventricles and occurring earlier than normal. PVCs may occur in healthy people without causing problems. PVCs may occur singly, in clusters of two or more, or in repeating patterns, such as bigeminy (every other beat) or trigeminy (every third beat). When PVCs occur in patients with underlying heart disease, they may indicate impending lethal ventricular arrhythmias.

How it happens

PVCs are usually caused by electrical irritability in the ventricular conduction system or muscle tissue. This irritability may be provoked by anything that disrupts normal electrolyte shifts during cell depolarization and repolarization. (See *Causes of PVCs.*)

This could get serious

PVCs are significant for two reasons. First, they can lead to more serious arrhythmias, such as ventricular tachycardia (with or without a pulse) or ventricular fibrillation. The risk of developing a more serious arrhythmia increases in patients with an ischemic or damaged heart.

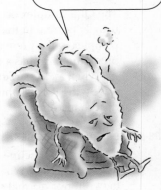

Because I'm weak, I'm at greater risk for developing a serious arrhythmia.

Causes of PVCs

Premature ventricular contractions (PVCs) may be caused by conditions that provoke electrical irritability in the ventricular conduction system or muscle tissue, including anything that disrupts normal electrolyte shifts during cell depolarization and repolarization. Conditions that may disrupt electrolyte shifts include the following:

• electrolyte imbalances, such as hypo-kalemia, hyperkalemia, hypomagnese-mia, and hypocalcemia
• metabolic acidosis
• hypoxia
• myocardial ischemia
• drug intoxication, particularly cocaine, amphetamines, and tricyclic antidepressants
• enlargement of the ventricular chambers
• increased sympathetic stimulation
• myocarditis.

PVCs also decrease cardiac output, especially if the ectopic beats are frequent or sustained. Decreased cardiac output is caused by reduced ventricular diastolic filling time and a loss of atrial kick. The clinical impact of PVCs hinges on how well perfusion is maintained and how long the abnormal rhythm lasts.

What to look for

On the ECG strip, PVCs look wide and bizarre and appear as early beats causing atrial and ventricular irregularity. The rate follows the underlying rhythm, which is usually regular. (See *Recognizing PVCs*.)

The P wave is usually absent. A PVC may trigger retrograde P waves, which can distort the ST segment. The PR interval and QT interval aren't measurable on a premature beat, only on the normal beats. There may be a compensatory pause following the PVC.

Complex configuration

The QRS complex occurs early. Configuration of the QRS complex is usually normal in the underlying rhythm. The duration of the QRS complex in the premature beat exceeds 0.12 second. The T wave in the premature beat has a deflection opposite that of the QRS complex.

When a PVC strikes on the downslope of the preceding normal T wave—the R-on-T phenomenon—it can trigger more serious rhythm disturbances.

The pause that compensates

A horizontal baseline called a *compensatory pause* may follow the T wave of the PVC. When a compensatory pause appears, the interval between two normal sinus beats containing a PVC equals two normal sinus intervals. (See *Recognizing compensatory pause*.) This pause occurs

Recognizing PVCs

This rhythm strip shows premature ventricular contractions (PVCs) on beats 1, 6, and 11. Note the wide and bizarre appearance of the QRS complex.

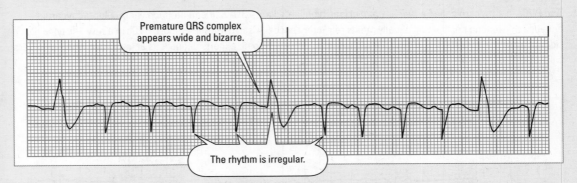

Premature QRS complex appears wide and bizarre.

The rhythm is irregular.

- *Rhythm:* Atrial and ventricular—irregular
- *Rate:* 120 beats/min
- *P wave:* None with PVC, but P wave present with other QRS complexes

- *PR interval:* 0.12 second in underlying rhythm
- *QRS complex:* Early, with bizarre configuration and duration of 0.14 second in PVC; QRS complexes are 0.08 second in underlying rhythm.

- *T wave:* Normal; opposite direction from QRS complex
- *QT interval:* 0.28 second with underlying rhythm
- *Other:* None

because the ventricle is refractory and can't respond to the next regularly timed P wave from the sinus node. When a compensatory pause doesn't occur, the PVC is referred to as *interpolated*.

PVCs all in a row

PVCs that look alike are called *unifocal* and originate from the same ectopic focus. These beats may also appear in patterns that can progress to more lethal arrhythmias. (See *When PVCs spell danger*, pages 144 and 145.)

Peak technique

Recognizing compensatory pause

You can determine if a compensatory pause exists by using calipers to mark off two normal P-P intervals. Place one leg of the calipers on the sinus P wave that comes just before the premature ventricular contraction. If the pause is compensatory, the other leg of the calipers will fall precisely on the P wave that comes after the pause.

When PVCs spell danger

Here are some examples of patterns of dangerous premature ventricular contractions (PVCs).

Paired PVCs

Two PVCs in a row are called a *pair* or *couplet* (see highlighted areas). A pair can produce ventricular tachycardia because the second contraction usually meets refractory tissue. A salvo—three or more PVCs in a row—is typically considered a run of nonsustained ventricular tachycardia. However, some experts define it as at least four, whereas others will not define the rhythm as ventricular tachycardia until many more are seen.

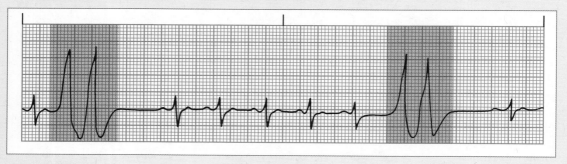

Multiform PVCs

PVCs that look different from one another arise from different sites or from the same site with abnormal conduction (see highlighted areas). Multiform PVCs may indicate severe heart disease or digoxin toxicity.

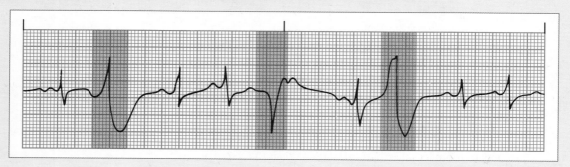

Ruling out trouble

To help determine the seriousness of PVCs, ask yourself these questions:

- How often do they occur? In patients with chronic PVCs, an increase in frequency or a change in the pattern of PVCs from the baseline rhythm may signal a more serious condition.

Bigeminy and trigeminy

PVCs that occur every other beat (bigeminy) or every third beat (trigeminy) can result in ventricular tachycardia or ventricular fibrillation (see highlighted areas).

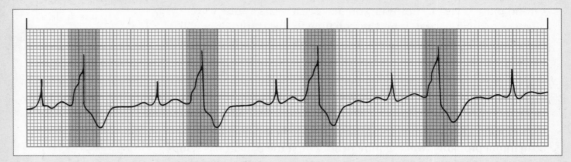

R-on-T phenomenon

In R-on-T phenomenon, the PVC occurs so early that it falls on the T wave of the preceding beat (see highlighted area). Because the cells haven't fully repolarized, ventricular tachycardia or ventricular fibrillation can result.

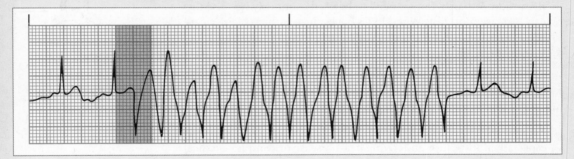

- In what pattern do they occur? If the ECG shows a dangerous pattern—such as paired PVCs, PVCs with more than one focus, bigeminy, or R-on-T phenomenon—the patient may require immediate treatment.
- Are they really PVCs? Make sure the complex you see is a PVC, not another, less dangerous arrhythmia. Don't delay treatment, however, if the patient is unstable.

Outward signs tell a story

The patient with PVCs has a much weaker pulse wave after the premature beat and a longer-than-normal pause between pulse waves. At times, you won't be able to palpate any pulse after the PVC. If the carotid pulse is visible, however, you may see a weaker pulse wave after the premature beat. When auscultating for heart sounds, you'll hear an abnormally early heart sound and diminished amplitude with each premature beat.

Patients with frequent PVCs may complain of palpitations and may also experience hypotension or syncope.

How you intervene

If the patient is asymptomatic and doesn't have heart disease, the arrhythmia probably won't require treatment. If the patient has symptoms or a dangerous form of PVCs, the type of treatment depends on the cause of the problem.

If the PVCs have a cardiac origin, the healthcare provider may order drugs to suppress ventricular irritability such as amiodarone or flecainide. Antiarrhythmics need to be used cautiously because they can increase mortality. When PVCs have a noncardiac origin, treatment aims to correct the cause, which may include adjusting drug therapy or correcting acidosis, electrolyte imbalances, hypothermia, or hypoxia. Beta-adrenergic blockers or calcium channel blockers may also be used.

The danger zone

Patients who have recently developed PVCs need prompt assessment, especially if they have underlying heart disease or complex medical problems. Those with chronic PVCs should be observed closely for the development of more frequent PVCs or more dangerous PVC patterns.

Until effective treatment begins, patients with PVCs accompanied by serious symptoms should have continuous ECG monitoring and ambulate only with assistance. If the patient is discharged from the hospital on antiarrhythmic medications, make sure family members know how to contact the emergency medical system (911) and how to perform cardiopulmonary resuscitation (CPR).

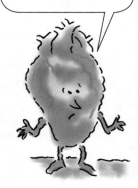

When evaluating PVCs, remember that an increase in frequency, a change in pattern, or a dangerous pattern may indicate a more serious condition.

Ventricular tachycardia

In ventricular tachycardia, commonly called *V-tach*, three or more PVCs occur in a row and the ventricular rate exceeds 100 beats/min. (Ventricular tachycardia of this low rate is generally considered to be a "slow ventricular tachycardia," even though it fits the definition of tachycardia.) Ventricular tachycardia is usually seen with a much higher rate. This arrhythmia usually precedes ventricular fibrillation and sudden cardiac death, especially in patients who aren't in the hospital.

Ventricular tachycardia is an extremely unstable rhythm. It can occur in short, paroxysmal bursts lasting fewer than 30 seconds and causing few or no symptoms. Alternatively, it can be sustained, requiring immediate treatment to prevent death, even in patients initially able to maintain adequate cardiac output.

How it happens

Ventricular tachycardia usually results from increased myocardial irritability, which may be triggered by enhanced automaticity or reentry within the Purkinje system or by PVCs initiating the R-on-T phenomenon. (See *Causes of ventricular tachycardia*.)

Running on empty

Ventricular tachycardia is significant because of its unpredictability and potential to cause death. A patient may be stable with a normal pulse and adequate hemodynamics or unstable with hypotension and no detectable pulse. Because of reduced ventricular filling time and the drop in cardiac output, the patient's condition can quickly deteriorate to ventricular fibrillation and complete cardiac collapse.

What to look for

On the ECG strip, the atrial rhythm and rate can't be determined. The ventricular rhythm is usually regular but may be slightly irregular. The ventricular rate is usually rapid—100 to 200 beats/min or more.

The P wave is usually absent but may be obscured by the QRS complex. Retrograde P waves may be present. Because the P wave can't be seen in most cases, you can't measure the PR interval. The QRS complex has a bizarre configuration, usually with an increased

Causes of ventricular tachycardia

Conditions that can cause ventricular tachycardia include the following:

- myocardial ischemia
- myocardial infarction
- coronary artery disease
- valvular heart disease
- heart failure
- cardiomyopathy

- electrolyte imbalances such as hypokalemia
- drug intoxication from digoxin (Lanoxin), procainamide (Pronestyl), quinidine, or cocaine
- pulmonary embolism
- tension pneumothorax.

amplitude and a duration of longer than 0.14 second. The T wave may also be difficult to visualize, thereby making it difficult or impossible to determine the QT interval.

Not everyone likes uniforms

QRS complexes in monomorphic ventricular tachycardia have a uniform shape. In polymorphic ventricular tachycardia, the shape of the QRS complex constantly changes. If the T wave is visible, it occurs opposite the QRS complex. The QT interval isn't measurable. (See *Recognizing ventricular tachycardia*, page 148.)

Torsades de pointes (a French term for twisting points) is a special variation of polymorphic ventricular tachycardia. (See *Understanding torsades de pointes*, page 149.)

Headed for trouble

Although some patients have only minor symptoms at first, the arrhythmia can quickly lead to cardiac collapse. Most patients with ventricular tachycardia have weak or absent pulses. Low cardiac output leads to hypotension and a decreased LOC, causing unresponsiveness. Ventricular tachycardia may precipitate angina, heart failure, or a substantial decrease in organ perfusion.

Recognizing ventricular tachycardia

Take a look at this example of how ventricular tachycardia appears on a rhythm strip. Notice its distinguishing characteristics.

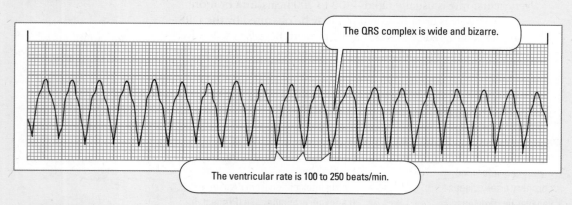

The QRS complex is wide and bizarre.

The ventricular rate is 100 to 250 beats/min.

- *Rhythm:* Atrial and ventricular—regular
- *Rate:* Atrial and ventricular—187 beats/min

- *P wave:* Absent
- *PR interval:* Unmeasurable
- *QRS complex:* 0.24 second; wide and bizarre

- *T wave:* Opposite direction of QRS complex
- *QT interval:* Unmeasurable
- *Other:* None

Understanding torsades de pointes

Torsades de pointes, which means "twisting about the points," is a special form of polymorphic ventricular tachycardia. The hallmark characteristics of this rhythm, shown below, are QRS complexes that rotate about the baseline, deflecting downward and upward for several beats. The rate is generally 150 to 250 beats/min, usually with an irregular rhythm, and the QRS complexes are wide. The P wave is usually absent.

Paroxysmal rhythm

This arrhythmia may be paroxysmal, starting and stopping suddenly, and may deteriorate into ventricular fibrillation. It should be considered when ventricular tachycardia doesn't respond to antiarrhythmic therapy or other treatments.

Reversible causes

The cause of this form of ventricular tachycardia is usually reversible. The most common causes are drugs

that lengthen the QT interval, such as the antiarrhythmics quinidine, procainamide (Pronestyl), and sotalol (Betapace). Opioids, such as methadone and buprenorphine, also increase the QT interval. Other causes include myocardial ischemia; hypoxemia; heart failure; and electrolyte abnormalities, such as hypokalemia, hypomagnesemia, and hypocalcemia.

Going into overdrive

Torsades de pointes is treated by correcting the underlying cause, especially if the cause is related to specific drug therapy. The healthcare provider may order mechanical overdrive pacing, which overrides the ventricular rate and breaks the triggered mechanism for the arrhythmia. Magnesium may also be effective. Electrical cardioversion may be used when torsades de pointes doesn't respond to other treatment.

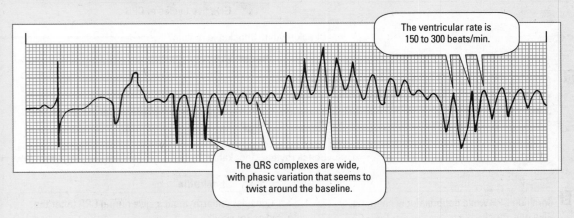

The ventricular rate is 150 to 300 beats/min.

The QRS complexes are wide, with phasic variation that seems to twist around the baseline.

How you intervene

Treatment depends on whether the patient's pulse is detectable or undetectable. Patients with pulseless ventricular tachycardia require immediate resuscitation using the pulseless arrest algorithm. (See *Treating pulseless arrest*, pages 150 and 151.)

Peak technique

Treating pulseless arrest

The following algorithm shows the critical steps to take during pulseless cardiac arrest.

1   **Pulseless arrest**
- Basic life support algorithm; call for help and give cardiopulmonary resuscitation (CPR).
- Give oxygen when available.
- Attach monitor and defibrillator when available.

3 **Ventricular fibrillation or ventricular tachycardia** ◄ **Shockable** **2** Check rhythm. Shockable rhythm?

Shockable

4
Give one shock.
- Manual biphasic: device specific (typically 120–200 J; if unknown, use maximum available)
- Automated external defibrillator (AED): device-specific
- Monophasic: 360 J
Resume CPR immediately after the shock.

When IV/IO available, give Epinephrine during CPR (generally after the first shock; 1 mg IV/IO). Repeat every 3–5 minutes.
- Consider advanced airway, capnography

Give five cycles of CPR

5 Check rhythm. Shockable rhythm?

Shockable

6
Continue CPR while defibrillator is charging. Give one shock.
- Manual biphasic: device-specific (higher dose, usually 300 J)

- AED: device-specific
- Monophasic: 360 J
Resume CPR immediately after the shock.

Give five cycles of CPR

7 Check rhythm. Shockable rhythm?

Shockable

8
Continue CPR while defibrillator is charging. Give one shock.
- Manual biphasic: device-specific (usually 360 J)
- AED: device specific
- Monophasic: 360 J
Resume CPR immediately after the shock.

- Consider antiarrhythmics; give during CPR (after the 2nd or 3rd shock):
– Amiodarone IV/IO dose: First dose: 300 mg bolus. Second dose: 150 mg.
– Lidocaine IV/IO dose: First dose: 1–1.5 mg/kg. Second dose: 0.5–0.75 mg/kg.
- After five cycles of CPR,*= go to Box 5.

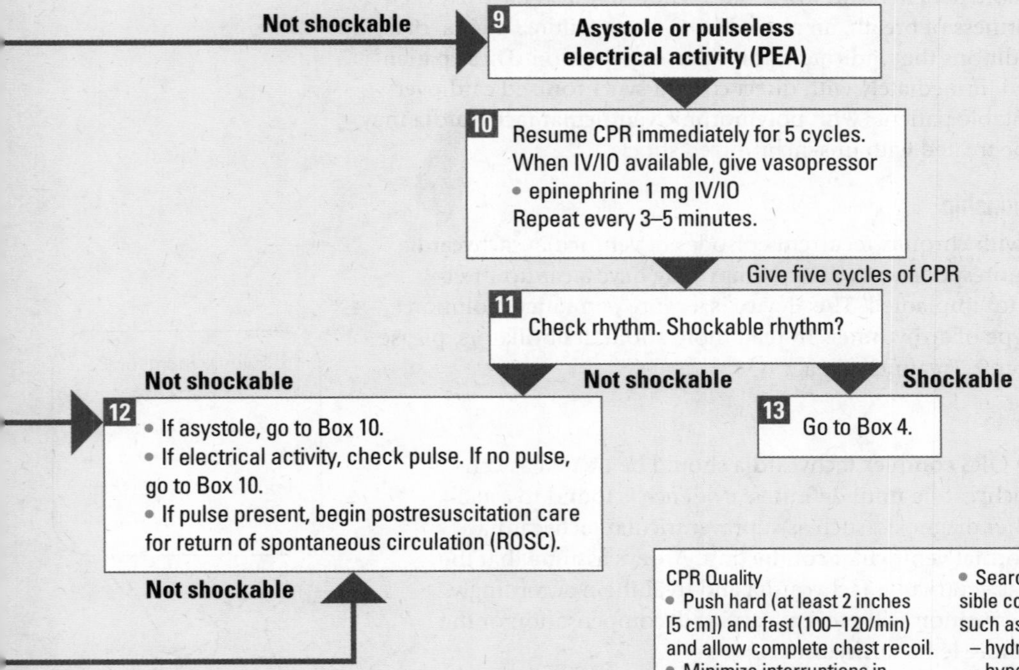

Not shockable →

9 **Asystole or pulseless electrical activity (PEA)**

↓

10 Resume CPR immediately for 5 cycles.
When IV/IO available, give vasopressor
• epinephrine 1 mg IV/IO
Repeat every 3–5 minutes.

↓ Give five cycles of CPR

11 Check rhythm. Shockable rhythm?

Not shockable   **Shockable**

Not shockable

12
• If asystole, go to Box 10.
• If electrical activity, check pulse. If no pulse, go to Box 10.
• If pulse present, begin postresuscitation care for return of spontaneous circulation (ROSC).

Not shockable

13 Go to Box 4.

CPR Quality
• Push hard (at least 2 inches [5 cm]) and fast (100–120/min) and allow complete chest recoil.
• Minimize interruptions in compressions.
• Avoid excessive ventilation.
• Change compressor every 2 minutes, or sooner if fatigued.
• If no advanced airway, 30:2 compression-ventilation ratio
• Quantitative waveform capnography
–If Petco2 is low or decreasing, reassess CPR quality.

• Search for and treat possible contributing factors, such as:
– hydrogen ion (acidosis)
– hypokalemia or hyperkalemia
– hypothermia
– hypovolemia
– hypoxia
– tamponade, cardiac
– tension pneumothorax
– thrombosis (coronary or pulmonary)
– toxins

---

*After an advanced airway is placed, rescuers no longer deliver "cycles" of CPR. Give continuous chest compressions without pauses for breaths. Give one breath every 6 seconds if rescue breathing only is needed. Check rhythm and check for a pulse every 2 minutes.
See also:
Advanced Cardiovascular Life Support: Provider Manual.
© 2020, American Heart Association.
Source: American Heart Association, Inc.

Looking for some stability

Treatment of patients with a detectable pulse depends on whether their condition is stable or unstable. A stable patient with a wide QRS complex tachycardia that is monomorphic may be treated with adenosine. If the patient has monomorphic ventricular tachycardia, IV doses of amiodarone, procainamide, or sotalol may be given. Medications that cause prolonged QT intervals and correct electrolyte imbalances should be discontinued. If the patient becomes clinically unstable, immediately perform synchronized cardioversion.

Unstable patients generally have heart rates greater than 150 beats/ min, although it is possible to have stable patients with higher rates and unstable patients with lower rates. They may also have hypotension, shortness of breath, an altered LOC, heart failure, angina, or MI—conditions that indicate cardiac decompensation. These patients are treated immediately with direct current synchronized cardioversion. Unstable patients with polymorphic ventricular tachycardia may need to be treated with unsynchronized shocks.

A permanent relationship

Patients with chronic, recurrent episodes of ventricular tachycardia who are unresponsive to drug therapy may have a cardioverter-defibrillator implanted. This device is a more permanent solution for this type of arrhythmia. To read more about defibrillators, please see chapter 9, Treatments, page 338.

Assume the worst

Any wide QRS complex tachycardia should be treated as ventricular tachycardia until definitive evidence is found to establish another diagnosis, such as supraventricular tachycardia with abnormal ventricular conduction. Always assume that the patient has ventricular tachycardia and treat them accordingly. Rapid intervention will prevent cardiac decompensation or the onset of more lethal arrhythmias.

Teacher, teacher

Be sure to teach patients and their families about the serious nature of this arrhythmia and the need for prompt treatment. If your patient is undergoing cardioversion, tell them they'll be given an analgesic or a sedative to help prevent discomfort.

If a patient will be discharged with an implanted cardioverter-defibrillator or a prescription for long-term antiarrhythmic medications, teach family members how to contact the emergency medical system and how to perform CPR.

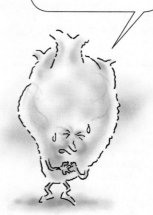

Family members of patients with ventricular tachycardia should learn how to perform CPR.

Ventricular fibrillation

Ventricular fibrillation, commonly called *V-fib*, is a chaotic pattern of electrical activity in the ventricles in which electrical impulses arise from many different foci. It produces no effective muscular contraction and no cardiac output. Untreated ventricular fibrillation causes most cases of sudden cardiac death in people outside of a hospital.

How it happens

With ventricular fibrillation, the ventricles quiver instead of contract, so cardiac output falls to zero. If fibrillation continues, it leads to ventricular standstill and death. (See *Causes of ventricular fibrillation*.)

What to look for

On the ECG strip, ventricular activity appears as fibrillatory waves with no recognizable pattern. Atrial rate and rhythm can't be determined or can ventricular rhythm because no pattern or regularity occurs. As a result, the ventricular rate, P wave, PR interval, QRS complex, T wave, and QT interval can't be determined. Larger, or coarse, fibrillatory waves are easier to convert to a normal rhythm than are smaller waves because larger waves indicate a greater degree of electrical activity in the heart. The baseline is wavy, chaotic, and generally indiscernible. (See *Recognizing ventricular fibrillation*.)

911 emergency

The patient in ventricular fibrillation is in full cardiac arrest, unresponsive, and without a detectable blood pressure or carotid or femoral pulse. Whenever you see a pattern resembling ventricular fibrillation, check the patient immediately, check the rhythm in another lead, and start treatment.

How you intervene

Defibrillation is the most effective treatment for ventricular fibrillation. (See *Treating pulseless arrest*, pages 150 and 151.) CPR must be performed until the defibrillator arrives to preserve oxygen supply to the brain and other vital organs. Epinephrine is administered for its vasoconstrictive effects. Amiodarone and lidocaine may be used for ventricular fibrillation that has not responded to defibrillation or to prevent reoccurrence. Magnesium is usually only given for torsades de pointes or for a known or suspected case of hypomagnesemia.

Jump start

During defibrillation, electrodes direct an electric current through the patient's heart. The current causes the myocardium to depolarize, which, in turn, encourages the SA node to resume normal control of

---

Causes of ventricular fibrillation

Ventricular fibrillation can be caused by the following:
- myocardial ischemia
- myocardial infarction
- untreated ventricular tachycardia
- underlying heart disease
- acid–base imbalance
- electric shock
- severe hypothermia
- electrolyte imbalances, such as hypokalemia, hyperkalemia, and hypercalcemia.

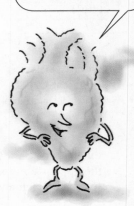

Defibrillation is the key to getting the heart back on track.

Recognizing ventricular fibrillation

The first rhythm strip shows coarse ventricular fibrillation; the second shows fine ventricular fibrillation. Fine ventricular fibrillation sometimes resembles asystole.

Coarse

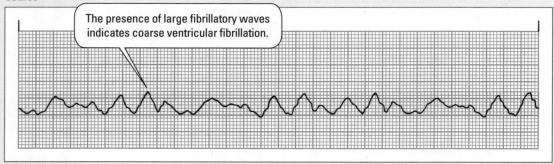

The presence of large fibrillatory waves indicates coarse ventricular fibrillation.

Fine

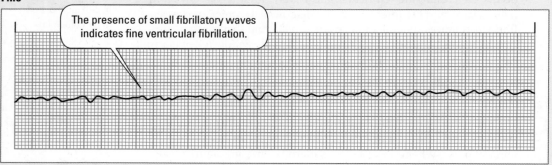

The presence of small fibrillatory waves indicates fine ventricular fibrillation.

- *Rhythm:* Chaotic
- *Rate:* Unmeasurable
- *P wave:* Absent
- *PR interval:* Not measurable
- *QRS complex:* Unable to distinguish (indiscernible)
- *T wave:* Unable to distinguish (indiscernible)
- *QT interval:* Not applicable
- *Other:* Waveform is a wavy line.

the heart's electrical activity. One electrode is placed to the right of the upper sternum, and one is placed over the fifth or sixth intercostal space at the left anterior axillary line.

ABCs of AEDs

Automated external defibrillators are increasingly being used to provide early defibrillation. In this method, electrode pads are placed on the patient's chest and a microcomputer in the unit interprets the cardiac rhythm, providing the caregiver with step-by-step instructions on how to proceed. These defibrillators can be used by people without medical experience. They generally do not display the rhythm but only interpret it internally. If the rhythm is determined to be ventricular fibrillation or pulseless ventricular tachycardia, a shock will be advised. The unit will charge itself up and notify the rescuer when to push the *shock* button and then to resume CPR. It will also usually count down the time until the next opportunity for rhythm analysis (2 minutes), during which time continuous CPR should be performed.

Speedy delivery

For the patient with ventricular fibrillation, successful resuscitation requires rapid recognition of the problem and prompt defibrillation. Many healthcare facilities and emergency medical systems have established protocols to help healthcare workers initiate prompt treatment. Make sure you know where your facility keeps its emergency equipment and how to recognize and deal with potentially lethal arrhythmias.

You'll also need to teach your patient and their family how to contact the emergency medical system. Family members need instruction in CPR. Teach them about long-term therapies that prevent recurrent episodes of ventricular fibrillation, including chronic antiarrhythmic drugs and implantation of a cardioverter-defibrillator.

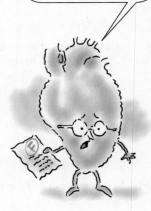

Oh no! My pacemaker failed. I'm at risk for idioventricular rhythms.

Idioventricular rhythms

Called the *rhythms of last resort*, idioventricular rhythms act as safety mechanisms to prevent ventricular standstill when no impulses are conducted to the ventricles from above the bundle of His. The cells of the His-Purkinje system take over and act as the heart's pacemaker to generate electrical impulses.

Idioventricular rhythms occur as ventricular escape beats, *idioventricular rhythm* (a term used to designate a specific type of idioventricular rhythm), or accelerated idioventricular rhythm.

How it happens

Idioventricular rhythms occur when all of the heart's other pacemakers fail to function or when supraventricular impulses can't reach the ventricles because of a block in the conduction system. (See *Causes of idioventricular rhythms*.)

Conduction shortcomings and pacemaker failures

Idioventricular rhythms signal a serious conduction defect with a failure of the primary pacemaker. The slow ventricular rate of these arrhythmias and the loss of atrial kick markedly reduce cardiac output. Patients require close monitoring because this problem can progress to more lethal arrhythmias. Idioventricular rhythms also commonly occur in dying patients.

Causes of idioventricular rhythms

Idioventricular rhythms may accompany third-degree heart block or may be caused by the following:

- myocardial ischemia
- myocardial infarction
- digoxin toxicity
- pacemaker failure
- metabolic imbalances.

What to look for

If just one idioventricular beat is generated, it's called a *ventricular escape beat*. The beat appears late in the conduction cycle, when the rate drops to 40 beats/min.

Consecutive ventricular beats on the ECG strip make up idioventricular rhythm. When this arrhythmia occurs, atrial rhythm and rate can't be determined. The ventricular rhythm is usually regular at 20 to 40 beats/min, the inherent rate of the ventricles. (See *Recognizing idioventricular rhythm*, page 156.) If the rate is faster, it's called an *accelerated idioventricular rhythm*. (See *Recognizing accelerated idioventricular rhythm*, page 157.)

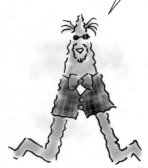

Bizarre QRS complexes characterize idioventricular rhythms.

An absent P...

Distinguishing characteristics of idioventricular rhythm include an absent P wave or one that has no relationship to the QRS complex. These factors make the PR interval unmeasurable (not measurable).

...and a bizarre QRS...

Because of abnormal ventricular depolarization, the QRS complex has a duration of longer than 0.12 second, with a wide and bizarre configuration. The T-wave deflection may be opposite the QRS complex. The QT interval is usually prolonged, indicating delayed depolarization and repolarization.

Recognizing idioventricular rhythm

Take a look at this example of how an idioventricular rhythm appears on a rhythm strip. Notice its distinguishing characteristics.

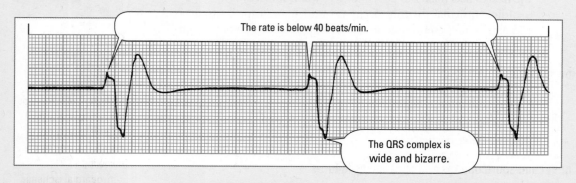

The rate is below 40 beats/min.

The QRS complex is wide and bizarre.

- *Rhythm:* Irregular
- *Rate:* Atrial—not measurable—30 beats/min
- *P wave:* Absent

- *PR interval:* Not measurable
- *QRS complex:* 0.36 second and bizarre

- *T wave:* Directly opposite last part of QRS complex
- *QT interval:* 0.60 second
- *Other:* None

Recognizing accelerated idioventricular rhythm

An accelerated idioventricular rhythm has the same characteristics as an idioventricular rhythm except that it's faster. The rate shown here varies between 40 and 100 beats/min.

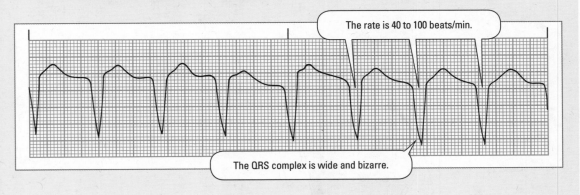

The rate is 40 to 100 beats/min.

The QRS complex is wide and bizarre.

. . . make for one dizzy patient

The patient may complain of palpitations, dizziness, or light-headedness, or they may have a syncopal episode. If the arrhythmia persists, hypotension, weak peripheral pulses, decreased urine output, or confusion can occur.

How you intervene

Treatment should be initiated immediately to increase the patient's heart rate, improve cardiac output, and establish a normal rhythm. Atropine may be prescribed to increase the heart rate. If atropine isn't effective or if the patient develops hypotension or other signs of instability, a pacemaker may be needed to reestablish a heart rate that provides enough cardiac output to perfuse organs properly. A transcutaneous pacemaker may be used in an emergency until a temporary or permanent transvenous pacemaker can be inserted. (See *Transcutaneous pacemaker*, page 158.)

Remember that the goal of treatment doesn't include suppressing the idioventricular rhythm because it acts as a safety mechanism to protect the heart from standstill. Idioventricular rhythm should never be treated with lidocaine or other antiarrhythmics that would suppress that safety mechanism.

Electronic surveillance

Patients with idioventricular rhythms need continuous ECG monitoring and constant assessment until treatment restores hemodynamic stability. Keep atropine and pacemaker equipment at the bedside. Enforce bed rest until a permanent system is in place for maintaining an effective heart rate.

Never give lidocaine or another arrhythmia suppressant to a patient with an idioventricular rhythm. Doing so could suppress the rhythm and lead to cardiac standstill.

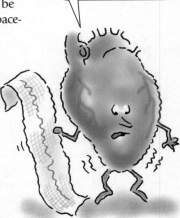

Peak technique

Transcutaneous pacemaker

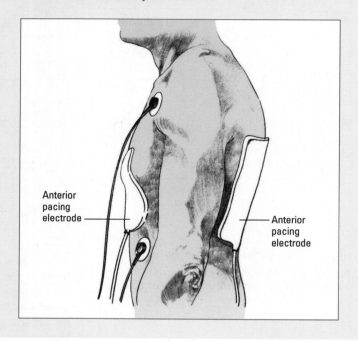

Anterior pacing electrode

Anterior pacing electrode

Be sure to tell the patient and their family members about the serious nature of this arrhythmia and all aspects of treatment. If a permanent pacemaker is inserted, teach the patient and their family how it works, how to recognize problems, when to contact the healthcare provider, and how pacemaker function will be monitored.

Asystole

Asystole is ventricular standstill. The patient is completely unresponsive, with no electrical activity in the heart and no cardiac output. This arrhythmia results most commonly from a prolonged period of cardiac emergency, such as ventricular fibrillation, without effective resuscitation. (Some experts do not consider asystole a "rhythm" because there is no rhythm or electrical activity present.)

Asystole has been called the *arrhythmia of death*. The patient is in cardiopulmonary arrest. Without rapid initiation of CPR and appropriate treatment, the situation quickly becomes irreversible.

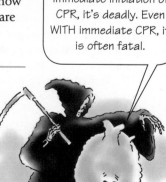

Asystole is sometimes called the arrhythmia of death because without immediate initiation of CPR, it's deadly. Even WITH immediate CPR, it is often fatal.

How it happens

Without ventricular electrical activity, ventricular contractions can't occur. As a result, cardiac output drops to zero and vital organs are no longer perfused. Asystole is typically considered to be a confirmation of death, rather than an arrhythmia to be treated. (See *Causes of asystole*.)

What to look for

A patient in asystole is unresponsive, without any discernible pulse or blood pressure.

On the ECG strip, asystole looks like a nearly flat line (except for changes caused by chest compressions during CPR). No electrical activity is evident, except possibly P waves for a time. Atrial and ventricular activity is at a standstill, so no intervals can be measured. In the patient with a pacemaker, pacer spikes may be evident on the strip, but no P wave or QRS complex occurs in response to the stimulus. (See *Recognizing asystole*.)

How you intervene

If the patient is already on a cardiac monitor, verify the presence of asystole in two or more leads. The immediate treatment for asystole is CPR. (See *Treating pulseless arrest*, pages 150 and 151.) Start CPR as soon as you determine that the patient has no pulse. Then verify the presence of asystole by checking two different ECG leads. Give repeated doses of epinephrine every 3 to 5 minutes or as ordered.

Subsequent treatment for asystole focuses on identifying and either treating or removing the underlying cause.

Causes of asystole

Anything that causes inadequate blood flow to the heart may lead to asystole, including:
- myocardial infarction
- severe electrolyte disturbances such as hyperkalemia
- massive pulmonary embolism
- prolonged hypoxemia
- severe, uncorrected acid–base disturbances
- electric shock
- overdoses of drugs such as heroin, oxycodone, and cocaine.

Recognizing asystole

This rhythm strip shows asystole, the absence of electrical activity in the ventricles. Except for a few P waves or pacer spikes, nothing appears on the waveform and the line is almost flat.

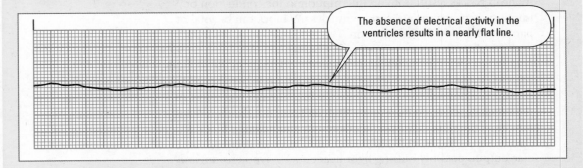

The absence of electrical activity in the ventricles results in a nearly flat line.

Now I get it!

Pulseless electrical activity

In pulseless electrical activity, the heart muscle loses its ability to contract even though electrical activity is preserved. As a result, the patient goes into cardiac arrest.

On an electrocardiogram, you'll see evidence of organized electrical activity, but you won't be able to palpate a pulse or measure the blood pressure.

Causes

This condition requires rapid identification and treatment.

Causes include the following:

• hypovolemia
• hypoxia
• acidosis
• tension pneumothorax
• cardiac tamponade
• massive pulmonary embolism
• hypothermia
• hypo- or hyperkalemia
• massive acute myocardial infarction
• overdose of drugs such as tricyclic antidepressants or other toxins.

Treatment

CPR is the immediate treatment, along with epinephrine. Subsequent treatment focuses on identifying and correcting the underlying cause.

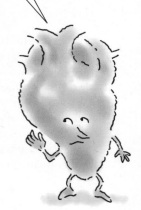

Treat any situation where you can't find the patient's pulse as an emergency—even if the monitor shows a waveform.

Start me up

Your job is to recognize this life-threatening arrhythmia and start resuscitation right away. Unfortunately, most patients with asystole can't be resuscitated, especially after a prolonged period of cardiac arrest.

Pulseless electrical activity can lead to asystole, so it is important to recognize and treat causes early.

Atrioventricular blocks

AV heart blocks result from an interruption in the conduction of impulses between the atria and ventricles. AV block can be total or partial or it may delay conduction. The block can occur at the AV node, the bundle of His, or the bundle branches.

The heart's electrical impulses normally originate in the SA node, so when those impulses are blocked at the AV node, atrial rates are commonly normal (60 to 100 beats/min). The clinical effect of the block depends on how many impulses are completely blocked, how slow the ventricular rate is as a result, and how the block ultimately affects the heart. A slow ventricular rate can decrease cardiac output, possibly causing light-headedness, hypotension, and confusion.

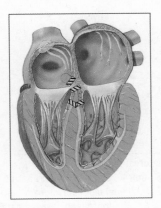

A troubled relationship

Factors that cause AV blocks include the following:

- *Myocardial ischemia* impairs cellular function, so cells repolarize more slowly or incompletely. The injured cells, in turn, may conduct impulses slowly or inconsistently. Relief of the ischemia can restore normal function to the AV node.
- In *MI*, cell death occurs. If the necrotic cells are part of the conduction system, they no longer conduct impulses, and a permanent AV block occurs.
- *Excessive dosage* of or an *exaggerated response* to a drug can cause AV block or increase the likelihood that a block will develop. Although many antiarrhythmic medications can have this effect, the drugs more commonly known to cause or exacerbate AV blocks include digoxin, beta-adrenergic blockers, and calcium channel blockers.
- *Congenital anomalies*, such as congenital ventricular septal defect, may involve cardiac structures and affect the conduction system. Anomalies of the conduction system, such as an AV node that doesn't conduct impulses, may occur in the absence of structural defects.
- *Injury during cardiac surgery or radiofrequency ablation therapy.* This is most likely to occur during surgical procedures that involve the mitral or tricuspid valve. If the injury involves tissues adjacent to the surgical site and the conduction system isn't physically disrupted, the block may be only temporary. If a portion of the conduction system itself is severed, a permanent block results.

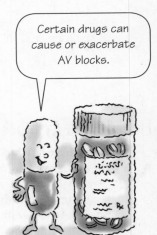

Certain drugs can cause or exacerbate AV blocks.

Class consciousness

AV blocks are classified according to their severity, not their location. That severity is measured according to how well the node conducts impulses and is separated by degrees—first, second, and third. In this section, we'll look at all four types of AV blocks.

Comparing degrees of AV block

Type	Distinguishing Characteristic	Possible Causes
First	• PR interval >0.20 s Considered a "delay" rather than a block	• Degenerative changes • Drugs: beta-adrenergic blockers, calcium channel blockers, digoxin • MI • Myocarditis
Type I second degree	• Progressive prolongation of PR interval until P wave occurs without a QRS complex (dropped beat)	• CAD • Drugs: beta-adrenergic blockers, calcium channel blockers, digoxin • Increased parasympathetic tone • Inferior wall MI • Rheumatic fever
Type II second degree	• Constant PR interval for conducted beats • Periodic nonconducted P wave (dropped beat)	• Anterior wall MI (LAD artery) • Degenerative changes in conduction system • Organic heart disease • Severe CAD
Third degree	• No relationship between P wave and QRS complex • Independent beating of atria and ventricles	**At AV node level** • AV node damage • Increased parasympathetic tone • Inferior wall MI • Drug toxicity **At infranodal level** • Extensive anterior wall MI

First-degree AV block

First-degree AV block occurs when impulses from the atria are consistently delayed during conduction through the AV node. Conduction eventually occurs; it just takes longer than normal. It's as if people are walking in a line through a doorway, but each person hesitates before crossing the threshold.

How it happens

First-degree AV block may be temporary, particularly if it stems from medications or ischemia early in the course of an MI. First-degree block is the least dangerous type of AV block, but it can progress to a more severe block, so it should be monitored. (See *Causes of first-degree AV block*.) However, many patients are asymptomatic with first-degree AV block, and it may go undetected or undiagnosed for years.

What to look for

In general, a rhythm strip with this block looks like a normal sinus rhythm except that the PR interval is longer than normal. The rhythm is regular, with one normal P wave for every QRS complex. The PR interval is greater than 0.20 second and is consistent for each beat. The QRS complex is usually normal, although sometimes, a bundle-branch block may occur along with first-degree AV block and cause a widening of the QRS complex. (See *Recognizing first-degree AV block*.)

Blocked but not bothered

Most patients with first-degree AV block show no symptoms of the block because cardiac output isn't significantly affected. If the PR interval is extremely long, a longer interval between S_1 and S_2 may be noted on cardiac auscultation.

How you intervene

Usually, just the underlying cause is treated, not the conduction disturbance itself. For example, if a medication is causing the block, the dosage may be reduced, or the medication discontinued. Close monitoring helps to detect progression of first-degree AV block to a more serious form of block.

Causes of first-degree AV block

First-degree atrioventricular (AV) block may appear normally in a healthy person or may result from:
• myocardial ischemia or infarction
• myocarditis
• degenerative changes in the heart
• medications, such as digoxin (Lanoxin), calcium channel blockers, and beta-adrenergic blockers.

Recognizing first-degree AV block

Take a look at this example of how first-degree atrioventricular (AV) block appears on a rhythm strip. Notice its distinguishing characteristics.

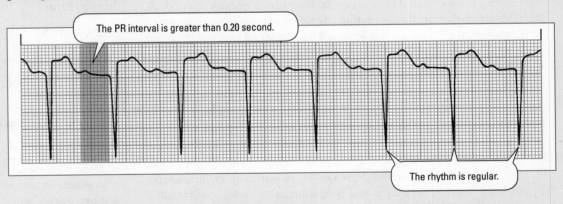

The PR interval is greater than 0.20 second.

The rhythm is regular.

• *Rhythm:* Regular
• *Rate:* 79 beats/min
• *P wave:* Normal

• *PR interval:* 0.32 second
• *QRS complex:* 0.08 second
• *T wave:* Normal

• *QT interval:* 0.40 second
• *Other:* None

When caring for a patient with first-degree AV block, evaluate for underlying causes that can be corrected. Observe the ECG for progression of the block to a more severe form of block. Administer digoxin, calcium channel blockers, and beta-adrenergic blockers cautiously.

Second-degree AV block, type I

Also called *Wenckebach* or *Mobitz type I block*, second-degree AV block, type I, occurs when each successive impulse from the SA node is delayed slightly longer than the previous impulse. That pattern continues until an impulse fails to be conducted to the ventricles and the cycle then repeats. It's like a line of people trying to get through a doorway, each one taking longer and longer until finally one can't get through.

How it happens

Second-degree AV block, type I, may occur normally in an otherwise healthy person. Almost always temporary, this type of block resolves when the underlying condition is corrected. Although an asymptomatic patient with this block has a good prognosis, the block may progress to a more serious form, especially if it occurs early during an MI. (See *Causes of second-degree AV block, type I*, page 164.)

What to look for

When monitoring a patient with second-degree AV block, type I, you'll note that because the SA node isn't affected by this lower block, it continues its normal activity. As a result, the atrial rhythm is normal. The PR interval gets gradually longer with each successive beat until finally a P wave fails to conduct to the ventricles. This lack of conduction makes the ventricular rhythm irregular, with a repeating pattern of groups of QRS complexes followed by a dropped beat in which the P wave isn't followed by a QRS complex. The QRS complexes are usually normal because the delays occur in the AV node. (See *Recognizing second-degree AV block, type I* and *Following the footprints*.)

When you're trying to identify second-degree AV block, type I, think of the phrase "longer, longer, drop," which describes the progressively prolonged PR intervals and the missing QRS complex.

Lonely Ps, light-headed patients

A patient with type I second-degree AV block is usually asymptomatic, although there may be signs and symptoms of decreased cardiac output, such as light-headedness and hypotension. Symptoms may be especially pronounced if ventricular rate is slow.

How you intervene

No treatment is needed for second-degree AV block, type I, if the patient is asymptomatic. For a symptomatic patient, atropine may

Causes of second-degree AV block, type I

Causes of second-degree atrioventricular (AV) block, type I include the following:
- coronary artery disease
- inferior-wall myocardial infarction
- rheumatic fever
- cardiac medications, such as beta-adrenergic blockers, digoxin (Lanoxin), and calcium channel blockers
- increased vagal stimulation.

Recognizing second-degree AV block, type I

Take a look at this example of how second-degree atrioventricular (AV) block, type I, appears on a rhythm strip. Notice its distinguishing characteristics.

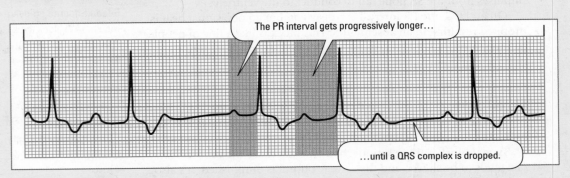

The PR interval gets progressively longer...

...until a QRS complex is dropped.

- *Rhythm:* Atrial—regular; ventricular—irregular
- *Rate:* Atrial—80 beats/min; ventricular—50 beats/min
- *P wave:* Normal
- *PR interval:* Progressively prolonged
- *QRS complex:* 0.08 second
- *T wave:* Normal
- *QT interval:* 0.46 second
- *Other:* Wenckebach pattern of grouped beats

improve AV node conduction. A temporary pacemaker may be required for long-term relief of symptoms until the rhythm resolves.

When caring for a patient with this block, assess tolerance for the rhythm and the need for treatment to improve cardiac output. Evaluate the patient for possible causes of the block, including the use of certain medications or the presence of ischemia.

Keep an eye on the ECG

Check the ECG frequently to see if a more severe type of AV block develops. Make sure the patient has a patent IV line and provide teaching about a temporary pacemaker if indicated.

Following the footprints

The pattern of grouped beating that accompanies second-degree atrioventricular (AV) block, type I, is sometimes referred to as the *footprints of Wenckebach.* Karel Frederik Wenckebach was a Dutch internist who, at the turn of the century and long before the introduction of the electrocardiogram (ECG), described the two forms of what's now known as second-degree AV block by analyzing waves in the jugular venous pulse. Following the introduction of the ECG, German cardiologist Woldemar Mobitz clarified Wenckebach's findings as type I and type II.

Second-degree AV block, type II

Second-degree AV block, type II, also known as *Mobitz type II block*, is less common than type I but more serious. It occurs when occasional impulses from the SA node fail to conduct to the ventricles.

On an ECG, the PR interval is consistent, but an occasional beat is dropped resulting in an absent QRS. This block is like a line of people passing through a doorway at the same speed, except that, periodically, one of them falls down and can't go through.

How it happens

Second-degree AV block, type II, indicates a problem at the level of the bundle of His or bundle branches. (See *Causes of second-degree AV block, type II*, page 166.)

Type II block is more serious than type I because the ventricular rate tends to be slower, and the cardiac output is diminished. It's also more likely to cause symptoms, particularly if the sinus rhythm is slow and the ratio of conducted beats to dropped beats is low, such as 2:1. (See *Recognizing second-degree AV block, type II*, page 166.)

Overall, the monitoring strip will look as if someone erased some QRS complexes. The PR interval will be constant for all conducted beats but may be prolonged in some cases. The QRS complex is usually wide, but normal complexes may occur. (See *2:1 Second-degree AV block.*) The more QRS complexes that are missing, the more serious the block.

Causes of second-degree AV block, type II

Second-degree atrioventricular (AV) block, type II, is usually caused by the following:
* anterior-wall myocardial infarction
* degenerative changes in the conduction system
* severe coronary artery disease.

Recognizing second-degree AV block, type II

Take a look at this example of how type II second-degree atrioventricular (AV) block appears on a rhythm strip. Notice its distinguishing characteristics.

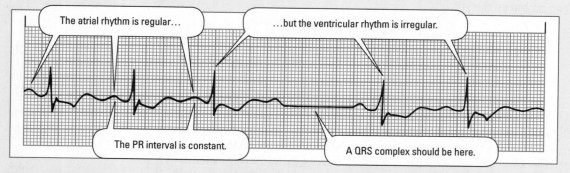

The atrial rhythm is regular...

...but the ventricular rhythm is irregular.

The PR interval is constant.

A QRS complex should be here.

* *Rhythm:* Atrial—regular; ventricular—irregular
* *Rate:* Atrial—60 beats/min; ventricular—50 beats/min

* *P wave:* Normal
* *PR interval:* 0.28 second
* *QRS complex:* 0.10 second
* *T wave:* Normal

* *QT interval:* 0.60 second
* *Other:* None

2:1 Second-degree AV block

In 2:1 second-degree atrioventricular (AV) block, every other QRS complex is dropped, so there are always two P waves for every QRS complex. The resulting ventricular rhythm is regular.

Type I or type II?

To help determine whether a rhythm is type I or type II block, look at the width of the QRS complexes. If they're wide and a short PR interval is present, the block is probably type II.

Keep in mind that type II block is more likely to impair cardiac output, lead to symptoms such as syncope, and progress to a more severe form of block. Be sure to monitor the patient carefully.

Jumpin' palpitations!

Most patients who experience a few dropped beats remain asymptomatic as long as cardiac output is maintained. As the number of dropped beats increases, a patient may experience palpitations, fatigue, dyspnea, chest pain, or light-headedness. On physical examination, you may note hypotension, and the pulse may be slow and regular or irregular.

How you intervene

If the dropped beats are infrequent and the patient shows no symptoms of decreased cardiac output, the healthcare provider may choose only to observe the rhythm, particularly if the cause is thought to be reversible. If the patient is hypotensive, treatment aims to improve cardiac output by increasing the heart rate. Because the conduction block occurs in the His-Purkinje system, transcutaneous pacing should be initiated quickly. Atropine is unlikely to be helpful.

Pick up the pace

Second-degree AV block, type II, commonly requires placement of a pacemaker. A temporary pacemaker may be used until a permanent pacemaker can be placed.

When caring for a patient with second-degree block, type II, assess their tolerance for the rhythm and the need for treatment to improve cardiac output. Evaluate for possible correctable causes such as ischemia.

Keep the patient on bed rest, if indicated, to reduce myocardial oxygen demands. Administer oxygen therapy as ordered. Observe the patient for progression to a more severe form of AV block. If the patient receives a pacemaker, teach them and their family about its use.

Third-degree AV block

Also called *complete heart block* or *AV dissociation* (see later description of true AV dissociation), third-degree AV block occurs when impulses from the atria are completely blocked at the AV node and can't be conducted to the ventricles. Maintaining our doorway analogy, this form of block is like a line of people waiting to go through a doorway, but no one can go through.

Beats of different drummers

Acting independently, the atria, generally under the control of the SA node, tend to maintain a regular rate of 60 to 100 beats/min. The ventricular rhythm can originate from the AV node and maintain a rate of 40 to 60 beats/min or from the Purkinje system in the ventricles and maintain a rate of 20 to 40 beats/min.

How it happens

Third-degree AV block that originates at the level of the AV node is most commonly a congenital condition. (See *Causes of third-degree AV block.*) It may be temporary or permanent.

Loss of productivity

Because the ventricular rate is so slow, third-degree AV block presents a potentially life-threatening situation because cardiac output can drop dramatically. In addition, the patient loses their atrial kick—that extra 30% of blood flow pushed into the ventricles by atrial contraction—as a result of the loss of synchrony between the atrial and ventricular contractions. The loss of atrial kick further decreases cardiac output. Any exertion on the part of the patient can worsen symptoms.

What to look for

When analyzing an ECG for this rhythm, you'll note regular atrial and ventricular rhythms. However, because the atria and ventricles beat independently of each other, PR intervals vary with no pattern or regularity.

Mixing up your Ps and Qs

Some P waves may be buried in QRS complexes or T waves. In fact, the rhythm strip of a patient with third-degree AV block looks like a strip of P waves laid independently over a strip of QRS complexes. (See *Recognizing third-degree AV block,* page 169.)

The site of the escape rhythm determines the appearance of the QRS complex. If it originates in the AV node, the QRS complex is normal, and the ventricular rate is 40 to 60 beats/min. If the escape

Causes of third-degree AV block

In addition to congenital causes, third-degree atrioventricular (AV) block may be caused by the following:
- coronary artery disease
- an anterior- or inferior-wall myocardial infarction
- degenerative changes in the heart
- digoxin toxicity
- calcium channel blockers
- beta-adrenergic blockers
- surgical injury.

Recognizing third-degree AV block

Take a look at this example of how third-degree atrioventricular (AV) block appears on a rhythm strip. Notice its distinguishing characteristics.

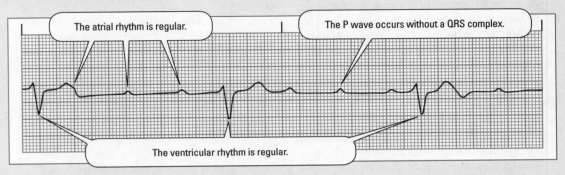

The atrial rhythm is regular.

The P wave occurs without a QRS complex.

The ventricular rhythm is regular.

- *Rhythm:* Atrial and ventricular—regular
- *Rate:* Atrial—90 beats/min; ventricular—30 beats/min
- *P wave:* Normal
- *PR interval:* Varies
- *QRS complex:* 0.16 second
- *T wave:* Normal
- *QT interval:* 0.56 second
- *Other:* None

rhythm originates in the Purkinje system, the QRS complex is wide, with a ventricular rate below 40 beats/min.

Third-degree block is a similar rhythm to complete AV dissociation; however, there are some key differences. (See *Recognizing complete AV dissociation*, page 170.)

Sinking spell

Most patients with third-degree AV block experience significant symptoms, including severe fatigue, dyspnea, chest pain, light-headedness, changes in mental status, and loss of consciousness. You may note hypotension, pallor, diaphoresis, bradycardia, and a variation in the intensity of the pulse.

A few patients will be relatively free from symptoms, complaining only that they can't tolerate exercise and that they're often tired for no apparent reason. The severity of symptoms depends to a great extent on the resulting ventricular rate.

How you intervene

When caring for a patient with third-degree heart block, immediately assess the patient's tolerance of the rhythm and the need for treatment to support cardiac output and relieve symptoms. Make sure the patient has a patent IV line. Administer oxygen therapy as ordered. Evaluate for possible correctable causes of the arrhythmia, such as

Recognizing complete AV dissociation

With third-degree atrioventricular (AV) block and complete AV dissociation, the atria and ventricles beat independently, each controlled by its own pacemaker.

However, there's a key difference between these two arrhythmias: In third-degree AV block, the atrial rate is faster than the ventricular rate. With complete AV dissociation, the two rates are usually about the same, with the ventricular rate slightly faster.

Rhythm disturbances

Never the primary problem, complete AV dissociation results from one of three underlying rhythm disturbances:
• slowed or impaired sinus impulse formation or sinoatrial conduction, as in sinus bradycardia or sinus arrest

• accelerated impulse formation in the AV junction or the ventricular pacemaker, as in junctional or ventricular tachycardia
• AV conduction disturbance, as in complete AV block.

When to treat

The clinical significance of complete AV dissociation—as well as treatment for the arrhythmia—depends on the underlying cause and its effects on the patient. If the underlying rhythm decreases cardiac output, the patient needs treatment to correct the arrhythmia.

Depending on the underlying cause, the patient may be treated with an antiarrhythmic, such as atropine or isoproterenol, to restore synchrony. Alternatively, the patient may be given a pacemaker to support a slow ventricular rate. If drug toxicity caused the original disturbance, the drug should be discontinued.

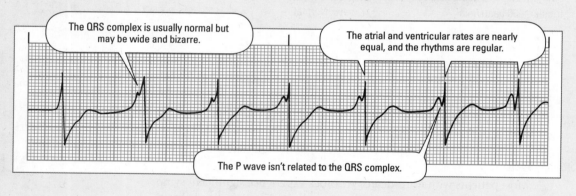

The QRS complex is usually normal but may be wide and bizarre.

The atrial and ventricular rates are nearly equal, and the rhythms are regular.

The P wave isn't related to the QRS complex.

medications or ischemia. Minimize the patient's activity and maintain bed rest.

If cardiac output isn't adequate or the patient's condition seems to be deteriorating, therapy aims to improve the ventricular rate. Atropine may be given, although according to current advanced cardiac life support guidelines, it is generally ineffective for new third-degree heart block with widened QRS complexes, and it may actually cause a slowing of the heart rate. More commonly, a pacemaker may be used to restore adequate cardiac output. Temporary pacing may continue until the cause of the block resolves or until a permanent pacemaker can be inserted. A permanent block requires placement of a permanent pacemaker.

Bundles of troubles

The patient with an anterior-wall MI is more likely to have permanent third-degree AV block if the MI involved the bundle of His or the bundle branches than if it involved other areas of the myocardium. Those patients commonly require prompt placement of a permanent pacemaker.

An AV block in a patient with an inferior-wall MI is more likely to be temporary, as a result of injury to the AV node. Placement of a permanent pacemaker is usually delayed in such cases to evaluate recovery of the conduction system.

Bundle–branch block

Bundle-branch block is a potential complication of MI. In this disorder, either the left or the right bundle branch fails to conduct impulses. A bundle-branch block that occurs low in the left bundle, in the posterior or anterior fasciculus, is called a *hemiblock*.

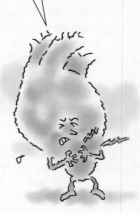

A pacemaker may be just what I need to get me out of this slump.

Impulsive behavior

In a bundle-branch block, the impulse travels down the unaffected bundle branch and then from one myocardial cell to the next to depolarize the ventricle. Because this cell-to-cell conduction progresses much slower than the conduction along the specialized cells of the conduction system, ventricular depolarization is prolonged.

Wide world of complexes

Prolonged ventricular depolarization means that the QRS complex will be widened. The normal width of the complex is 0.06 to 0.10 second. If the width increases to greater than 0.12 second, a bundle-branch block is present.

After you identify a bundle-branch block, examine lead V_1, which lies to the right of the heart, and lead V_6, which lies to the left of the heart. You'll use these leads to determine whether the block is in the right or the left bundle.

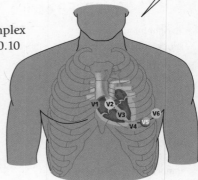

Use leads V_1 and V_6 to determine whether a block is in the right or the left bundle.

Right bundle-branch block

When the right bundle branch fails to conduct impulses, the patient has a right bundle-branch block (RBBB).

How it happens

RBBB may occur in patients with CAD or pulmonary embolism or patients who have recently had an anterior-wall MI. However, it can also occur without the presence of cardiac disease. If this block develops as the heart rate increases, it's called *rate-related right bundle-branch block*. (See *How RBBB occurs*.)

What to look for

On an ECG, RBBB is characterized by a QRS complex that's greater than 0.12 second and has a different configuration, sometimes resembling rabbit ears or the letter "M." Septal depolarization isn't affected in lead V_1, so the initial small R wave remains. The R wave is followed by an S wave, which represents LV depolarization, and a tall R wave (called *R prime*, or *R'*), which represents late right ventricular depolarization. The T wave is negative in this lead. However, that deflection is called a *secondary T-wave change* and is of no clinical significance.

Opposing moves

The opposite occurs in lead V_6. A small Q wave is followed by depolarization of the left ventricle, which produces a tall R wave. Depolarization of the right ventricle then causes a broad S wave. In lead V_6, the T wave should be positive. (See *Recognizing RBBB*, page 173.)

How you intervene

Some blocks require treatment with a temporary pacemaker. Others are monitored only to detect whether they progress to a more complete block.

Now I get it!

How RBBB occurs

In right bundle-branch block (RBBB), the initial impulse activates the interventricular septum from left to right, just as in normal activation (arrow 1). Next, the left bundle branch activates the left ventricle (arrow 2). The impulse then crosses the interventricular septum to activate the right ventricle (arrow 3).

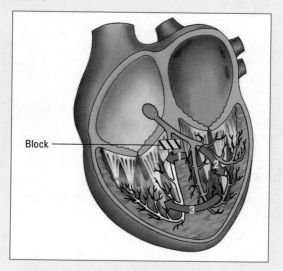

Block

Recognizing RBBB

This 12-lead electrocardiogram shows the characteristic changes of right bundle-branch block (RBBB). In lead V_1, note the rsR′ pattern and T-wave inversion. In lead V_6, see the widened S wave and the upright T wave. Also note the prolonged QRS complexes.

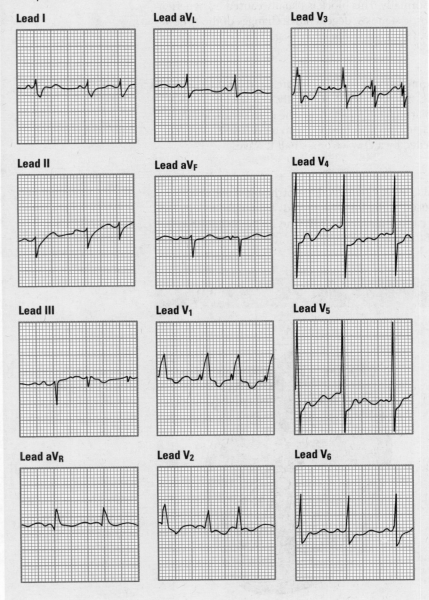

Lead I Lead aV_L Lead V₃

Lead II Lead aV_F Lead V₄

Lead III Lead V₁ Lead V₅

Lead aV_R Lead V₂ Lead V₆

Left bundle-branch block

When the left bundle branch fails to conduct, the patient has a left bundle-branch block (LBBB).

How it happens

LBBB never occurs normally. This block is usually caused by hypertensive heart disease, aortic stenosis, degenerative changes of the conduction system, or CAD. (See *How LBBB occurs*, page 174.)

What to look for

In LBBB, the QRS complexes on an ECG are greater than 0.12 second because the ventricles are activated sequentially, not simultaneously. As the wave of depolarization spreads from the right ventricle to the left, a wide S wave is produced in lead V_1, with a positive T wave. The S wave may be preceded by a Q wave or a small R wave.

Slurring your R waves

In lead V_6, no initial Q wave occurs. A tall, notched R wave, or a slurred one, is produced as the impulse spreads from right to left. This initial positive deflection is a sign of LBBB. The T wave is negative. (See *Recognizing LBBB*, page 175.)

Now I get it!

How LBBB occurs

In left bundle-branch block (LBBB), the impulse first travels down the right bundle branch (arrow 1). Then the impulse activates the interventricular septum from right to left (arrow 2), the opposite of normal activation. Finally, the impulse activates the left ventricle (arrow 3).

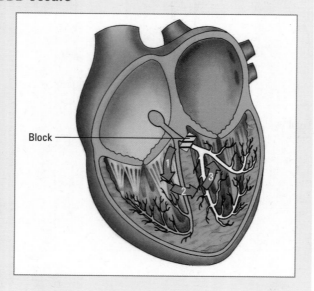

Block

Recognizing LBBB

This 12-lead electrocardiogram shows characteristic changes of left bundle-branch block (LBBB). All leads have prolonged QRS complexes. In lead V_1, note the QS wave pattern. In lead V_6, you'll see the slurred R-wave and T-wave inversion. The elevated ST segments and upright T waves in leads V_1 to V_4 are also common in LBBB.

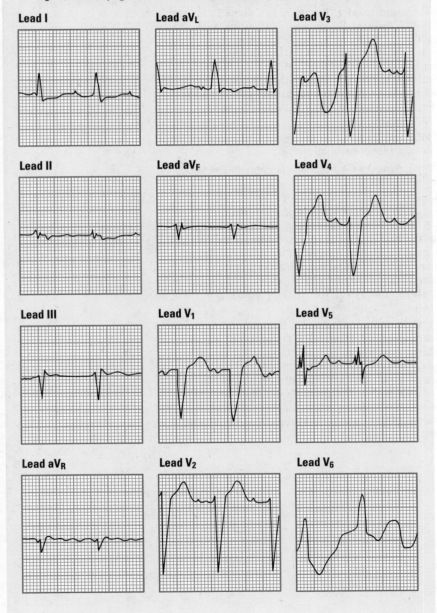

Lead I

Lead aV_L

Lead V_3

Lead II

Lead aV_F

Lead V_4

Lead III

Lead V_1

Lead V_5

Lead aV_R

Lead V_2

Lead V_6

How you intervene

When LBBB occurs along with an anterior-wall MI, it usually signals complete heart block, which requires insertion of a pacemaker.

Suggested references

Al-Khatib, S. M., Stevenson, W. G., Ackerman, M. J., Bryant, W. J., Callans, D. J., Curtis, A. B., Deal, B. J., Dickfeld, T., Field, M. E., Fonarow, G. C., Gillis, A. M., Granger, C. B., Hammill, S. C., Hlatky, M. A., Joglar, J. A., Kay, G. N., Matlock, D. D., Myerburg, R. J., & Page, R. L. (2018). 2017 AHA/ACC/HRS guideline for management of patients with ventricular arrhythmias and the prevention of sudden cardiac death: A report of the American College of Cardiology/American Heart Association task force on clinical practice guidelines and the heart rhythm society. *Circulation, 138*(13), e272–e391. https://doi.org/10.1161/CIR.0000000000000549

American Heart Association. (2015). *2015 Handbook of Emergency Cardiovascular Care for Healthcare Providers*. American Heart Association.

American Heart Association. (2020). *Advanced Cardiovascular Life Support Provider Manual*. American Heart Association.

January, C. T., Wann, L. S., Calkins, H., Chen, L. Y., Cigarroa, J. E., Cleveland, J. C., Ellinor, P. T., Ezekowitz, M. D., Field, M. E., Furie, K. L., Heidenreich, P. A., Murray, K. T., Shea, J. B., Tracy, C. M., & Yancy, C. W. (2019). 2019 AHA/ACC/HRS focused update of the 2014 AHA/ACC/HRS guideline for the management of patients with atrial fibrillation: A report of the American College of Cardiology/American Heart Association task force on clinical practice guidelines and the heart rhythm society in collaboration with the society of thoracic surgeons. *Circulation, 140*(2), e125–e151. https://doi.org/10.1161/CIR.0000000000000665

Page, R. L., Joglar, J. A., Caldwell, M. A., Calkins, H., Conti, J. B., Deal, B. J., Estes, N. A. M., Field, M. E., Goldberger, Z. D., Hammill, S. C., Indik, J. H., Lindsay, B. D., Olshansky, B., Russo, A. M., Shen, W., Tracy, C. M., Al-Khatib, S. M., & Evidence Review Committee Chair. (2016). 2015 ACC/AHA/HRS guideline for the management of adult patients with supraventricular tachycardia: A report of the American College of Cardiology/American Heart Association task force on clinical practice guidelines and the heart rhythm society. *Circulation, 133*(14), e506–e574. https://doi.org/10.1161/CIR.0000000000000311

Chapter 6

Hemodynamic monitoring

Arterial blood pressure monitoring

Hemodynamic monitoring is used to assess cardiac function and to determine the effectiveness of therapy. In arterial blood pressure monitoring, a healthcare provider inserts a catheter into the patient's radial or femoral artery to measure systolic, diastolic, and mean pressures or to obtain samples for arterial blood gas studies. A transducer transforms the flow of blood during systole and diastole into a waveform, which appears on a monitor screen.

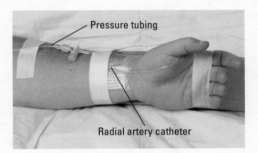

Pressure tubing

Radial artery catheter

Normal arterial pressure parameters

In general, arterial **systolic pressure** reflects the peak pressure generated by the left ventricle. It also indicates compliance of the large arteries, or the *peripheral resistance*.

Arterial **diastolic pressure** reflects the runoff velocity and elasticity of the arterial system, particularly the arterioles.

Mean arterial pressure (MAP) is the average pressure in the arterial system during systole and diastole. It reflects the driving, or *perfusion*, pressure and is determined by arterial blood volume and blood vessel elasticity and resistance.

$$MAP = \frac{\text{systolic pressure} + 2(\text{diastolic pressure})}{3}$$

Arterial waveform configuration

Normal arterial blood pressure produces a characteristic waveform, representing ventricular systole and diastole. The waveform has five distinct components, as shown below.

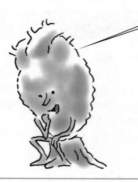

Knowing the components of an arterial waveform keeps you ahead of the game on arterial pressure monitoring.

Normal arterial waveform

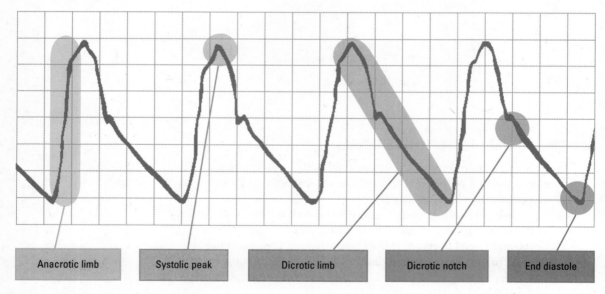

Anacrotic limb	Systolic peak	Dicrotic limb	Dicrotic notch	End diastole

The *anacrotic limb* marks the waveform's initial upstroke, which occurs as blood is rapidly ejected from the ventricle through the open aortic valve into the aorta.

Arterial pressure then rises sharply, resulting in the *systolic peak*—the waveform's highest point.

As blood continues into the peripheral vessels, arterial pressure falls and the waveform begins a downward trend, called the *dicrotic limb*. Arterial pressure usually keeps falling until pressure in the ventricle is less than pressure in the aortic root.

When ventricular pressure is lower than aortic root pressure, the aortic valve closes. This event appears as a small notch on the waveform's downside, called the *dicrotic notch*.

When the aortic valve closes, diastole begins, progressing until aortic root pressure gradually falls to its lowest point. On the waveform, this is known as *end diastole*.

Recognizing abnormal waveforms

Understanding a normal arterial waveform is relatively straightforward. Unfortunately, an abnormal waveform isn't so easy to decipher. Abnormal patterns and markings, however, may provide important diagnostic clues to the patient's cardiovascular status, or they may simply signal trouble in the monitor. Use this chart to help you recognize waveform abnormalities. *Always check the patient when an abnormal waveform is noted*.

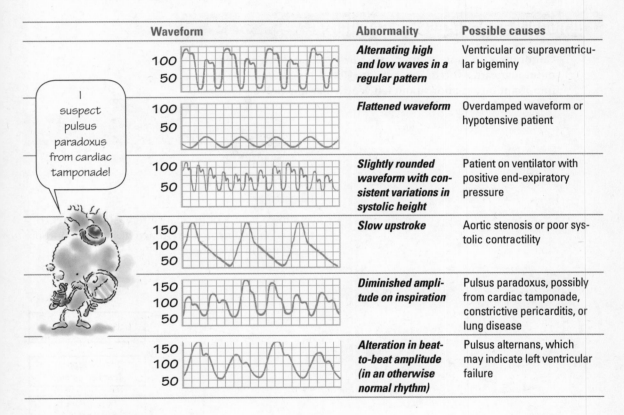

Waveform	Abnormality	Possible causes
100 / 50	**Alternating high and low waves in a regular pattern**	Ventricular or supraventricular bigeminy
100 / 50	**Flattened waveform**	Overdamped waveform or hypotensive patient
100 / 50	**Slightly rounded waveform with consistent variations in systolic height**	Patient on ventilator with positive end-expiratory pressure
150 / 100 / 50	**Slow upstroke**	Aortic stenosis or poor systolic contractility
150 / 100 / 50	**Diminished amplitude on inspiration**	Pulsus paradoxus, possibly from cardiac tamponade, constrictive pericarditis, or lung disease
150 / 100 / 50	**Alteration in beat-to-beat amplitude (in an otherwise normal rhythm)**	Pulsus alternans, which may indicate left ventricular failure

I suspect pulsus paradoxus from cardiac tamponade!

Nursing considerations

- Explain the procedure to the patient and their family, including the purpose of arterial pressure monitoring.
- After catheter insertion, observe the pressure waveform to assess arterial pressure. The catheter will be attached to a pressure monitor transducer setup, and pressure waveforms will appear on the monitor.
- Assess the insertion site for signs of infection, such as redness and swelling. Notify the healthcare provider immediately if you note such signs.

- Carefully assess the neurovascular status of the extremity distal to the catheter insertion. Notify the healthcare provider of diminished pulses; pale, cool skin; and decreased movement. Also notify the healthcare provider if the patient reports numbness or tingling in that area.
- Document the date, time, and site of catheter insertion; type of flush solution used; type of dressing applied; and the patient's tolerance of the procedure.

Pulmonary artery pressure monitoring

Continuous pulmonary artery pressure (PAP) and intermittent pulmonary artery occlusion pressure (PAOP) measurements provide important information about left ventricular function and preload.

Come equipped

PA catheter

As shown here, a pulmonary artery (PA) catheter contains several lumens. Each lumen has its own purpose (indicated in parentheses).

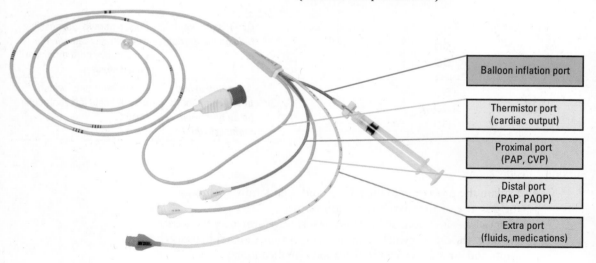

Balloon inflation port

Thermistor port (cardiac output)

Proximal port (PAP, CVP)

Distal port (PAP, PAOP)

Extra port (fluids, medications)

Normal PAP values

Right atrial pressure	1–6 mm Hg
Systolic right ventricular pressure	20–30 mm Hg
End-diastolic right ventricular pressure	Less than 5 mm Hg
Systolic PAP	20–30 mm Hg
Diastolic PAP	10–15 mm Hg
Mean PAP	Less than 20 mm Hg
PAOP	6–12 mm Hg

Normal pulmonary artery waveforms

After insertion into a large vein (usually the subclavian, jugular, or femoral vein), a PA catheter is advanced through the vena cava into the right atrium, through the right ventricle, and into a branch of the PA. As the catheter advances through the heart chambers during insertion, the monitor shows various waveforms, as shown below.

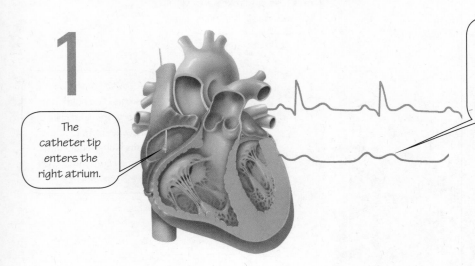

1

The catheter tip enters the right atrium.

When the catheter tip enters the right atrium, this waveform appears on the monitor, representing right atrial pressure.

2

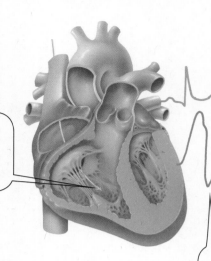

Next, the catheter tip reaches the right ventricle.

Remember to watch the patient's ECG monitor closely. Ventricular arrhythmias can occur as the catheter passes through the right ventricle.

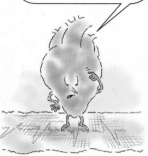

As the catheter tip reaches the right ventricle, you'll see a waveform with sharp systolic upstrokes and lower diastolic dips.

3

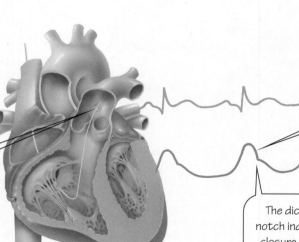

The catheter floats into the pulmonary artery.

As the catheter reaches the pulmonary artery, the upstroke of the waveform becomes smoother than that of the right ventricular waveform.

The dicrotic notch indicates closure of the pulmonic valve.

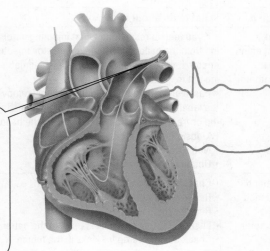

4

The catheter's balloon floats into a distal branch of the pulmonary artery. The balloon occludes the vessel because it is too narrow for it to pass.

The monitor now shows a PAOP waveform with two small uprises. The balloon is then passively deflated by simply removing the syringe, and the catheter is left in the pulmonary artery.

Identifying hemodynamic pressure monitoring problems

Problem	What might cause it	What to do about it
Line fails to flush	• Inadequate pressure from pressure bag • Blood clot in catheter	• Make sure the pressure bag gauge reads 300 mm Hg. • Try to aspirate the clot with a syringe. If the line still won't flush, notify the doctor and prepare to replace the line. ***Never use a syringe to flush a hemodynamic line.***
Damped waveform	• Air bubbles • Blood flashback in line • Incorrect transducer position • Malpositioned arterial catheter (out of blood vessel or pressed against vessel wall) • Incorrect pressure scale setting	• Secure all connections. • Remove air from the lines and the transducer. • Check for and replace cracked equipment. • Make sure stopcock positions are correct; tighten loose connections and replace cracked equipment, if necessary. • Flush the line with the fast-flush valve/pig tail. • Replace the transducer if blood backs up into it. • Make sure the transducer is kept at the level of the right atrium at all times. Improper levels give false-high or false-low pressure readings. • Reposition the catheter if it's against the vessel wall. • Try to aspirate blood to confirm proper placement in the vessel. If you can't aspirate blood, notify the doctor and prepare to replace the line. ***Note: Bloody drainage at the insertion site may indicate catheter displacement. Notify the doctor immediately.*** • Ensure that the scale is set for the appropriate pressure.

Problem	What might cause it	What to do about it
PAOP tracing unobtainable	• Ruptured balloon • Incorrect amount of air in balloon • Malpositioned catheter	• If you feel no resistance when injecting air or if you see blood leaking from the balloon inflation lumen, stop injecting air and notify the doctor. If the catheter is left in, label the inflation lumen with a warning not to inflate. • Passively deflate the balloon by simply removing the syringe. Check the label on the catheter for correct volume. Reinflate slowly with the correct amount. To avoid rupturing the balloon, always utilize a PA-designated syringe. • Notify the doctor. • Obtain a chest X-ray.
No waveform	• Defective equipment • Incorrectly positioned stopcock • Clot or kink in catheter	• Check all connections. • Replace the monitor cable. • Replace the transducer. • Ensure that the stopcock is open to the patient. • Check the line setup for kinks in the tubing. If none are noted, slowly aspirate for blood return. If none is noted, notify the physician.

Nursing considerations

- Tell the patient that they will be conscious during catheterization and that they may feel temporary local discomfort from the administration of the local anesthetic. Catheter insertion takes about 30 minutes. The PA catheter is inserted through a large central venous access, such as the internal jugular or subclavian veins, or least preferred the femoral vein.
- After catheter insertion, you may inflate the balloon with a syringe to take pulmonary artery wedge pressure (PAWP) readings. Don't inflate the balloon with more than 1.5 mL of air because overinflation could distend the PA, causing vessel rupture. Never leave the balloon wedged for a prolonged period; doing so may lead to a pulmonary infarction, ischemia, or a rupture.
- After each PAWP reading, flush the line; if you encounter difficulty, notify the healthcare provider.
- Maintain 300 mm Hg pressure in the pressure bag to permit a flush flow of 3 to 6 mL/hour.
- If fever develops when the catheter is in place, inform the healthcare provider; they may remove the catheter and send its tip to the laboratory for culture.

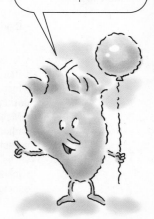

When taking PAWP readings, don't inflate the balloon with more than 1.5 cc of air. Overinflation could cause the vessel to rupture.

Tight is right

Make sure stopcocks are properly positioned and connections are secure. Loose connections may introduce air into the system or cause blood backup, leakage of deoxygenated blood, or inaccurate pressure readings. Also, make sure the lumen hubs are properly identified to serve the appropriate catheter ports.

Cardiac output monitoring

Measuring cardiac output (CO)—the amount of blood (in liters) ejected by the heart in 1 minute—helps evaluate cardiac function. Common methods for monitoring CO are the bolus thermodilution method, continuous cardiac output (CCO) monitoring PA catheter, and arterial pressure-based CO (APCO) monitoring.

Bolus thermodilution method

In the bolus thermodilution method, a solution colder than the patient's blood is injected into the right atrium through a port on a PA catheter. The catheter detects changes in temperature as the blood flows, and a computer uses these data to calculate CO.

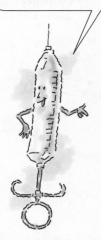

Repeat the injection procedure at least three times to obtain a mean CO value.

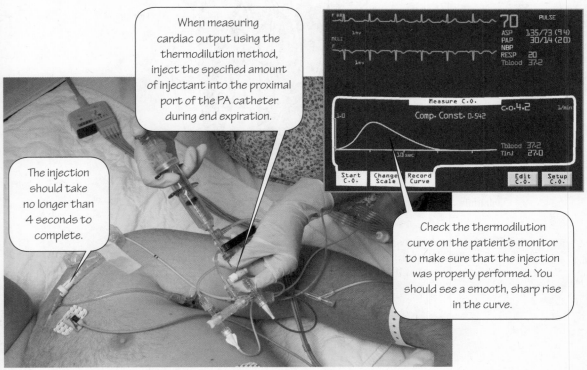

When measuring cardiac output using the thermodilution method, inject the specified amount of injectant into the proximal port of the PA catheter during end expiration.

The injection should take no longer than 4 seconds to complete.

Check the thermodilution curve on the patient's monitor to make sure that the injection was properly performed. You should see a smooth, sharp rise in the curve.

A closer look at the thermodilution method

Performed at the bedside, the thermodilution method is the most practical way of evaluating the cardiac status of critically ill patients and those suspected of having cardiac disease. This illustration shows the path of the injectate solution through the heart during thermodilution CO monitoring.

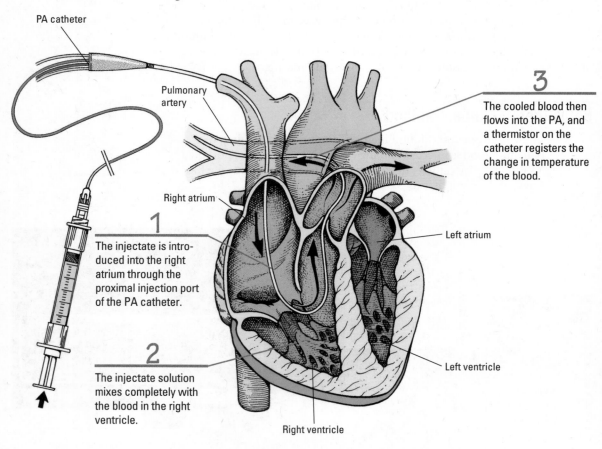

PA catheter

Pulmonary artery

3

The cooled blood then flows into the PA, and a thermistor on the catheter registers the change in temperature of the blood.

Right atrium

1

The injectate is introduced into the right atrium through the proximal injection port of the PA catheter.

Left atrium

2

The injectate solution mixes completely with the blood in the right ventricle.

Left ventricle

Right ventricle

CCO PA catheters have a heating filament in them, which heats the blood in the right ventricle, and the temperature change is sensed by the thermistor at the distal end of the catheter.

Analyzing thermodilution curves

The thermodilution curve provides valuable information about CO, injection technique, and equipment problems. When studying the curve, keep in mind that the area under the curve is inversely proportionate to CO: the smaller the area under the curve, the higher the CO; the larger the area under the curve, the lower the CO.

In addition to providing a record of CO, the curve may indicate problems related to technique, such as erratic or slow injectate instillations, or other problems, such as respiratory variations or electrical interference. The curves shown here correspond to those typically seen in clinical practice.

Normal thermodilution curve

In a patient who has adequate CO, the thermodilution curve begins with a smooth, rapid upstroke (representing proper injection technique) and is followed by a smooth, gradual downslope. The height of the curve varies, depending on whether you use a room temperature or an iced injectate.

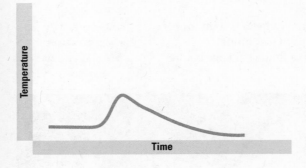

Cardiac index
*Measurement of CO per unit of time that takes into account the patient's body surface area (BSA)
*Normally calculated in $L/min/m^2$
Cardiac index = CO ÷ BSA

Normal ranges
For nonpregnant adults: 2.5 to 4.2 $L/min/m^2$
For pregnant females: 3.5 to 6.5 $L/min/m^2$

High CO curve

A high CO curve has a rapid, smooth upstroke. Because the ventricles are ejecting blood too forcefully, the injectate moves through the heart quickly and the curve returns to baseline more rapidly. The smaller area under the curve suggests high CO.

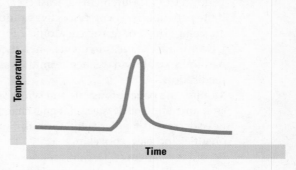

Low CO curve

A low CO curve has a rapid, smooth upstroke. However, because blood is being ejected less efficiently from the ventricles, the injectate warms slowly and takes longer to be ejected. Consequently, the curve takes longer to return to baseline. This slow return produces a larger area under the curve, corresponding to low CO.

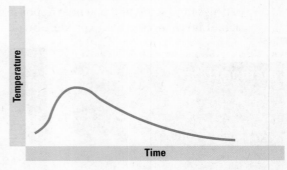

Nursing considerations

- Make sure the patient doesn't move during the procedure because movement can cause an error in measurement. Use the same position, whether supine or semi-Fowler, every time a measurement is performed. Allow the patient to stabilize for 5 to 15 minutes after a position change before obtaining measurements.
- Perform CO measurements at least every 2 to 4 hours, especially if the patient is receiving vasoactive or inotropic agents or if fluids are being added or restricted. Monitor for changes.
- Discontinue CO measurements when the patient is hemodynamically stable and weaned from the vasoactive and inotropic medications.
- Monitor the patient for signs and symptoms of inadequate perfusion, including restlessness; fatigue; changes in level of consciousness; decreased capillary refill time; diminished peripheral pulses; oliguria; and pale, cool skin.
- Record the patient's CO, cardiac index, and other hemodynamic values and vital signs at the time of measurement. Also, note the patient's position during measurement. Note also the measurement marking on the catheter at the insertion site, recorded in cm. (Following the same marking helps assess catheter position.)

APCO monitoring

In APCO monitoring, a patient's existing arterial catheter is used to continuously calculate and display CO. It helps to determine a patient's fluid status and potential response to a fluid challenge before significant changes in blood pressure occur.

> The arterial catheter and line connect to a sensor, transducer, and monitor.

memory board

Important equations:

CO = Stroke volume × Heart rate
(normal CO is 4–8 L/min)

Pulse pressure = Systolic pressure – Diastolic pressure

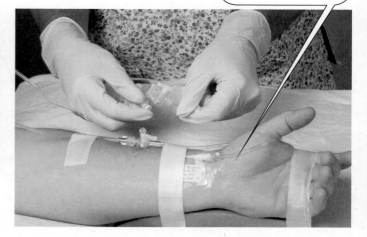

The sensor measures variations in the patient's systolic and diastolic blood pressures to calculate pulse pressure, which is proportional to stroke volume (the volume of blood ejected by the ventricle with each contraction). Stroke volume and heart rate determine CO.

The patient's age, gender, height, and weight are entered into a computer and are used to determine vascular compliance and resistance.

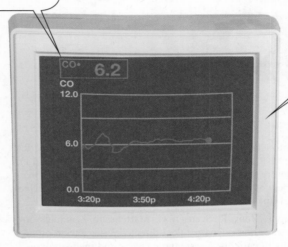

CO• 6.2
CO
12.0

6.0

0.0
3:20p 3:50p 4:20p

Pulse oximetry monitoring

Performed intermittently or continuously, pulse oximetry is a simple procedure used to noninvasively monitor arterial oxygen saturation. Two light-emitting diodes send red and infrared light through a pulsating arterial vascular bed, commonly in the fingertip or earlobe. A photodetector measures the transmitted light as it passes through the vascular bed, detects the relative amount of color absorbed by arterial blood, and calculates the exact arterial oxygen saturation.

Arterial oxygen saturation values obtained by pulse oximetry are indicated by the symbol SpO_2, whereas invasively measured arterial oxygen saturation values are indicated by the symbol SaO_2.

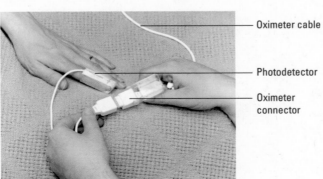

Oximeter cable

Photodetector

Oximeter connector

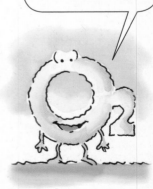

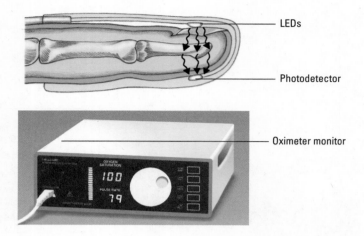

LEDs

Photodetector

Oximeter monitor

OXYGEN
SATURATION

I00

PULSE RATE

79

Suggested references

Cecconi, M., De Backer, D., Antonelli, M., Beale, R., Bakker, J., Hofer, C., Jaeschke, R., Mebazaa, A., Pinsky, M. R., Teboul, J. L., Vincent, J. L., & Rhodes, A. (2014). Consensus on circulatory shock and hemodynamic monitoring. Task force of the European Society of Intensive Care Medicine, *Intensive Care Medicine*, *40*(12), 1795–1815. https://doi.org/10.1007/s00134-014-3525-z

Cronhjort, M., Wall, O., Nyberg, E., Zeng, R., Svensen, C., Martensson, J., & Joelsson-Alm, E. (2018). Impact of hemodynamic goal-directed resuscitation on mortality in adult critically ill patients: A systematic review and meta-analysis. *Journal of Clinical Monitoring and Computing*, *32*(3), 403–414. https://doi.org/10.1007/s10877-017-0032-0

Furer, A., Wessler, J., & Burkhoff, D. (2017). Hemodynamics of cardiogenic shock, *Interventional Cardiology Clinics*, *6*(3), 359–371. https://doi.org/10.1016/j.iccl.2017.03.006

Magder, S. (2015). Invasive hemodynamic monitoring. *Critical Care Clinics*, *31*(1), 67–87.

Chapter 7

Common cardiovascular disorders

Just the facts

In this chapter, you'll learn:

◆ disorders that alter blood flow and cardiovascular function

◆ pathophysiology and treatments related to these disorders

◆ diagnostic tests, assessment findings, and nursing interventions for each disorder.

A look at cardiovascular disorders

Structural cardiac disorders can cause degenerative cardiac disorders and vice versa! Structural cardiac disorders are conditions in which there is a deformity in one of the areas of the heart such as the heart muscle, valves, chambers (atria or ventricles), the walls of the heart chambers, and coronary arteries. Examples of structural conditions are valvular disorders, hypertrophic cardiomyopathy (HCM), and infections.

Degenerative cardiac disorders, which are disorders that cause damage over time, include acute coronary syndromes (ACS), restrictive cardiomyopathy heart failure (HF), hypertension, and pulmonary hypertension (PH). Several degenerative disorders presented in this chapter are a direct result of a buildup of cholesterol or sclerotic plaque in the arteries, also known as atherosclerotic cardiovascular disease (ASCVD). These plaques can cause ischemic heart disease (IHD), peripheral arterial disease (PAD), and stroke. It is important to note that the onset of some of these disorders can be gradual, triggering symptoms only after the disease has progressed. Early recognition and screening are critical to preventing the progression of the disease and poor health outcomes for the patient.

Ischemic heart disease

IHD occurs because of an inadequate blood supply to the myocardium (the muscle tissue of the heart) via the coronary arteries. Blood flow to the coronary arteries can be restricted by plaque formation (atherosclerosis), vasoconstriction, and clot formation (embolism).

ACS commonly occurs when plaque (an unstable and lipid-rich substance) ruptures or erodes inside a coronary artery. The rupture results in platelet adhesions, fibrin clot formation, and activation of thrombin. A thrombus occludes blood flow. The effect is an imbalance in myocardial oxygen supply and demand.

Depending on the degree of occlusion, the syndrome is defined as unstable angina, ST-segment elevation myocardial infarction (STEMI), or non–ST-segment elevation myocardial infarction (NSTEMI). Coronary artery disease (CAD) is the leading cause of mortality in the United States.

Other, less common causes of myocardial ischemia are coronary vasospasm (with cocaine use or coronary dissection) and an embolism in the coronary arteries.

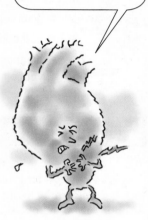

Owww! An MI is just one kind of acute coronary syndrome.

Risks you can and can't change
Modifiable and non-modifiable factors are assessed to determine a patient's risk of heart disease over their lifetime. Nurses and the health-care team members should assess patients for risk factors and provide education and resources to promote changes in health behaviors. Early intervention for modifiable risk factors is key to reduce the chances of a patient developing cardiovascular diseases, thus prolonging their life (Wong et al., 2022).

What they can't change
- Age—most common over the age of 50 years
- Male gender
- Ethnicity—different ethnic groups are at higher risk of disorders in metabolic syndrome
- Family history of ASCVD at an early age of a first-degree male relative
- Past medical history of chronic inflammation disorders such as rheumatoid arthritis, chronic kidney disease, HIV, and other auto-immune disorders

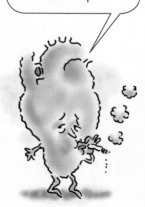

Smoking is a risk factor for acute coronary syndromes. I better quit!

What they can change
- Smoking
- Metabolic syndrome
  - High blood pressure—control hypertension
  - Obesity—lose weight and reduce insulin resistance
  - Elevated blood sugar—control diabetes
  - High cholesterol, high triglycerides, high low-density cholesterol (LDL; bad cholesterol), and low high-density cholesterol (HDL; good cholesterol) blood levels—diet change and lipid-lowering medications to reduce levels

Types of ACS

ACS means the patient has irreversible cardiac ischemia or death of the cardiac tissue. Complications of ACS include HF, chronic activity intolerance, and death.

- If the patient has unstable angina, a thrombus partially occludes a coronary vessel. This thrombus is full of platelets. The partially occluded vessel may have distal microthrombi that cause necrosis in some myocytes. The patient typically experiences symptoms of myocardial ischemia, but there are no changes on electrocardiogram (ECG) or cardiac enzymes.
- A STEMI means that there is an ST segment elevation on two or more contiguous leads of an ECG associated with a myocardial infarction (MI). A STEMI results when reduced blood flow through one of the coronary arteries causes myocardial ischemia, injury, and necrosis. The damage extends through all myocardial layers.
- If smaller vessels infarct, the patient is at higher risk of MI, which may progress to a non-STEMI or NSTEMI. With an NSTEMI, there are symptoms of myocardial ischemia without ECG changes. Usually, only the innermost layer of the heart is damaged.

What to look for

A patient with chest pain associated with ACS typically experiences pain described as burning, squeezing, crushing, or tightness in the following locations:

Typical
- Retrosternal
- Precordial

Atypical
- Epigastric area
- Upper back
- Left shoulder or arm
- Right arm or shoulder
- Neck or jaw

Associated symptoms

Patients are likely to experience the following symptoms along with chest pain:
- Dyspnea or shortness of breath at rest or with activity
- Sweating
- Nausea and indigestion
- Dread or anxiety—"I feel like I am going to die."
- Syncope or presyncope
- Palpitations (See *Atypical chest pain in women*.)

Atypical chest pain in women

Women are more likely than men to present with atypical chest pain. The pain may be vague or less severe. It may be referred to the neck, back, and left shoulder or arm. Women will also experience more associated symptoms of ACS such as dyspnea, sweating, palpitations, nausea, weakness, and syncope.

It hurts when I do this

Angina most frequently follows physical exertion but may also follow emotional excitement, exposure to cold, or a large meal. Angina symptoms may be relieved by nitroglycerin. It's less severe and is shorter lived than the pain of acute MI.

Four forms of angina

Angina has four major forms:
1. Stable—predictable pain, in frequency and duration, which can be relieved with nitrates and rest
2. Unstable—easily induced, increased pain, or change in pain pattern that may occur or is unrelieved at rest
3. Prinzmetal or a variant—pain from unpredictable coronary artery spasm
4. Microvascular—angina-like chest pain due to impairment of vasodilator reserve (ability of the arteries to dilate) in a patient with normal coronary arteries.

My, my, MI pain

A patient with MI may experience severe, persistent typical or atypical chest pain that isn't relieved by rest or sublingual nitroglycerin.

What tests tell you

These tests are used to diagnose ACS:
- ECG during an anginal episode may show ischemia. Serial 12-lead ECGs may be normal or inconclusive during the first few hours after an MI. Abnormalities include serial ST-segment depression in an NSTEMI and ST-segment elevation and Q waves, representing scarring and necrosis, in a STEMI. (See *Pinpointing infarction.*)
- Coronary angiography reveals coronary artery stenosis or occlusion and collateral circulation and shows the condition of the arteries beyond the narrowing.
- Myocardial perfusion imaging with Persantine thallium during treadmill exercise (stress test) discloses ischemic areas of the myocardium, visualized as "cold spots."
- With MI, serial serum cardiac marker measurements show elevated creatine kinase (CK), especially the CK-MB isoenzyme (the cardiac muscle fraction of CK), troponin T and I, and myoglobin.
- With a STEMI, echocardiography shows ventricular wall dyskinesia.
- Cardiac magnetic resonance imaging (MRI) can assess the structure and function of the cardiac structures and myocardial viability.
- High-sensitivity troponin (hs-Tn) assays can detect lower levels of troponin, eliminating the need of serial testing and shortening the time for the diagnosis of an MI.

Now I get it!

Pinpointing infarction

The site of an MI depends on the vessels involved:

• Occlusion of the circumflex branch of the left coronary artery causes a lateral wall infarction.

• Occlusion of the anterior descending branch of the left coronary artery leads to an anterior wall infarction.

• True posterior or inferior wall infarctions generally result from occlusion of the right coronary artery or one of its branches.

• Right ventricular infarctions can also result from right coronary artery occlusion, can accompany inferior infarctions, and can cause right-sided HF.

• In an ST-segment-elevation MI, tissue damage extends through all myocardial layers; in a non–ST-segment-elevation MI, damage occurs only in the innermost layer.

Initial approach in the evaluation of chest pain

Most complaints of chest pain are not ACS. It is important to assess the patient quickly because if the patient is experiencing an MI, some lifesaving interventions need to be started within hours of presentation.

• Obtain an ECG within 10 minutes of patient's presentation of chest pain. This is to assess for ECG changes indicating an MI.

• If there are no changes, assess the cardiac troponin levels for elevations at initial presentation, 3 and 6 hours after symptom onset. The patient may also have serial ECGs to assess for changes. If changes occur during serial testing, then the patient is admitted and managed for myocardial ischemia.

• When all serial testing is completed and indicate no changes, then the patient may undergo cardiac stress testing.

How it's treated

For patients with angina, the goal of treatment is to reduce myocardial oxygen demand or increase oxygen supply.

These treatments are used to manage angina:

• Nitrates reduce myocardial oxygen consumption in the acute phase of chest pain. They are the first-line therapy and appropriate to treat vasospastic-related angina.

• Beta-adrenergic blockers (BBs) may be administered to reduce cardiac workload and oxygen demands of the heart muscle.

• Calcium channel blockers may be given if angina is caused by coronary artery spasm.

- Antiplatelet drugs decrease platelet aggregation and the danger of coronary artery occlusion.
- Lipid-lowering drugs such as statins can reduce elevated serum cholesterol or triglyceride levels to prevent CAD.
- Obstructive lesions may necessitate coronary artery bypass grafting (CABG) or percutaneous transluminal coronary angioplasty (PTCA). Other alternatives include laser angioplasty, minimally invasive surgery, rotational atherectomy, or stent placement.
- Reducing oxygen demands of the heart muscle will be enhanced by providing oxygen therapy during acute episodes of chest pain.

MI relief

The goals of treatment for MI are to relieve pain, stabilize heart rhythm, revascularize the coronary artery, preserve myocardial tissue, and reduce cardiac workload.

Here are some guidelines for treatment:

- Emergency medical service providers or emergency department staff should give 160 to 325 mg of aspirin unless the patient has signs of active or recent gastrointestinal (GI) bleeding. Clopidogrel 300 mg can be used if the patient has an allergy to aspirin (Woo & Robinson, 2020).
- Thrombolytics can be used within 3 hours of the onset of symptoms (unless contraindications exist). Thrombolytic therapy involves administration of streptokinase (Streptase), alteplase (Activase), or reteplase (Retavase).
- Oxygen is administered to increase oxygenation of the blood to the heart.
- Nitroglycerin is administered sublingually to relieve chest pain unless systolic blood pressure (BP) is less than 90 mm Hg or heart rate is less than 50 beats/minute or greater than 100 beats/minute.
- Morphine is administered as analgesia because pain stimulates the sympathetic nervous system, leading to an increase in heart rate and vasoconstriction. Additionally, morphine is a vasodilator that reduces ventricular preload and oxygen requirements of the heart.
- Intravenous (IV) heparin is given to patients who have received tissue plasminogen activator to increase the chances of patency in the affected coronary artery.
- Physical activity is limited for the first 12 hours to reduce cardiac workload, thereby limiting the area of necrosis.
- Lidocaine, amiodarone (Pacerone), transcutaneous pacing patches (or a transvenous pacemaker), defibrillation, or epinephrine may be necessary if arrhythmias are present.

A daily, low dose of aspirin is recommended to patients with high risk of MI or those that had a previous MI. Patients should not be advised to initiate aspirin therapy on their own but consult with their healthcare provider.

- IV nitroglycerin is administered for 24 to 48 hours in patients without hypotension, bradycardia, or excessive tachycardia to reduce afterload and preload and to relieve chest pain.
- Glycoprotein IIb/IIIa inhibitors (such as abciximab [ReoPro]) are administered to patients with continued unstable angina or acute chest pain to reduce platelet aggregation. They're also administered after invasive cardiac procedures.
- An IV BB is administered early to patients with evolving acute MI; it's followed by oral therapy to reduce heart rate and contractility and to reduce myocardial oxygen requirements.
- Angiotensin-converting enzyme (ACE) inhibitors are administered to those with evolving MI with ST-segment elevation or left bundle branch block to reduce afterload and preload and to prevent heart muscle remodeling.
- Laser angioplasty, angioplasty, atherectomy, or stent placement may be initiated. PTCA and stent placement are options for opening blocked or narrowed arteries.
- Percutaneous coronary intervention is performed in the cardiac catheterization lab. A catheter tube and dye are injected to locate the blockage. Once the site of the blockage is located, a balloon or a stent is inserted to break up the clot in the coronary artery.
- Cardiac surgery may be performed for emergencies that are unable to be addressed in the percutaneous intervention. CABG may restore blood flow to occluded arteries by sewing a patent vein or artery beyond the infarct site, thus restoring blood flow to the cardiac muscle. Patients meeting criteria may undergo minimally invasive bypass surgery to allow for a faster recovery.
- Lipid-lowering drugs are administered to patients with elevated low-density lipoprotein and cholesterol levels.

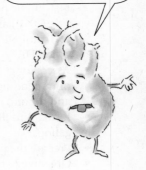

Treatment for MI can take many forms, depending on the patient's symptoms and the extent of damage.

What to do

- Collaborate care with a skilled team, which may include emergency medical personnel, a cardiologist, a cardiothoracic surgeon, a nutritionist, and a cardiac rehabilitation team.
- During anginal episodes, assess BP and heart rate. Take an ECG before administering nitroglycerin or other nitrates. The immediate effect of nitroglycerin is vasodilation, which can alter the ECG results. Record the duration of pain, the amount of medication required to relieve it, and accompanying symptoms.
- On admission to the coronary care unit, monitor and record the patient's ECG, BP, temperature, and heart and breath sounds. Also, assess and record the severity, location, type, and duration of pain. Assess fluid input and output for any signs of fluid overload.

Status checks

- Monitor the patient's hemodynamic status closely. Be alert for signs of decreased cardiac output, such as decreased BP, increased heart rate, increased pulmonary artery pressure (PAP), increased pulmonary artery wedge pressure (PAWP), decreased cardiac output measurements, and decreased right atrial pressure.
- Assess urine output hourly.
- Monitor the patient's oxygen saturation levels and notify the health-care provider if oxygen saturation falls below 92%.
- Check the patient's BP after giving nitroglycerin, especially after the first dose.
- Frequently monitor ECG rhythm strips to detect heart rate changes and arrhythmias.

Take action

- During episodes of chest pain, monitor ECG, BP, and pulmonary artery (PA) catheter readings (if applicable) to determine changes.
- Obtain serial measurements of cardiac enzyme levels as ordered.
- Natriuretic peptides (NPs), such as B-type natriuretic peptide (BNP) assay or N-terminal pro-B-type natriuretic peptide (NT-proBNP), may be ordered to determine if the patient is developing HF.
- Assess for crackles cough, tachypnea, and peripheral edema—signs of impending left-sided HF. Carefully monitor daily weight, intake and output, respiratory rate, serum enzyme levels, ECG waveforms, and BP. Auscultate for third or fourth heart sound (S_3 or S_4) gallops.
- Prepare the patient for reperfusion therapy as indicated.
- Organize patient care and activities to allow rest periods. If the patient is immobilized, turn them often and use intermittent compression devices. Gradually increase the patient's activity level as tolerated.
- Provide a clear-liquid diet until nausea subsides. Anticipate a possible order for a low-cholesterol, low-sodium diet without caffeine.
- Provide a stool softener to prevent straining and increased workload on the heart during defecation.
- If your patient is a smoker, evaluate nicotine dependence and consult with the patient, family, and providers about appropriate smoking-cessation techniques.
- Recommend that the patient receives influenza and pneumococcal vaccines prior to discharge when appropriate.
- Document the patient's response to treatment, vital signs, cardiac rhythm, episodes of pain and pain relief, and understanding of teaching.
- Discuss lifestyle modifications with the patient and family

- ○ Stop smoking.
- ○ Follow a low-sodium (1500 mg per day), low-cholesterol diet. Maintain 60 mEq of potassium per day as the heart needs potassium for contractility.
- ○ Limit alcohol intake to no more than one drink per day.
- ○ Increase physical activity as ordered.
- Teach the patient about the typical and atypical signs of ACS.
  - ○ Instruct the patient to take their prescribed nitroglycerin once if experiencing any signs or symptoms of ACS. Call emergency medical services after 5 minutes if the signs and symptoms do not resolve—don't delay (Robinson, 2020).
- Review the administration directions and possible adverse effects of the patient's medications.
- Teach about ASCVD risk factors and how to reduce them, as appropriate.
- Encourage family members to learn cardiopulmonary resuscitation and how to use an automated external defibrillator.

Cardiomyopathy

Cardiomyopathy generally refers to the disease of the heart muscle fibers. In most cases, the heart muscle weakens, resulting in an alteration in blood flow and electrical conduction. Most patients with cardiomyopathy have an idiopathic or a primary disease, but some cases are secondary to identifiable causes. The primary categories of cardiomyopathy are acquired, genetic, and mixed. Acquired cardiomyopathies are myocarditis, takotsubo (stress induced), and the rare peripartum. Genetic cardiomyopathies are hypertrophic and arrhythmogenic right ventricular dysplasia. A family history of cardiomyopathy, HF, and sudden cardiac arrest can raise your risk of cardiomyopathy. The most common cardiomyopathies are dilated, hypertrophic, and restrictive. The causes of secondary cardiomyopathy are varied. Some of the more common causes of secondary cardiomyopathy include the following:

- Endocrine disorders such as thyroid disease, diabetes syndrome, and obesity
- Infections such as hepatitis C, HIV, viral, and mycobacterial infections.
- Cardiotoxic chemicals such as long-term alcohol abuse, anabolic steroids, chemotherapy, heavy metal poisoning, and excess iron (hemochromatosis)
- Autoimmune disorders such as sarcoidosis, scleroderma, and systemic lupus erythematosus
- Neuromuscular disease such as muscular dystrophy and neurofibromatosis.

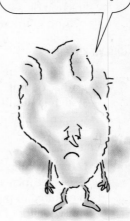

Peripartum cardiomyopathy is a rare form of dilated cardiomyopathy that occurs in women in the last month of pregnancy or within 5 months of delivery.

Complications of cardiomyopathy

Complications include HF, arrhythmias, hypoxemia, pulmonary edema, valvular dysfunction, hepatomegaly, and multiple organ dysfunction syndrome (MODS) resulting from low cardiac output. Sudden cardiac death can occur before the cardiomyopathy is even diagnosed.

Diagnostic testing for cardiomyopathy

- An ECG can identify ventricular arrhythmias.
- A 24-hour Holter monitor can identify arrhythmias.
- A treadmill test is used to see how well your heart handles work.
- Stress test and BP monitoring are used to evaluate the severity.
- A transthoracic echocardiogram is used to assess blood flow through the heart.
- A transesophageal echocardiogram (TEE) is ordered prior to surgical myomectomy.

Dilated cardiomyopathy

Dilated cardiomyopathy (DCM) is considered a mixed etiology. There is an inherited autosomal dominant pattern and environment factors. Most commonly, symptoms of DCM occur during the middle age years of adults. DCM is the leading reason for heart transplantation.

In DCM, the ventricles are enlarged, the wall of the left ventricle is normal, and there is systolic dysfunction. As systolic function declines, stroke volume, ejection fraction, and cardiac output decrease. As end-diastolic volumes increase, pulmonary congestion may occur. The elevated end-diastolic volume is a compensatory response to preserve stroke volume despite a reduced ejection fraction. It results from extensively damaged myocardial muscle fibers.

Ejection fraction is measured on echocardiogram to assess the percentage of blood that is pumped out of the ventricle during contraction or systole. The lower the percentage is, the more blood is left behind in the ventricles after a contraction.

Kidneys kick in

The kidneys are stimulated to retain sodium and water to maintain cardiac output, and vasoconstriction occurs as the renin-angiotensin system is stimulated. When these compensatory mechanisms can no longer maintain cardiac output, the heart begins to fail.

Detrimental dilation

Left ventricular dilation occurs as venous return and systemic vascular resistance increase. Eventually, the atria also dilate because more work is required to pump blood into the full ventricles. Cardiomegaly is a consequence of dilation of the atria and ventricles. Blood pooling in the ventricles increases the risk of thrombus formation and emboli. Dilation of the left ventricle may lead to mitral valve regurgitation.

DCM: Presenting signs and symptoms

For a patient with DCM, presenting signs and symptoms may be overlooked until left ventricular failure occurs. Be sure to evaluate the patient's current condition and then compare it with their condition over the past 6 to 12 months.

Presenting signs and symptoms distinctive to DCM

- Cardiac assessment—pansystolic murmur associated with mitral and tricuspid insufficiency, arrhythmias, S_3 and S_4 gallop
- Respiratory assessment—shortness of breath, orthopnea, dyspnea on exertion (DOE), paroxysmal nocturnal dyspnea (PND), fatigue, and a dry cough at night due to left-sided HF
- Peripheral vascular—signs and symptoms of thromboembolic event (extremity warmth, erythema, swelling)
- Diagnostic testing—a low ejection fraction and left ventricular enlargement that is found on echocardiogram to establish the diagnosis; cardiomegaly or an enlarged cardiac silhouette that is seen on a chest x-ray

DCM: How it's treated

DCM is treated based on the current HF treatment guidelines. The use of ACE inhibitors (ACEis) and angiotensin receptor blockers (ARBs) demonstrated a reduced mortality rate for patients. BBs are used to decrease the workload on the heart.

Hypertrophic cardiomyopathy

HCM is regarded as one of the most common inherited cardiac diseases. HCM primarily affects diastolic function. The features of HCM include left ventricular and intraventricular septum hypertrophy, obstruction of ventricular blood flow, dysfunction of ventricular relaxation and chamber stiffness, inability for the BP to rise during exercise (exercise intolerance), arrhythmias, and MI.

HCM: Signs and symptoms

Signs and symptoms vary widely among patients with HCM. Some patients are asymptomatic, and HCM is an incidental finding during a routine exam. Presenting symptoms of HCM are commonly **syncope or sudden cardiac death**. Other possible signs and symptoms include the following:

- Cardiovascular assessment—atypical chest pain, systolic murmur, sustained ventricular tachycardia (VT)
- Respiratory—exertional dyspnea, PND
- Diagnostic testing—decreased ejection fraction on echocardiogram, arrhythmias or atrial fibrillation on ECG (Geske et al., 2018).

Sudden cardiac death with HCM is most common among the young, including competitive athletes. Preparticipation exams (PPE) screen for HCM in athletes. Ask about a family history of HCM and early death due to a cardiac disease and the symptoms of HCM including complaints of chest pain, near syncope, palpitations, and dizziness with extreme heat or exercise. Physicals signs of HCM include an elevated BP, presence of a murmur on exertion, displacement of the point of maximal intensity on palpation, and signs of Marfan syndrome (+thumb sign, chest bone deformities, tall stature with long extremities, scoliosis, eye disorders, and a long face with a recessed jaw).

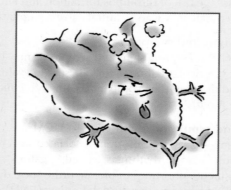

HCM: How it's treated

The goal is identification and prevention of patients at risk of sudden cardiac death from HCM. Genetic testing for patients with a history of sudden cardiac death at an early age is available to identify young people at risk of inheritance. Treatment options include the following:

- When identified early enough, implantable cardioverter-defibrillators (ICDs) can be inserted to prevent sudden death due to arrhythmias.
- Surgical cardiac myomectomy can repair the outflow obstruction and prevent HF symptoms in young, healthy adults (Geske et al., 2018).
- Nonsurgical interventions include percutaneous alcohol septal ablation to resolve arrhythmias in older adults with comorbidities.
- Medications that control HF symptoms such as exertional dyspnea and chest pain can also be used in the management of HCM.

Restrictive cardiomyopathy

Restrictive cardiomyopathy is the least common cardiomyopathy. It is characterized by impaired ventricular filling despite a normal systolic phase of ventricular contraction. This results in stiffness and thickening of the left ventricle. The ability of the ventricle to relax and fill during diastole is reduced. Furthermore, the rigid myocardium fails to contract completely during systole. As a result, cardiac output decreases. Restrictive cardiomyopathy is typically caused by autoimmune disorders such as sarcoidosis and scleroderma as well as amyloidosis, radiation therapy, and exposure to toxins.

Restrictive cardiomyopathy: Presenting signs and symptoms
A patient with restrictive cardiomyopathy presents with signs and symptoms of right-sided HF:

- Ascites
- Peripheral edema
- Hepatomegaly
- Jugular vein distention
- Weight gain
- Dyspnea.

Restrictive cardiomyopathy: Treatment
For the patient with restrictive cardiomyopathy, treatment may involve the following:

- Management of the underlying cause such as toxin exposure or management of autoimmune disorders
- Diuretics, aldosterone antagonists, and a restricted sodium diet to reduce fluid overload
- A pacemaker to control the atrioventricular block (first-, second-, and third-degree heart blocks).

What to look for

Generally, for patients with dilated or restrictive cardiomyopathy, the onset is gradual. As the disease progresses, exacerbations and hospitalizations are common regardless of the type of cardiomyopathy.

What tests tell you

These tests are used to diagnose cardiomyopathy:

- Echocardiography confirms the diagnosis of restrictive cardiomyopathy showing biatrial enlargement and diastolic dysfunction while systolic function and wall thickness is normal.
- Chest x-ray may reveal pulmonary congestion with a normal cardiac silhouette.
- ECG may reveal a prolonged PR segment and diffuse reduced voltage.

How it's treated

There's no known cure for cardiomyopathy. Treatment is individualized based on the type and cause of cardiomyopathy and the patient's condition. Heart transplantation may be required for HCM.

What to do

- Collaborate care with a skilled team, which may include a cardiologist, a cardiothoracic surgeon, a nutritionist, physical and occupational therapists, social workers, and a cardiac rehabilitation team.

- Assess hemodynamic status every 2 hours and as needed to identify systolic hypotension (less than 90 mm Hg), elevated heart rate, and tachypnea (respiratory rate over 20 breaths/minute).
- Monitor intake and output closely and obtain daily weights; institute fluid restrictions as ordered.
- Institute continuous cardiac monitoring to evaluate for arrhythmias.
- Assess for signs and symptoms of thromboembolic events such as sudden-onset chest pain, shortness of breath, erythema, swelling and pain in extremities, sudden-onset vision loss, and severe headache.
- Assess the patient for cardiovascular status—irregular heart rhythm, murmurs, extra heart sounds, grading pitting edema, erythema and tenderness of the extremities, jugular vein distention.
- Assess the patient for respiratory issues—shortness of breath at rest or with activity, fatigue, crackles or wheezing on auscultation of lung fields.
- Assess the patient for GI issues—enlarged liver, hepatojugular reflex.
- Administer medications, as ordered, to promote adequate heart function and reduce fluid overload.
- Prevent thromboembolic events with range of motion (ROM) exercises. Apply antiembolism stockings.
- Administer oxygen therapy to promote oxygenation. Assess for changes in level of consciousness, such as restlessness or decreased responsiveness, indicating diminished cerebral perfusion. If the patient has a PA catheter in place, evaluate mixed venous oxygen saturation levels; if not, monitor oxygen saturation levels using pulse oximetry.
- Assist the patient with activities of daily living (ADLs) to decrease oxygen demand. Organize care to promote periods of rest for the patient.

When to call

- Teach the patient about their diagnosis, signs and symptoms, diagnostic tests, and treatment. Be sure to cover the patient's medications, administration, and potential adverse effects.
- Teach the patient and caregivers to monitor weight and BPs at home. Keep a log for visits with their providers.
- Remind them to notify their health-care provider with early symptoms of weight gain, exercise intolerance, swelling of extremities, or shortness of breath.
- Review dietary and fluid restrictions. Verify that the patient has access to food and meal preparation to follow the dietary restrictions. Refer to social work to assist with access.

Heart failure

When the myocardium cannot pump effectively enough to meet the body's metabolic needs, HF occurs. Pump failure usually occurs in a damaged left ventricle but may also happen in the right ventricle. (See *Understanding left- and right-sided heart failure and Different types of heart failure* on pages 205 and 206.)

Now I get it!

Understanding left- and right-sided heart failure

These illustrations show how myocardial damage leads to HF.

Left-sided HF

1. Increased workload and end-diastolic volume enlarge the left ventricle (see illustration below). Because of lack of oxygen, the ventricle enlarges with stretched tissue rather than functional tissue. The patient may experience increased heart rate, pale and cool skin, tingling in the extremities, decreased cardiac output, and arrhythmias.

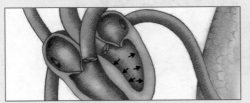

2. Diminished left ventricular function allows blood to pool in the ventricle and the atrium and eventually back up into the pulmonary veins and capillaries (as shown below). At this stage, the patient may experience DOE, confusion, light-headedness, orthostatic hypotension, decreased peripheral pulses and pulse pressure, cyanosis, and an S_3 gallop.

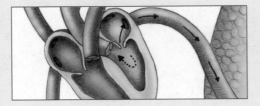

3. As the pulmonary circulation becomes engorged, rising capillary pressure pushes sodium (Na) and water (H_2O) into the interstitial space (as shown below), causing pulmonary edema. You'll note coughing, subclavian retractions, crackles, tachypnea, elevated PAP, diminished pulmonary compliance, and increased partial pressure of carbon dioxide.

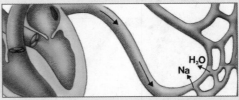

4. When the patient lies down, fluid in the extremities moves into the systemic circulation. Because the left ventricle can't handle the increased venous return, fluid pools in the pulmonary circulation, worsening pulmonary edema (see illustration below). You may note decreased breath sounds, dullness on percussion, crackles, and orthopnea.

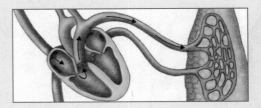

(Continued)

Understanding left- and right-sided heart failure *(continued)*

5. The right ventricle may now become stressed because it's pumping against greater pulmonary vascular resistance and left ventricular pressure (see illustration below). When this occurs, the patient's symptoms worsen.

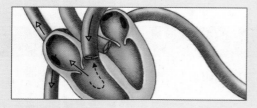

Right-sided HF
6. The stressed right ventricle enlarges with the formation of stretched tissue (see illustration below). Increasing conduction time and deviation of the heart from its normal axis can cause arrhythmias. If the patient doesn't already have left-sided HF, they may experience increased heart rate, cool skin, cyanosis, decreased cardiac output, palpitations, and dyspnea.

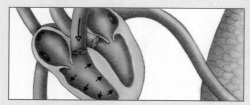

7. Blood pools in the right ventricle and right atrium. The backed-up blood causes pressure and congestion in the vena cava and systemic circulation (see illustration below). The patient will have elevated central venous pressure, jugular vein distention, and hepatojugular reflux.

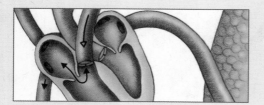

8. Backed-up blood also distends the visceral veins, especially the hepatic vein. As the liver and spleen become engorged (see illustration below), their function is impaired. The patient may develop anorexia, nausea, abdominal pain, palpable liver and spleen, weakness, and dyspnea secondary to abdominal distention.

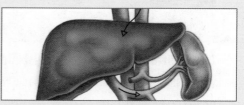

9. Rising capillary pressure forces excess fluid from the capillaries into the interstitial space (see illustration below). This causes tissue edema, especially in the lower extremities and abdomen. The patient may experience weight gain, pitting edema, and nocturia.

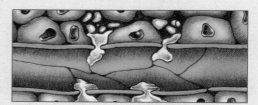

Different types of heart failure

HF is diagnosed according to its pathophysiology. As discussed earlier, it may be left-sided or right-sided. It may be systolic or diastolic, acute or chronic, and have a preserved or reduced ejection fraction.

Systolic or diastolic

In systolic HF, the left ventricle can't pump enough blood out to the systemic circulation during systole, and the ejection fraction falls. Consequently, blood backs up into the pulmonary circulation, pressure rises in the pulmonary venous system, and cardiac output falls.

In diastolic HF, the left ventricle can't relax and fill properly during diastole, and the stroke volume falls. Therefore, larger ventricular volumes are needed to maintain cardiac output.

Acute or chronic

The term *acute* refers to the timing of the onset of symptoms and whether compensatory mechanisms kick in. Typically, in acute HF, fluid status is normal or low, and sodium and water retention do not occur.

In chronic HF, signs and symptoms have been present for some time, compensatory mechanisms have taken effect, and fluid volume overload persists. Drugs, diet changes, and activity restrictions usually control symptoms.

Preserved or reduced ejection fraction

Ejection fraction is measured on echocardiogram to assess the percentage of blood that is pumped out of the left ventricle (LVEF) during contraction or systole. The lower the percentage, the more blood is left behind in the ventricles after a contraction. Ejection fraction can also be measured by invasive and noninvasive hemodynamic monitoring at rest or with exercise in hospital setting. The classifications of HF by ejection fraction help to guide treatment plans and evaluate the potential recovery (Heidenreich et al., 2022).

HF with preserved ejection fraction (HFpEF) means the patient has diagnostic markers and signs and symptoms of HF, but the ejection fraction remains at or above 50%. In the case of HFpEF, the signs and symptoms can be provoked or spontaneous, and because dyspnea has other noncardiac causes, they need to be ruled out before a diagnosis of HFpEF is determined. (See *It's not all heart* on page 208.) Other factors in determining the diagnosis of HFpEF are the presence of risk factors such as obesity and diabetes.

HF with a reduced ejection fraction have three subclassifications. For HF with reduced ejection fraction (HFrEF), the threshold for the LVEF is below 40%. Patients with an LVEF between 41% and 49% have a mildly reduced HF (HFmrEF). Once a patient is determined to have a reduced ejection fraction, they cannot be classified again as HFpEF even if their EF improves with therapy. Patients with HF that have improved ejection fractions above 40% are HFimpEF.

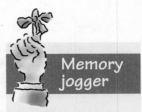

Memory jogger

During systole, the ventricles contract, the atria relax, and the aortic and pulmonic valves open as oxygenated blood is pumped to the lungs and body.

During diastole, the atria contract, the mitral and tricuspid valves open, and the ventricles dilate to allow blood in.

Quality time

Symptoms of HF may restrict a person's ability to perform ADLs, resulting in activity intolerance, and may severely affect quality of life. Also, medications to treat HF such as beta-blockers can compound activity intolerance since they lower the patient's heart rate and workload. Advances in diagnostic and therapeutic techniques have improved outcomes for these patients. However, prognosis still depends on the underlying cause and its response to treatment.

Daunting difficulties

Complications of HF include cardiomyopathy, arrhythmias, valvular dysfunction, mental status changes, exercise intolerance, MODS, and death.

What causes it

Cardiovascular disorders that lead to HF include the following:
- Atherosclerotic heart disease
- IHD (MI, restrictive cardiomyopathy, DCM, myocarditis)
- Hypertension
- Rheumatic heart disease
- Congenital heart defects
- Valvular diseases
- Arrhythmias.

It's not all heart

Noncardiovascular causes of HF include the following:
- Sleep apnea
- Obesity
- Severe anemia
- Diabetes
- Severe lung diseases (chronic obstructive pulmonary disease [COPD], pulmonary embolism [PE])
- Hyperthyroidism.

How it happens

The patient's underlying condition determines whether HF is acute or chronic. HF is commonly associated with systolic or diastolic overloading and myocardial weakness. As stress on the heart muscle reaches a critical level, the muscle's contractility is reduced, and cardiac output declines. Venous input to the ventricle remains the same, however.

The body's responses to decreased cardiac output include the following:
- Reflex increase in sympathetic nervous system activity
- Release of renin from the juxtaglomerular cells of the kidney
- Anaerobic metabolism by affected cells
- Increased extraction of oxygen by the peripheral cells.

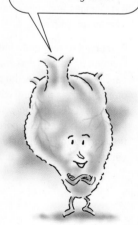

I can sometimes compensate for the increased workload, delaying symptoms for a long time.

Adept at adaptation

When blood in the ventricles increases, the heart compensates or adapts. Compensation may occur for prolonged periods of time before signs and symptoms develop. Adaptations may include:

- *Short term*—As the end-diastolic fiber length increases, the ventricular muscle responds by dilating and increasing the force of contractions. (This is called the *Frank-Starling curve* or ventricular remodeling.)
- *Long term*—Ventricular hypertrophy increases the heart muscle's ability to contract and push its volume of blood into the circulation.

What to look for

Physical signs of left-sided HF include the following:
- Shortness of breath
- Orthopnea (difficulty breathing when lying down)
- DOE
- PND (episodes of severe shortness of breath and coughing at night)
- A dry cough
- Tachycardia and hypotension
- Peripheral edema and cool extremities
- Crackles auscultated at the lung bases
  The patient with right-sided HF may develop:
- Exercise intolerance
- Peripheral edema and cool extremities
- Jugular vein distention
- Hepatomegaly (enlarged liver)
- Weight gain
- Ascites
- Anasarca—an accumulation of fluid in the interstitial spaces and a sign of acute HF

What tests tell you

- Blood tests may show elevated blood urea nitrogen (BUN) and creatinine levels, elevated serum norepinephrine levels, and elevated transaminase and bilirubin levels if hepatic function is impaired. Low hemoglobin, hematocrit, and mean corpuscular volume demonstrate anemia, a common comorbidity with HF.
- Elevated blood levels of cardiac biomarkers BNP or NT-proBNP can be useful in outpatient settings to rule in or rule out a diagnosis of HF. Any patients presenting with dyspnea unrelated to other causes should have these tests performed. These tests can also be used to monitor the emergence of HF in at-risk patients. In acute care settings, BNP levels can predict the prognosis of recovery in acutely ill patients with HF.

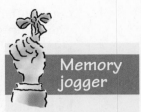

Memory jogger

Remember left-sided HF causes an accumulation of fluid in the lungs, so most of the signs and symptoms involve the respiratory system. Right-sided HF involves a "backup" of blood in the extremities, liver, and other organs, so these symptoms center around increased venous pressure and the GI system.

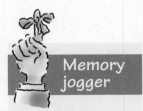

Memory jogger

Advice from Experts

There are other noncardiac conditions that can cause elevated NP levels such obstructive sleep apnea, pneumonia, bacterial sepsis, and advanced age. Obesity is associated with lower levels of BNP and NT-proBNP.

- Complete blood count (CBC) assesses anemia, which is associated with an increased mortality in cases of HF.
- ECG reflects heart strain or ventricular enlargement (ischemia). It may also reveal atrial enlargement, tachycardia, and extrasystoles, suggesting HF.
- Genetic testing for inherited cardiomyopathies is recommended for first-degree relatives to detect and manage cardiac diseases and to slow the progression of HF.
- Chest x-ray shows increased pulmonary vascular markings, interstitial edema, or pleural effusion and cardiomegaly.
- Cardiac catheterization may show ventricular dilation, coronary artery occlusion, and valvular disorders (such as aortic stenosis and mitral valve insufficiency) in both left- and right-sided HF.
- Echocardiography and transesophageal echocardiography (TEE) may show ventricular hypertrophy, decreased contractility, and valvular disorders in both left- and right-sided HF. Serial echocardiograms may help assess the patient's response to therapy.
- Cardiopulmonary exercise testing to evaluate the patient's ventricular performance during exercise may show decreased oxygen uptake. This test can be used by health-care providers to assess the stage of HF and to predict prognosis as patient disease worsens.

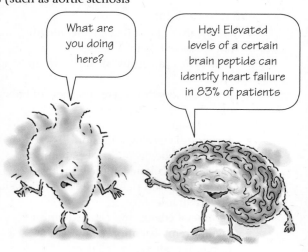

How it's treated

Diagnosis and management of HF is determined by the patient's symptoms and structural defects in the heart. Cardiac biomarkers such as the BNP or NT-proBNP guide the treatment plan for HF. Monitoring a decrease in ejection fraction with an echocardiogram is helpful, but a patient can have symptomatic HF with a normal ejection fraction. Some examples of guidelines used are the New York Heart Association (NYHA) classification system and the American College of Cardiology/American Heart Association guidelines (ACC/AHA). (See *Comparison of ACC/AHA stages of HF and NYHA functional classifications*.) (McDonagh et al., 2021)

A quadruple threat...

Drug therapy begins with an angiotensin receptor-neprilysin inhibitor (ARNI) + a BB + a mineralocorticoid receptor antagonist (MRA) + sodium glucose cotransporter-2 inhibitors (SGLT2i). An ACE or ARB can be used if the patient cannot tolerate the ARNI. Other medications can be added to control the symptoms and slow disease progression.

Comparison of ACC/AHA stages of HF and NYHA functional classifications

ACCF/AHA stages of HF		NYHA functional classification	
A	At risk for HF but without a structural heart disease, cardiac biomarkers, symptoms of HF	None	
B	Structural heart disease, increased filling pressures with diagnostic testing, or cardiac biomarkers present but without signs or symptoms of HF	I	No limitation of physical activity Ordinary physical activity does not cause symptoms of HF
C	Structural heart disease with prior or current symptoms of HF	I	No limitation of physical activity Ordinary physical activity does not cause symptoms of HF
		II	Slight limitation of physical activity Comfortable at rest, but ordinary physical activity results in HF symptoms
		III	Significant limitation of physical activity Comfortable at rest, but less-than-ordinary activity causes HF symptoms
		IV	Unable to carry on any physical activity without discomfort and symptoms of HF at rest
D	Marked HF symptoms that interfere with ADLs and result in repeated hospitalizations despite guideline-directed medical therapy	IV	Unable to carry on any physical activity without discomfort and symptoms of HF at rest

Abbreviations: ACC, American College of Cardiology; ADLs, activities of daily living; AHA, American Heart Association; HF, heart failure; NYHA, New York Heart Association.

Heidenreich et al., 2022.

- ACE or ARBs: Either an ACE or an ARB is a recommended therapy for HF. Both medications block the renin-angiotensin-aldosterone system and will reduce vasoconstriction and lower the workload on the heart.
- ARNI: Neprilysin inhibition is believed to reduce remodeling and hypertrophy in the heart muscle. It promotes diuresis and vasodilation and inhibits aldosterone. This combination drug is recommended for HF patients with a reduced ejection fraction (Shim et al., 2020).
- BBs will reduce the workload on the heart.
- MRAs will block sodium retention, myocardial fibrosis, and vascular inflammation.
- SGLT2i is a drug class to treat type 2 diabetes. This drug class is recommended to treat HF with preserved and reduced ejection fraction. SGLT2i drugs act on the distal tubules of the kidneys to prevent reabsorption of glucose and sodium. It is believed this drug is beneficial in the

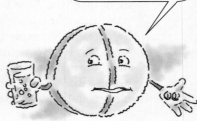

An ARNI and an ACE should never be given together due to the risk of angioedema. Separate dosages by 36 hours (about 1 and a half days) when changing medications.

treatment of HF because it reduces cardiac preload and after load, BP, and intraglomerular pressure. SGLT2is can be used for HF patients regardless of whether they have diabetes (Heidenreich et al., 2022).

- Sinoatrial node modulator ivabradine may be beneficial for hospitalized, acutely ill patients in HF.
- Diuretics reduce preload by decreasing total blood volume and circulatory congestion.
- Isosorbide dinitrate is a nitrate that causes vasodilation and reduces the workload on the heart. This is given with the diuretic hydralazine.
- ICD or cardiac resynchronization therapy corrects arrhythmias.
- In NYHA classes III to IV or stage D HF, treatment includes heart transplantation for eligible patients; left ventricular assist device, which is an implantable pump that acts on the left ventricle to strengthen contraction; or palliative care.

Caution

ACEs and ARNIs can cause angioedema! Assess for a new-onset dry cough that can present any time from days to weeks after starting an ACE or ARNI drug. Do not give the medication if the patient has a history of angioedema.

What to do

- Collaborate care with a skilled team, which may include a cardiologist, a cardiovascular surgeon, a hematologist, a pulmonologist, a nutritionist, physical and occupational therapists, social workers, a cardiac rehabilitation team, and social services.
- Frequently monitor CBC; BUN; serum creatinine; and potassium, sodium, chloride, magnesium, and BNP levels.
- Provide and monitor oxygen therapy as ordered.
- Reinforce the importance of adhering to a low-sodium diet and to eat small, frequent meals to allow rest periods.
- If fluid restrictions have been ordered, arrange a mutually acceptable schedule for allowable fluids.
- Assess the patient's progress by monitoring daily weights, BP, and pulse oximetry; auscultating lung fields and heart sounds; and assessing for dyspnea and peripheral edema.
- Prevent thromboembolic events with ROM exercises and ambulation. Apply antiembolism stockings.
- Document cardiac and respiratory status and response to treatment. Document patient teaching and the patient's understanding of the information.

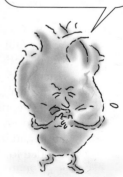

ACEs and ARNIs can cause angioedema! Assess for a new onset dry cough that can present any time from days to weeks after starting an ACE or ARNI drug. Do not give the medication if the patient has a history of angioedema.

Preparing for discharge: Sodium down, potassium up

- Teach the patient about lifestyle changes. Advise them to avoid foods high in sodium to help curb fluid overload. Explain that the potassium that is lost through diuretic therapy must be replaced by a prescribed potassium supplement and eating high-potassium foods. Stress the benefits of balancing activity and rest.
- Assist the patient in making follow-up appointments with their health-care providers including their primary care provider, cardiologist, and cardiac rehabilitation provider.

- Educate the patient about the actions and side effects of their medications. Emphasize that some medications can cause activity intolerance due to a low heart rate and low BP. Also, patients that are initiated with ARNIs and ACE should be educated on the symptoms of angioedema and to immediately report a new-onset cough.
- Teach the patient how to assess their radial pulse. Notify their health-care provider if their pulse is unusually irregular or less than 60 beats/min.
- Teach the patient about worsening signs and symptoms of HF. Notify the health-care provider if the patient experiences dizziness, shortness of breath, PND, swollen ankles, or decreased urine output or a weight of 3 to 5 lb (1.5 to 2.5 kg) in 1 week.

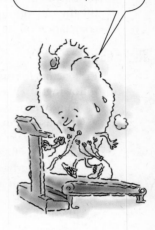

With heart failure, cardiopulmonary exercise testing may show decreased oxygen uptake.

Hypertension

Hypertension is the most common condition seen in primary care. Uncontrolled hypertension may lead to stroke, MI, HF, PAD, retinopathy, and renal failure. Detecting and treating it before complications develop greatly improves the patient's prognosis. Severely elevated BP may become fatal.

Essential (idiopathic) hypertension is the most common form. Secondary hypertension results from several disorders. Malignant hypertension is a severe form of hypertension common to both types.

BP is classified as normal, prehypertension, stage 1, or stage 2. The severity of hypertension helps to guide treatment. (See *Blood pressure classifications*.)

One thing leads to another

What causes it

Scientists haven't been able to identify a single cause for essential hypertension. The disorder probably reflects an interaction of multiple homeostatic forces, including changes in renal regulation of

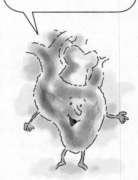

High potassium foods help fight heart failure.

Blood pressure classifications (ACC/AHA, 2017)

	Systolic mm Hg		Diastolic mm Hg
Normal	<120	and	<80
Prehypertension	120-139	or	80-89
Stage I	140-159	or	90-99
Stage II	≥160	or	≥100

Whelton et al. (2018).

sodium and extracellular fluids, aldosterone secretion and metabolism, norepinephrine secretion and metabolism, and arterial walls.

Secondary hypertension may be caused by obstructive sleep apnea; chronic kidney disease; medications (hormonal contraception, antidepressants, caffeine, decongestants, stimulants); pheochromocytoma; primary hyperaldosteronism; Cushing syndrome; or dysfunction of the thyroid, pituitary, or parathyroid glands. It may also result from coarctation of the aorta, pregnancy, and neurologic disorders.

Risky business

Risk factors for primary or essential hypertension include the following:
- Family history of hypertension
- Increased age
- Race (more common in blacks)
- Sex (males have a higher risk than premenopausal females)
- Obesity and weight gain
- Excessive salt intake
- Tobacco use
- Physical inactivity
- Excessive alcohol use.

How it happens

Essential hypertension usually begins insidiously as a benign disease, slowly progressing to a malignant state. If left untreated, even mild cases can cause major complications and death.

Why? Why? Why?

Several theories help to explain the development of hypertension. (See *Blood vessel damage.*) It's thought to arise from the following:
- Changes in the arteriolar bed, causing increased resistance
- Abnormally increased tone in the sensory nervous system that originates in the vasomotor system centers, causing increased peripheral vascular resistance
- Increased blood volume resulting from renal or hormonal dysfunction
- Increased arteriolar thickening caused by genetic factors, leading to increased peripheral vascular resistance
- Abnormal renin release resulting in the formation of angiotensin II, which constricts the arterioles and increases blood volume.

Secondary isn't small

The pathophysiology of secondary hypertension is related to the underlying disease. For example, consider these points:
- The most common cause of secondary hypertension is chronic renal disease. Insult to the kidney from chronic glomerulonephritis or renal artery stenosis interferes with sodium excretion, the

Blood vessel damage

Sustained hypertension damages blood vessels. Vascular injury begins with alternating areas of dilation and constriction in the arterioles. The following illustrations show how damage occurs.

1. Increased intra-arterial pressure damages the endothelium.

2. Angiotensin II induces endothelial wall contraction, allowing plasma to leak through interendothelial spaces.

3. Plasma constituents deposited in the vessel wall cause medial necrosis.

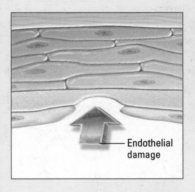

Endothelial damage

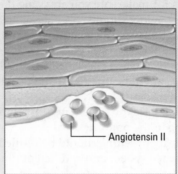

Angiotensin II

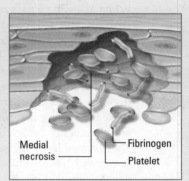

Medial necrosis

Fibrinogen

Platelet

renin-angiotensin-aldosterone system, or renal perfusion. This disruption causes BP to rise.

- In obstructive sleep apnea, the upper airways close off when the patient is lying down typically due to increased weight or loss of muscle control around the chest and neck. This results in pauses in breathing. The sympathetic nervous system is activated; there is deoxygenation of the blood, an increase in inflammation, and peripheral vascular resistance. At first, the patient experiences nocturnal hypertension and then progresses to all-day hypertension.
- In Cushing's syndrome, increased cortisol levels raise BP by increasing renal sodium retention, angiotensin II levels, and vascular response to norepinephrine.
- In primary aldosteronism, increased intravascular volume, altered sodium concentrations in vessel walls, or very high aldosterone levels cause vasoconstriction (increased resistance).
- Pheochromocytoma is a secreting tumor of chromaffin cells, usually of the adrenal medulla. It causes hypertension due to increased secretion of epinephrine and norepinephrine. Epinephrine functions mainly to increase cardiac contractility and rate; norepinephrine to increase peripheral vascular resistance.

Hypertension: The silent killer

Almost half of the American population older than 20 years has hypertension, and they do not know it. Hypertension is referred to as the "silent killer" because there are no signs and symptoms. To screen for hypertension, patients need to have their BP taken any time they present for healthcare. Hypertension is diagnosed by increased BP measurements based on the Eighth Joint National Committee (JNC 8) guidelines on two or more readings taken at two or more visits after an initial screening. (See *Blood pressure classifications*, page 213.)

Follow up after an elevated BP reading

- When assessing a patient's BP, make sure you are using the correct-size cuff. The width of the bladder should cover about 40% of the circumference of the upper arm. The length of the cuff should cover about 80% of the length of the upper arm.
- Note the position of the patient when checking the BP. When the patient is sitting, their legs should be uncrossed and feet flat on the floor for the most accurate reading.
- If the BP reading is elevated, have the patient rest for 5 minutes and then verify the reading in the opposite arm.
- The elevated BP in an outpatient setting should be verified at home with a home automated system and at different times of the day (Whelton et al., 2018).

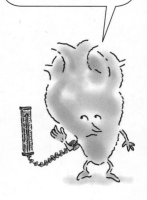

With secondary hypertension, you'll need to look for manifestations of the primary disease.

Problems plus

Expect a patient with secondary hypertension to have clinical manifestations of the primary disease. Other clinical effects don't appear until complications develop because of vascular changes in target organs. These effects include the following:

- left ventricular hypertrophy
- angina
- MI
- HF
- stroke
- transient ischemic attack
- nephropathy
- PAD
- retinopathy.

What tests tell you

Along with patient history, these tests may show predisposing factors and help identify an underlying cause:

- Chronic kidney disease due to end-organ damage from uncontrolled hypertension would show an elevated glomerular filtration rate.
- A BUN level that's normal or elevated to more than 20 mg/dL and a creatinine level that's normal or elevated to more than 1.5 mg/dL suggests renal disease.
- Protein, red blood cells (RBCs), and white blood cells in urinalysis may indicate glomerulonephritis.

- A sleep study with oxygen saturation monitoring would show if obstructive sleep apnea were a secondary cause of elevated BP readings.
- Elevated blood glucose levels may indicate diabetes.
- Anemia may cause a high-output state resulting in hypertension. Polycythemia increases the risk of hypertension and stroke.
- Elevated total cholesterol and low-density lipoprotein levels increase the risk of atherosclerosis.
- A 24-hour urine for metanephrine and normetanephrine can identify pheochromocytoma.
- A serum thyroid-stimulating hormone and parathyroid hormone can assess for thyroid and parathyroid disease.
- A 24-hour urine for aldosterone levels can assess for primary hyperaldosteronism.

Detecting heart damage

Other tests help detect cardiovascular damage and other complications:
- ECG may show left ventricular hypertrophy or ischemia.
- Echocardiography may show left ventricular hypertrophy.
- Chest x-ray may show cardiomegaly.

How it's treated

Treatment of secondary hypertension includes correcting the underlying cause and controlling hypertensive effects. Although essential hypertension has no cure, lifestyle modifications and drug therapy can help to control it.

Time for a change

In early stages, lifestyle changes such as regular exercise may prevent hypertension from developing. Lifestyle modifications can be initiated in all patients at any stage of hypertension.
- Dietary Approaches to Stop Hypertension (DASH): Follow a DASH diet pattern combined with reduced sodium (no more than 1,500 mg per day) and sugars, low saturated fats, and no trans fats.
- Break a sweat: Exercise at least 3 to 4 times per week for 40 minutes at a moderate to vigorous intensity.
- Smoking cessation screening and counseling

Pharming out therapy

The need for drug therapy is determined by BP and the presence of target organ damage, risk factors, and other coexisting disorders such as diabetes. Drug therapy for uncomplicated hypertension usually begins with a thiazide diuretic, an ACEi, or a BB. Other antihypertensive drugs include angiotensin II receptor blockers, alpha-receptor blockers, direct arteriole dilators, and calcium channel blockers. (See *Managing antihypertensive therapy*, page 218.)

Managing antihypertensive therapy

This flowchart is based on the approach to antihypertensive therapy endorsed by the Joint National Committee on Prevention, Detection, Evaluation, and Treatment of High BP.

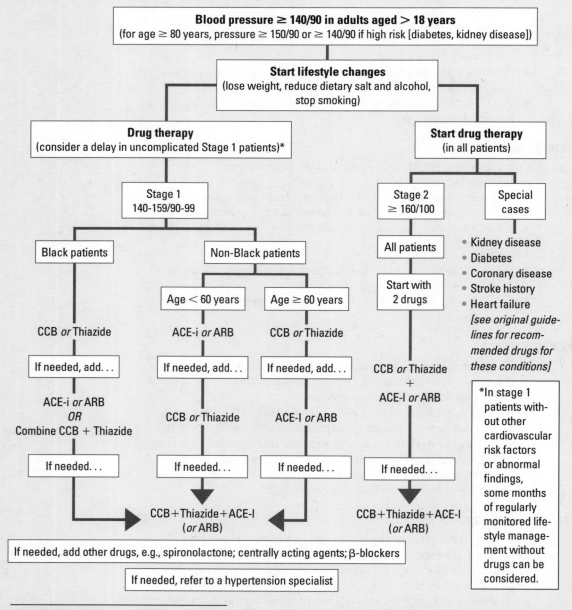

Source: Reprinted with permission from Hinkle, J. L., Cheever, K. H. *Brunner & Suddarth's Textbook of Medical-Surgical Nursing* (14th ed.). Philadelphia, PA: Wolters Kluwer Health, 2017.

Comparing BP Classifications by Key Guidelines for Adults of Age 18 Years or Older

Systolic BP (mm Hg)		Diastolic BP (mm Hg)	ACC/AHA (2017) Guideline[a]	JNC 7[b] and JNC 8[c] Guidelines
<120	-and-	<80	Normal	Normal
120–129	-and-	<80	Elevated	Prehypertension
130–139	-or-	80–89	Stage 1 hypertension	Prehypertension
140–159	-or-	90–99	Stage 2 hypertension	Stage 1 hypertension
≥160	-or-	≥100	Stage 2 hypertension	Stage 2 hypertension

Note: For each guideline, if the patient's systolic and diastolic BPs fall into different categories, then the patient is classified according to the highest category.

Abbreviations: ACC, American College of Cardiology; AHA, American Heart Association; BP, blood pressure; JNC 7, Seventh Joint National Committee; JNC 8, Eighth Joint National Committee.

[a]Adapted from Whelton, P. K., Carey, R. M., Aronow, W. S., Casey, D. E., Collins, K. J., Himmelfarb, C. D., DePalma, S. M., Gidding, S., Jamerson, K. A., Jones, D. W., McLaughlin, E. J., Munter, P., Ovbiagele, B., Smith, S. C. Jr, Spencer, C. C., Stafford, R. S., Taler, S. J., Thomas, R. J., Williams K. A. Sr, ... Wright, J. J. T. (2017). 2017 ACC/AHA/AAPA/ABC/ACPM/AGS/APhA/ASH/ASPC/NMA/PCNA guideline for the prevention, detection, evaluation, and management of high blood pressure in adults: A report of the American College of Cardiology/American Heart Association Task Force on Clinical Practice Guidelines. *Hypertension, 71*(6), e13–e115.

[b]Adapted from Chobanian, A. V., Bakris, G. L., Black, H. R., Cushman, W. C., Green, L. A., Izzo, J. L., Jones, D. W., Materson, B. J., Oparil, S., Wright, J. T. Jr, Rocella, E. J. et al.; National High Blood Pressure Education Program Coordinating Committee. (2003). Seventh Report of the Joint National Committee on prevention, detection, evaluation, and treatment of high blood pressure: The JNC 7 Report. *JAMA, 289*(19), 2560–2572.

[c]Adapted from James, P. A., Oparil, S., Carter, B. L., Cushman, W. C., Dennison-Himmelfarb, C., Handler, J., Lackland, D. T., Le Fevre, M. L., MacKenzie, T. D., Ogedegbe, O., Smith, S. C. Jr, Svetkey, L. P., Taler, S. J, Townsend, R. R., Wright, J. T. Jr, Narwa, A. S., & Ortiz, E. (2014). 2014 evidence-based guideline for the management of high blood pressure in adults: Report from the panel members appointed to the Eighth Joint National Committee (JNC 8). *JAMA, 311*(5), 507–520.

What to do
- Screen all patients for hypertension, especially those at high risk, at every health-care visit.
- Coordinate care with a health-care team, which may include a primary care provider, cardiologist, a nephrologist, an endocrinologist, a pharmacist, a nutritionist, social services, and an athletic trainer.
- Complete a thorough medication reconciliation when a patient is admitted to your facility. Verify all prescription and over-the-counter (OTC) medications and herbal supplements the patient is taking and the ones they are prescribed but not taking.
- If the patient is not taking their medications for hypertension, assess the reason (cost, lack of access to refills, bothersome side effects). Collaborate with the appropriate health-care team

member to resolve issues surrounding the lack of adherence to their medication.

- Refer all patients to a nutritionist and athletic trainer to assist with lifestyle modifications.
- If the patient smokes, encourage cessation and refer them to a smoking-cessation program.
- Teach the patient to use a self-monitoring BP cuff and to record readings at the same time of the day at least twice weekly to review with their health-care provider.

Patient instructions for at-home BP monitoring

- Do not smoke, exercise, or drink caffeinated beverages 30 minutes before BP reading.
- Alternate daytime and night-time readings. Night-time BP readings will be lower than daytime.
- Sit quietly for 5 minutes before checking BP.
- Sit up straight with your back against the chair and feet flat on the floor while checking BP. Keep your arm still on a flat surface at the level of your heart.
- Wait 5 minutes before rechecking BP.
- Record readings and bring record to every appointment.

(Whelton et al., 2018.)

- Review the signs and symptoms of the complications of hypertension related to chronic kidney disease, HF, cardiomyopathy, and ACS.
- To encourage adherence with drug therapy, suggest that the patient establish a daily routine for taking medication. Educate the patient on the adverse effects of the medications and encourage them to report these effects to their provider.

Don't suffer in silence

Some side effects of BP medication can be bothersome, causing patients to avoid or stop taking their medications. Educate your patients on the potential side effects of their medication. The most common side effects are dizziness, lack of energy, and even erectile problems. Encourage your patients to report these bothersome side effects as hypertension medications can be adjusted or changed. This will promote adherence to drug therapy and decrease the risk of target organ damage due to poorly controlled hypertension.

- Advise them to avoid OTC medications that can raise BP such as high-sodium antacids (sodium bicarbonate), cold and sinus medications, and stimulants found in dietary supplements and herbals. The use of nonsteroidal anti-inflammatory drugs (NSAIDs) should be avoided to decrease damage to the kidneys and the risk of BP medication interactions.
- Document vital signs and intake and output. Note cardiac and respiratory status and response to treatment. Document patient teaching and the patient's understanding of the information.
- Reassess the patient 1 to 3 months after initiating lifestyle modifications and antihypertensive therapy. After successful treatment for hypertension, the patient will demonstrate BP within range based on the JNC 8 guidelines. (See *Blood pressure classifications*, page 213.) Assess the patient's DASH diet patterns, lifestyle modifications, and adherence to drug therapy.

Pulmonary hypertension

PH is prevalent in 1% of the global population. The most common cause is left-sided heart disease followed by respiratory disease. The prevalence is increasing among older adults due to the degenerative nature of the disease. The pulmonary blood vessels are constricted due to arterial wall thickening and pressures builds. Less blood pumps through the lungs to become oxygenated. Complications of PH include right- and left-sided HF, valvular dysfunction, hypoxemia, arrhythmias, and death (Humbert et al., 2023).

Common cardiac causes of PH are left-sided HF, mitral valve disease, and aortic stenosis. Common respiratory causes of PH are caused by hypoxemic conditions, advanced COPD, sleep apnea, and pulmonary fibrosis.

Other rare causes of PH
Primary, or idiopathic, PH is rare and has no known cause. It's most common in women between ages 20 and 40 years and is usually fatal within 3 to 4 years. Mortality is highest in pregnant women. Secondary causes include connective tissue disorders (scleroderma), congenital heart disease (ventricular septal defect, patent ductus arteriosus, atrial septal defect), and portal hypertension. Drugs such as methylamphetamines and some seizure medications are associated with PA hypertension. A patient history of deep vein thrombosis (DVT) or pulmonary emboli can cause chronic thromboembolic pulmonary hypertension (CTEPH).

Pulmonary arterial hypertension (PAH) is one type of PH. Causes are hereditary, idiopathic, medication induced, HIV, connective tissue disease, and portal hypertension. Congenital disorders of the heart and liver can induce PAH in newborns.

What happens

In primary PH, the intimal lining of the pulmonary arteries thickens, narrowing the lumen of the artery, impairing distensibility, and increasing vascular resistance.

Alveolar hypoventilation can result from diseases causing alveolar destruction or diseases that prevent the chest wall from expanding sufficiently to allow air into the alveoli. The resulting decreased ventilation increases pulmonary vascular resistance.

Hypoxemia resulting from the ventilation-perfusion mismatch causes vasoconstriction, further increasing vascular resistance and resulting in PH.

Sans treatment

If a patient with PH doesn't receive treatment, here's what happens:
- Hypertrophy occurs in the medial smooth-muscle layer of the arterioles, worsening their ability to stretch and dilate. This will restrict blood flow.
- Increased pressure in the lungs is transmitted to the right ventricle (which supplies the PA).
- The ventricle becomes hypertrophic and eventually fails (cor pulmonale).
- Impaired distensibility due to hypertrophy can cause arrhythmias.

What to look, listen, and feel for

Symptoms of PH:
- DOE progressing to dyspnea with simple activities such as bending forward (bendopnea)
- Fatigue, exhaustion with activity
- Palpitations
- Hemoptysis
- Weight gain (fluid retention)
- Nausea and abdominal distension worse with activity
- A decreased O_2 saturation

In late stages of the disease, these symptoms of PH will occur even with rest.
- Shortness of breath
- Easily fatigued
- Wheezing
- Chest pain on exertion
- Syncope or presyncope on exertion
- Abdominal distention, ascites, anasarca, and jugular vein distention (signs of right-sided HF)
- A palpable precordial heave or lift and a reduced carotid pulse
- Dry crackles on lung auscultation indicating atelectasis (Humbert et al., 2023)

What tests tell you

Not all testing has a predictive value in diagnosing PH. The diagnosis and monitoring of PH includes history and physical examination and a combination of normal and abnormal findings of these diagnostic studies:

- ECG changes such as right or sagittal axis deviation, right bundle branch block, and ST depression with T wave inversion.
- Chest x-ray shows an enlarged cardiac silhouette due to the right ventricular hypertrophy.
- Echocardiography allows assessment of ventricular wall motion and possible valvular dysfunction. It's also used to identify right ventricular enlargement and dysfunction.
- Pulmonary function testing (PFT) with carbon monoxide diffusing capacity (or DLCO) is recommended as an initial evaluation of PH. Restrictive and obstructive changes on PFTs are indicative of respiratory-related PH and PA hypertension. They may show decreased flow rates and increased residual volume in case of the underlying obstructive disease. For the underlying restrictive disease, they may show reduced total lung capacity.
- Arterial blood gas analysis reveals hypoxemia, and the results help to monitor oxygen therapy.
- Routine CBC, BNP or NT-BNP, electrolytes, kidney function, uric acid and liver function tests, HIV and hepatitis status, iron status, and thyroid function tests will rule out secondary causes of PH.
- Exercise, vasoreactivity, and fluid challenge testing such as cardiopulmonary exercise tests or right catheterization testing are helpful to monitor activity intolerance and fatigue associated with PH.
- Genetic screenings test mutations that cause PH.
- High-resolution computed tomography (CT) scan is recommended for all patients with suspected PH. A CT scan without contrast can identify lung disease, and a CT scan with contrast can track blood flow.
- PA catheterization reveals increased PAP, with systolic pressure above 25 mm Hg. It may also show an increased PAWP if the underlying cause is left atrial myxoma, mitral stenosis, or left-sided HF; otherwise, PAWP is normal.
- An abdominal ultrasound detects portal hypertension.
- Pulmonary ventilation (V) and perfusion (Q) lung scans will show the air and blood flow patterns through the lungs, which will identify CTEPH (Humbert et al., 2023).

How it's treated

Early diagnosis for at-risk patients is helpful to avoid the progression of PH. Genetic testing for patients with first-degree relatives with primary PH is recommended. At-risk patients for the other causes of

PH include patients with portal hypertension, HIV, connective tissue disease, and a history of pulmonary emboli. Early screening tests for at-risk patients include NT-proBNP, ECG, echocardiogram, PFTs, and cardiopulmonary exercise stress testing.

Treatment measures include oxygen therapy to correct hypoxemia and fluid restriction to decrease preload and minimize workload of the right ventricle. In severe cases with irreversible changes, heart-lung transplantation may be necessary.

It is recommended that patients of childbearing age with PH should avoid pregnancy due to the increased fluid volume and workload on the heart. Supervised exercise training will assist the patient to safely avoid physical deconditioning and provide an outlet for socialization. The patient and caregivers should be referred for psychosocial support because PH can lead to social isolation due to the activity intolerance. As with all patients with chronic diseases, influenza and pneumococcal immunizations should be provided. Patients are counseled about the risk of travel by plane or to high-altitude areas due to hypoxia. Oxygen therapy may need to be modified when necessary for travel. Finally, elective surgeries and surgeries with general anesthesia are not recommended.

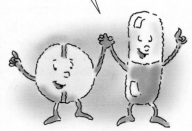

Medications can increase cardiac output, reduce workload, relax muscles, and help in other ways.

Diverse therapies

A patient with PH may be treated with the following measures:

- Physical activity and cardiac rehabilitation to increase exercise capacity and quality of life.
- Diuretics to prevent fluid retention, increase blood flow through the kidneys, and activate the RAAS. Use diuretics and fluid restrictions together.
- Continuous oxygen therapy to avoid hypoxia.
- Treatment of anemia with iron supplementation
- Bronchodilators to relax smooth muscles and increase airway patency when PH is associated with respiratory disease.
- Anticoagulant therapy in case of concurrent hypercoagulability (CTEPH)
- Cardiovascular drugs (ACEi, ARBs, ARNIs, BB, SGLT2) that are used to treat HF may be used for patients with PH, but there is a greater risk of a rapid drop in BP and heart rate. Use with caution.
- Phosphodiesterase type 5 inhibitors (PHE5) sildenafil and tadalafil work by opening the blood vessels in the lungs to increase blood flow in pulmonary arterial hypertension.

PH: Nursing interventions

- Collaborate care with a skilled team, which may include a cardiologist, pulmonologist, psychologist, a nutritionist, athletic trainer, and a cardiac rehabilitation team.
- Assess cardiopulmonary status. Auscultate heart and breath sounds, being alert for S_3 heart sounds, murmurs, or crackles indicating HF. Monitor vital signs, oxygen saturation, and heart rhythm.
- Assess hemodynamic status, including PAP and PAWP, every 2 hours or more often depending on the patient's condition and report any changes.
- Monitor intake and output closely and obtain daily weights. Institute fluid restriction as ordered.
- Administer medications as ordered to promote adequate heart and lung function. Assess for potential adverse reactions, such as orthostatic hypotension and bradycardia.
- Administer supplemental oxygen as ordered and organize care to allow rest periods. Monitor ABGs and pulse oximetry.
- Teach the patient about their diagnosis, medications, and treatments. Discuss adverse reactions of medications.
- Review a low-salt diet and fluid restrictions. Teach the patient to maintain an intake and output log.
- Teach the patient about signs and symptoms of HF such as increased shortness of breath, with activity or at rest, and increased fluid retention. Notify the health-care provider if signs or symptoms occur.
- Promote adherence to therapies. Facilitate access to care and medications in collaboration with the health-care team. Monitor medication use and adverse reactions. Assess patient's psychological status and motivation to participate in care.
- Document cardiac and respiratory status, vital signs, daily weight, intake and output, and pulse oximetry readings. Note the patient's response to treatment and document the patient's understanding of the teaching.

Inflammatory disorders

Inflammatory cardiac disorders include endocarditis, myocarditis, and pericarditis. In patients with these conditions, scar formation and otherwise normal healing processes can cause debilitating structural damage to the heart.

Endocarditis

Endocarditis is an inflammation of the endocardium, the heart valves, or prosthetic heart valves. It is typically caused by a bacterial invasion and, therefore, may also be referred to as *infective endocarditis* (IE). In IE, the leaflets of the heart valve begin to deteriorate and are eventually destroyed by bacterial invasion. Common organisms that cause endocarditis include staphylococci, especially *S. aureus*; streptococci; and *Candida albicans*. *Noninfective endocarditis* occurs when sterile blood clots develop on the valve in the absence of infection. It is often referred to as *nonbacterial thrombotic endocarditis* (NBTE).

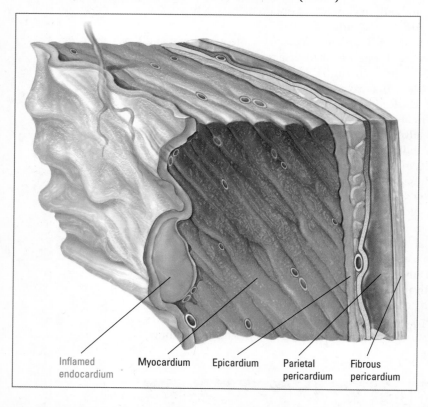

Inflamed endocardium   Myocardium   Epicardium   Parietal pericardium   Fibrous pericardium

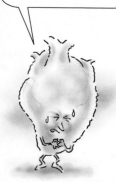

Untreated endocarditis usually proves fatal. However, with proper treatment, the cure rate ranges from 60% to 98%.

Location, location, location

Native valve endocarditis involves the aortic and mitral valves (left sided).

When IV drugs used and indwelling catheters induce endocarditis, the tricuspid valve is commonly affected (right side of the heart).

What to look for

- Fever occurs in 90% of patients
- New murmur or a change in existing murmur

IE—What's in a name?

The terminology used to describe IE changes as the causes of the disease become better understood. Some common names include the following:

- **acute bacterial endocarditis (ABE)**—describes a rapidly progressive disease process
- **subacute bacterial endocarditis (SBE)**—describes a disease process that lasts several months
- **rheumatic IE**—describes disease caused by rheumatic fever-related damage to heart valves caused by unresolved group A beta hemolytic streptococcal pharyngitis (strep throat)

- **native valve IE**—affects original heart valves
- **prosthetic valve IE**—affects artificial heart valves
- **IVDA IE**—affects IV drug users
- **nosocomial IE**—describes a disease that's associated with hospitalization.
- **Libman-Sacks endocarditis**—noninfective endocarditis found in people with systemic lupus erythematous

- Osler's nodes (tender purple lesions on the finger and toe tips)
- Janeway lesions (nontender erythematous papules or macules on the palms and soles)
- Splinter hemorrhages (on the distal portion of nails)
- Conjunctival petechiae

What to do

- Blood cultures—the diagnosis requires blood cultures to be drawn three times from different sites at least 1 hour apart.
- Additional labs—CBC with differential, C-reactive protein and rheumatoid factor (inflammation), kidney function (glomerulonephritis), and additional cultures from other body sources to identify the cause of the infection.
- Echocardiogram to evaluate the valve function.
- Provide IV antibiotics as ordered.
- Provide anticoagulant therapy as ordered.
- Assess and document the patient's vital signs, presence and worsening of a heart murmur, signs and symptoms of a blood clot, and hematuria.
- Promote activity and apply antiembolism stockings as ordered to prevent blood clots.

Myocarditis and pericarditis

Myocarditis is focal or diffuse inflammation of the cardiac muscle (myocardium). It can be acute, subacute, or chronic and can occur at any age. Pericarditis is inflammation of the sac or membrane around the heart. Both disorders are typically caused by a viral infection but can also be bacterial, protozoal, parasitic, or fungal in nature. Other noninfectious causes include autoimmune disorders. Pericarditis can be triggered by cancer treatments, recent cardiac surgery (when the pericardium was opened), or a recent MI (Dressler syndrome) (Barish & Hildalgo, 2021).

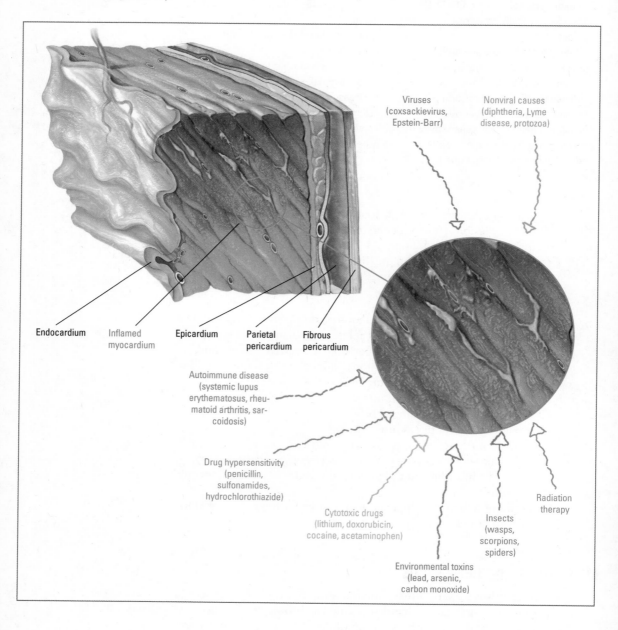

Viral myocarditis

Viral infections are the most common cause of myocarditis in the United States.

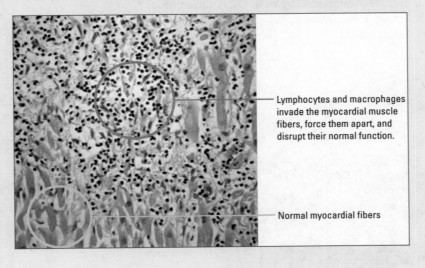

Lymphocytes and macrophages invade the myocardial muscle fibers, force them apart, and disrupt their normal function.

Normal myocardial fibers

What to look for

- Viral symptoms (fever, chills, myalgias)
- DOE and fatigue
- Palpitations
- Chest pain (possible and mild in severity)
- Severe disease—arrhythmias, signs and symptoms of HF

What to do

- Initial bed rest then a progressive return to physical activity
- Management of the underlying cause (antibiotics, immunotherapy)
- HF management in severe cases
- Continuous cardiac monitoring for arrhythmias
- Avoid NSAIDS for pain or fever control due to increased damage to the heart muscle
- Assess and document for arrhythmias, HF signs and symptoms, fevers, chills, malaise, and response to therapeutic interventions.

  Physical activity should not resume until the myocarditis symptoms are resolved. Young athletes must be removed or have limited participation in physical education and sports for at least 6 months.

Pericarditis

Pericarditis is an inflammation of the pericardium. Most cases are considered idiopathic and are presumed to be viral. Other causes of pericarditis include infection, inflammation, radiation therapy, trauma, renal failure, cancer, and MI.

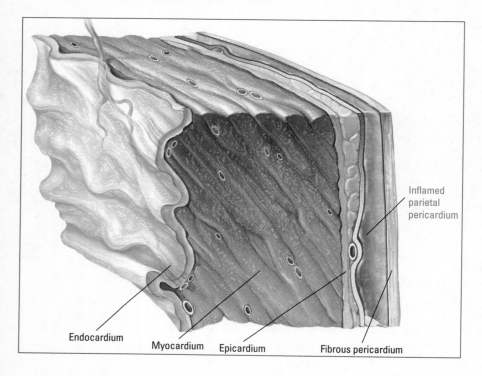

Inflamed parietal pericardium

Endocardium

Myocardium Epicardium Fibrous pericardium

What to look for

- Chest pain—severe and constant in nature, radiating to the neck and left scapula, worsened by deep inspirations and body movement
- Friction rub on auscultation over the left sternal border of the chest
- Fever
- Cough or hiccup
- Signs and symptoms of HF such as dyspnea, tachycardia, and peripheral edema
- Signs and symptoms of cardiac tamponade such as hypotension, muffled heart sounds, and jugular vein distention (Bickley, 2020a, 2020b)
- Pulsus paradoxus is a drop in systolic BP by more than 10 mm Hg with inspiration and indicates that a pericardial effusion is causing cardiac tamponade.

The inflammatory process in pericarditis

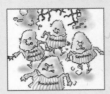 Pericardial tissue damaged by bacteria or other substances releases chemical mediators of inflammation into the surrounding tissue.

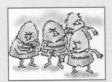 Friction occurs as the inflamed pericardial layers rub against each other.

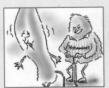 Histamines and other chemical mediators dilate vessels and increase vessel permeability.

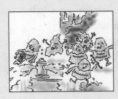 Fluids and protein (including fibrinogen) leak into the tissues, causing extracellular edema. Macrophages, neutrophils, and monocytes in the tissue begin to phagocytose the invading bacteria.

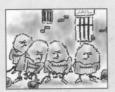 Gradually, the space fills with an exudate composed of necrotic tissue, dead and dying bacteria, neutrophils, and macrophages. These products are eventually reabsorbed into healthy tissue. Buildup of fluid can cause pericardial effusion. If the effusion builds too rapidly, cardiac tamponade may occur.

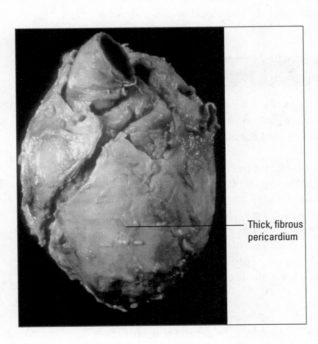

Thick, fibrous pericardium

What to do

- Maintain bedrest until symptoms subside.
- Identify pericardial effusion and inflammation surrounding the heart with an echocardiogram.
- Pericardiocentesis (needle inserted to remove fluid from the pericardium) to help with the diagnosis of pericarditis and relieve the pressure around the heart muscle and coronary arteries. Send fluid for analysis to identify the cause of the accumulation. After the procedure, insert a catheter in the pericardium so that drainage can continue until symptoms improve.
- NSAIDs are prescribed for pain. Corticosteroids can be used if the patient is allergic to NSAIDs or aspirin.
- Colchicine is prescribed if pain is not relieved with NSAIDs.
- Treatment for the underlying cause (infection).
- Assess and document cardiac friction rub, signs and symptoms of infection, cardiac tamponade, and HF.
- Assess the patient's pain and response to pain control. Assist with activities and positioning of the patient to decrease painful triggers.
- Gradually increase activities as the friction rub, fever, and pain subside.
- In severe cases, a pericardial resection is necessary to release the pressure surrounding the heart muscle and blood vessels (Barish & Hildalgo, 2021).

Valvular disorders

The opening and closing of heart valves generate the S1 and S1 heart sounds or "lub-dub." Valvular disorders can cause distinct types of murmurs and will be heard loudest over the affected valve and can cause extra heart sounds (S3, S4).

Stenotic valves narrow the opening between the heart chambers and obstruct blood flow. This narrowing can be caused by calcifications (or hardening) and scarring of the heart valves, which sometimes leads to fusion of the leaflets on the valve.

Valves that do not close completely cause a regurgitation of blood flow backwards into the previous heart chamber. A prolapsed valve or fallen valve can cause a regurgitation of blood flow. Myxomatous degeneration or a weakening of a valve closure is an expected finding related to aging.

Other possible causes of valvular disorders

- Calcified degeneration of the valves due to "wear and tear," inflammatory processes, and atherosclerosis
- Endocarditis (rheumatic, infectious)

- HCM
- Connective tissue disorder such as lupus
- Congenital abnormalities

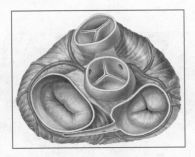

Potential complications of valvular disorders
- Syncope (exertional)
- HF
- Arrhythmias—atrial fibrillation
- Angina (Barish & Hildalgo, 2021)

Mitral valve prolapse and mitral valve regurgitation

Generally, a benign disorder, mitral valve prolapse causes the valve to bulge into the left atrium. Mitral valve prolapse can be made worse at times of increased fluid volume, such as pregnancy.

When mitral valve prolapse leads to regurgitation or a leaking of blood back into the left atrium. This is called mitral valve regurgitation. Mitral valve regurgitation is also caused by degeneration of the valve due to endocarditis, rheumatic heart disease, and calcifications (Keller, Sabatino, Winland-Brown, & Porter, 2022).

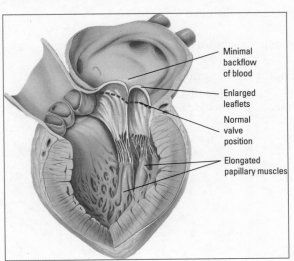

Minimal backflow of blood

Enlarged leaflets

Normal valve position

Elongated papillary muscles

Mitral regurgitation

Mitral regurgitation occurs when the mitral valve doesn't close completely, allowing blood to flow back through the valve.

1

Blood from the left ventricle flows back into the left atrium during systole, causing the atrium to enlarge to accommodate the backflow.

2

As a result, the left ventricle dilates to accommodate the increased blood volume from the atrium and to compensate for diminished cardiac output.

3

Ventricular hypertrophy and increased back-pressure in the left atrium result in increased PAP, eventually leading to left-sided and right-sided HF.

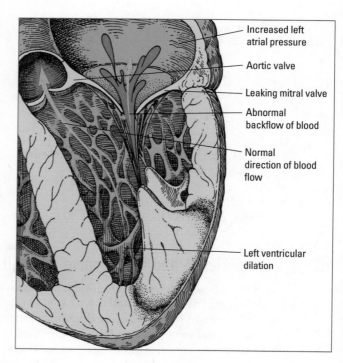

Increased left atrial pressure

Aortic valve

Leaking mitral valve

Abnormal backflow of blood

Normal direction of blood flow

Left ventricular dilation

What to look for

- Murmur—heard loudest at the apex of the heart while the patient is lying on their left side
- Mitral valve prolapse—midsystolic click heard between the "lub" and the "dub"
- Mitral valve regurgitation—a holosystolic murmur or a murmur heard from the end of the "lub" to the beginning of the "dub"
- Severe cases of mitral regurgitation may include signs and symptoms of HF or shock.

Management

- Most patients are asymptomatic, so management includes using echocardiograms to monitor the worsening of the disease over time
- Valve replacement or repair in severe cases
- Some patients may be on antithrombotic medications to prevent emboli.

Mitral valve stenosis

Mitral valve stenosis is hardening of the mitral valve caused by fibrosis or calcification. This hardening results in narrowing of the valve opening, which obstructs blood flow from the left atrium to the left ventricle. Consequently, left atrial volume and pressure increase, and the chamber dilates.

Mitral stenosis typically occurs in females. It most commonly results from rheumatic fever and may also be associated with congenital anomalies.

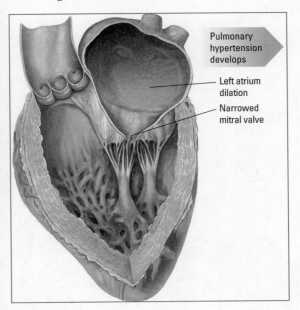

Pulmonary hypertension develops

Left atrium dilation

Narrowed mitral valve

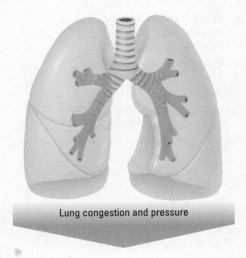

Lung congestion and pressure

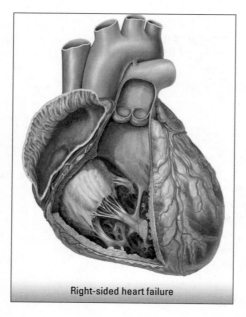

Right-sided heart failure

What to look for

- DOE, PND, and orthopnea
- Fatigue and weakness
- Right-sided HF and cardiac arrhythmias
- Crackles on auscultation

Management

Medications to manage the complications such as arrhythmias and HF valve surgery in severe cases

Aortic regurgitation

Aortic regurgitation occurs when the aortic semilunar valve doesn't close completely. In this condition, blood flows back through the valve into the left ventricle. It can result from IE or aortic dissection or it may be idiopathic.

Marfan syndrome, an inherited connective tissue disease, can cause valvular disorders such as mitral valve prolapse, aortic stenosis, aortic regurgitation, and aortic dissection. (For more on findings of Marfan syndrome, see *Hypertrophic cardiomyopathy* on page 201.)

What to look for

- Blowing, high-pitched murmur or S_3 heart sound
- Orthopnea and PND
- Angina
- Signs of left-sided HF
- Wide pulse pressure (low diastolic BP)
- Bounding carotid pulse (de Musset's sign—bobbing of the head with every pulse)

What to do

- No interventions are required for asymptomatic, mild, and moderate cases.
- Serial echocardiograms to monitor the disease progression.
- Valve replacement in severe cases. (See *Treatments* chapter.)

Aortic stenosis

Older patients are at increased risk of aortic stenosis due to atherosclerosis, which results in calcification of the valves. Patients are usually asymptomatic, and aortic stenosis is found on a routine cardiac examination. The prognosis decreases as symptoms develop and worsen. Exertional activities may provoke symptoms.

What to look for

Physical examination—heart sounds
- Ejection "click"
- High-pitched, harsh, blowing murmur heard loudest at the second ICS right sternal border—a sign of turbulent blood flow through the valve
- S_2 heart sound may split producing a gallop sound

Early symptoms
- Exertional dyspnea or decreased exercise tolerance
- Syncope, presyncope, or exertional dizziness
- Exertional angina

Classic or end-stage symptoms
- Angina
- Left-sided HF
- Syncope, exertional

What to do
- No interventions are required for asymptomatic, mild, and moderate cases.
- Serial echocardiograms to monitor the disease progression.
- Aortic valve replacement (AVR) is recommended in severe cases. (See *Treatment* chapter.)
- Educate the patient to avoid rigorous physical activity unless cleared to participate.

Promote medication adherence and lifestyle modifications to manage hypertension, HF, and atherosclerosis as these conditions can worsen aortic stenosis.

Vascular disorders

Vascular disorders can affect both arteries and veins. Arterial disorders include aneurysms, which result from weakening of the arterial wall, with dilation of the aorta, and arterial occlusive disease, which commonly results from atherosclerotic narrowing of the artery's lumen. Thrombophlebitis results from inflammation or occlusion of the veins. Patients with PAD also experience compromised blood flow from atherosclerosis much like CAD. The same risk factors for CAD apply to PAD. Risk factors include stroke, MI, and cardiovascular death. PAD can be life threatening if blockages in the vessels compromise circulation and oxygen delivery.

Aortic aneurysms

An aortic aneurysm is a potentially life-threatening condition. An aortic rupture is caused by a continued weakening of the aortic wall resulting in loss of tissue integrity and thus blood loss outside the aorta. The aorta begins to dilate with increased age. The average size of the aorta is 2 to 3 cm (about 1.18 inches). The abdominal aorta is the most common site for an aneurysm.

Aneurysms arise from a defect in the middle layer of the arterial wall (tunica media or medial layer). When the elastic fibers and collagen in the middle layer are damaged and stretched, segmental dilation occurs. As a result, the medial layer loses some of its elasticity, and it fragments. Smooth muscle cells are lost, and the wall thins. There are two types or shapes of aneurysms. The uniform shape includes dilation of the whole circumference of the aortic wall. The sacculated aneurysm is more localized and appears as a pouch, or saclike portion, of the aortic wall and may be caused by plaque hemorrhage or infection and is more likely to rupture.

A treatment for all ages

Valve repair, over replacement, is recommended for children.

Bioprosthetic valves are recommended for ages 50 and below.

Mechanical valves are recommended for ages 65 and above.

Either bioprosthetic or mechanical valve replacement for ages 50–65 years.

Thin and thinner

The thinned wall may contain calcium deposits and atherosclerotic plaque, making the wall brittle. As a person ages, the elastin in the wall decreases, further weakening the vessel. If hypertension is present, dilation of the arterial wall occurs more quickly, resulting in additional weakening.

Wide vessel, slow flow

When an aneurysm begins to develop, lateral pressure increases, causing the vessel lumen to widen and blood flow to slow. A thrombus may form within the dilated area. Over time, mechanical stressors contribute to elongation of the aneurysm.

Blood forces

Hemodynamic forces (hypertension, thrombus formation) may also play a role, causing pulsatile stresses on the weakened wall and pressing on the small vessels that supply nutrients to the arterial wall. In aortic aneurysms, this causes the aorta to become bowed and tortuous.

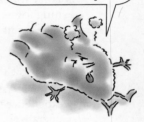

An aneurysm generally produces no symptoms, at least in the beginning. If it ruptures, however, immediate treatment is necessary.

Deadly complications

Major complications of an aortic aneurysms include hemorrhage, MI, renal failure, embolus, cerebrovascular insufficiency, hemodynamic collapse, and death. These complications can occur without any warning. Fortunately, there are screening recommendations for at-risk patients to avoid these poor outcomes.

Abdominal Aortic aneurysm

An aneurysm is an abnormal dilation in a weakened arterial wall. Abdominal aortic aneurysms (AAAs) typically occur in the abdominal aorta between the renal arteries and the iliac branches, but the thoracic aorta may also be affected. During AAA formation, a thrombus builds up along the weakened wall and may be dispersed with the rupturing of the aneurysm.

Risk factors of AAA

The exact cause of an AAA is unclear, but several factors place a person at risk:
- Older age (prevalence increases at age 50 years and over)
- Male gender
- Smoker
- Caucasian race
- Family history of AAA

Potential risk factors of an AAA:

- Hypertension
- Taller height
- CAD
- Atherosclerosis and hyperlipidemia
- Stroke

No warning

Since an AAA is typically asymptomatic, the prognosis is poor for patients that present with symptoms. There are national screening recommendations from the U.S. Preventive Services Health Task Force for at-risk patients to avoid complications. A one-time screening for a AAA with an ultrasound is recommended for all men between the ages of 65 and 75 years who are current or former smokers.

What to look for

Most AAAs are asymptomatic, and if the patient has symptoms, they may experience the following:

- Generalized, steady abdominal pain described as tearing, severe, throbbing
- Lower back pain, flank, or chest pain that's unaffected by movement
- Nausea and gastric or abdominal fullness
- A palpable, pulsating mass in the periumbilical area
- Bruit over the abdominal aorta or femoral arteries on auscultation of the abdomen
- Hypotension and cyanosis in the lower extremities (with aneurysm rupture).

Thoracic aortic aneurysm

Most thoracic aortic aneurysms (TAAs) are caused by atherosclerosis. They typically occur in males from ages 50 to 70 years. Risk factors include a strong familial history of aneurysm, genetic disposition, renal cysts, or connective tissue diseases (e.g., Marfan syndrome, Ehlers-Danlos syndrome, Turner syndrome, or Loeys-Dietz syndrome; Monaro & Walsh, 2021).

Some cases of TAAs are asymptomatic. The characteristics of the symptoms depend on the location and severity of the dilation of the TAA. If the aneurysm is closer to the laryngeal nerve and esophagus, the symptoms involve the throat. Difficulty in breathing and coughing present if the aneurysm blocks the lower respiratory tract. If the aneurysm is pressing on the cervical sympathetic nerve chain, there can be abnormalities of the pupil.

Symptoms of a TAA
- Pain—chronic deep aching in chest wall worsened when supine
- Respiratory symptoms—dyspnea, sudden, hoarse coughing attacks, stridor
- Throat symptoms—weak voice or loss of voice, difficulty swallowing
- Eyes—unequal pupils

What tests tell you
Most aneurysms are found incidentally during a physical examination or during testing for other medical problems.
- In a suspected leaking aneurysm, a CBC may reveal leukocytosis, and a decrease in hemoglobin and hematocrit, elevated levels of fibrinogen, D-dimer, and thrombin may indicate thrombin formation in or around the aneurysm.
- Abdominal ultrasound is the recommended choice to diagnosis a AAA. It is noninvasive, inexpensive, and accurate. Serial ultrasounds are performed every 6 months to monitor the size of a smaller aneurysm found while screening or as an incidental exam finding. TEE allows visualization of a TAA. It's combined with Doppler flow studies to provide information about blood flow. Computed tomography angiography (CTA) provides a more detailed view to identifying the size and location of the aneurysm. Contrast dye is injected to visualize the vasculature to test for an aneurysm. Anteroposterior and lateral x-rays of the chest or abdomen can be used to detect thoracic aortic calcification, widened mediastinal, enlarged aortic knob, and displaced trachea from a large TAA. MRI can disclose the aneurysm's size in detail and the effect on nearby organs.

How it's treated
Aneurysm treatment usually involves open surgery or an endovascular approach. The choice of repair is dependent on presenting symptoms and the urgency of the condition. The risk of dissection or rupture increases with the size of the aneurysm. A ruptured aneurysm is usually fatal if left untreated or treatment is delayed.

Aortic and thoracic aneurysms doubling in size or a ruptured aneurysm requires immediate open surgical resection and replacement of the aortic section using a vascular or Dacron graft. Treatment for a ruptured aneurysm includes fluid resuscitation and blood replacement. However, keep these points in mind:
- If the aneurysm is small and produces no symptoms, surgery may be delayed, with regular physical examination and ultrasound to monitor aneurysm progression.

- Large aneurysms and those in symptomatic patients, who are at risk for rupture, need immediate surgical repair.
- A nonsurgical procedure called an endovascular aneurysm repair (EVAR) grafting may be an option for a patient with an AAA. (See *Endovascular aneurysm repair grafting for AAA.*)
- Medications to control BP, to decrease the workload of the heart, to treat dyslipidemia, to relieve anxiety, and to control pain are also prescribed.

Rush to respond to rupture

Rupture of an aortic aneurysm is a medical emergency requiring prompt treatment, including the following:

- Resuscitation with IV fluids and prepare for massive transfusions (packed red blood cells [PRBCs], fresh frozen plasma [FFP])
- BBs to reduce BP and maintain a systolic BP of 80 to 100 mm Hg
- Analgesics to relieve pain
- An arterial line and indwelling urinary catheter to monitor the patient's condition preoperatively.

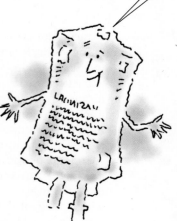

Treatment for a ruptured aortic aneurysm includes fluid resuscitation, blood replacement, and IV drugs.

Endovascular aneurysm repair grafting for AAA

EVAR grafting, shown at right, is a noninvasive procedure in which the walls of the aorta are reinforced to prevent expansion and rupture of an AAA. The stent graft is threaded through the femoral or iliac artery and placed within the AAA. Blood circulation is then routed through the graft and doesn't enter the aneurysm sac. The procedure can be done using local or regional anesthesia. Because the procedure is performed percutaneously, it's less invasive than an open surgical repair and associated with reduced mortality risk.

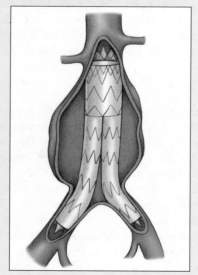

What to do

- Collaborate care with a skilled team, which may include emergency medical personnel, a vascular surgeon, cardiologist, nutritionist, and physical therapists.
- Assess the patient's vital signs, especially BP, frequently. Monitor BP and all pulses in the extremities and compare findings bilaterally.
- New studies suggest keeping the BP in the "permissive hypotension" (systolic 80 to 100 mm Hg) state, which may prevent further tearing of the aneurysm and lessen blood loss.
- Assess cardiovascular status frequently, including heart rate, rhythm, ECG, and cardiac enzyme levels. An MI is one of the most common complications.
- Obtain blood samples to evaluate kidney function by assessing BUN, creatinine, and electrolyte levels. Measure intake and output.
- Monitor CBC for evidence of blood loss, including decreased hemoglobin level, hematocrit, and RBC count.
- If the patient's condition changes acutely, obtain an arterial blood sample for arterial blood gas analysis, as ordered, and monitor cardiac rhythm. Assist with arterial line insertion to allow for continuous BP monitoring. Assist with insertion of a PA catheter to assess hemodynamic status.
- Administer beta-blockers to control hypertension. Provide analgesics to relieve pain, if present.
- Discuss screening recommendations for AAA with at-risk patients.
- Observe the patient for signs of rupture, which may be immediately fatal. Watch closely for any signs of acute blood loss: hypotension; tachycardia; tachypnea; cool, clammy skin; restlessness; and decreased level of consciousness.
- Explain the surgical procedure and the expected postoperative care to the patient and family.
- Reinforce instructions for controlling BP. Stress the importance of medications and diet therapy and the need for smoking cessation.

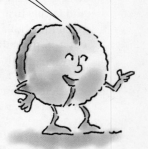

Analgesics can help relieve pain.

Rupture response

- If rupture occurs, insert two large-bore IV catheters, begin fluid resuscitation, and prepare for massive blood transfusion.
- If the patient is experiencing acute pain, administer pain medication as ordered.
- Prepare the patient for emergency surgery.

Peripheral arterial disease

PAD is a marker of systemic atherosclerosis. Most patients who have peripheral arterial or vascular disease also have CAD. It may affect large vessels, such as the aorta and its branches, or the subclavian, mesenteric, renal, or peripheral vessels. It may be acute or chronic. Ischemia occurs when there is an imbalance between blood supply and demand to the vessel. PAD usually affects the lower extremities, and patients are initially asymptomatic. An ulcer on an extremity can be an obvious indication of limb ischemia, but limb pain with ambulation or pain at rest, claudication, and diminished pulses can be a clinical sign of PAD. Major complications of PAD include severe pain, limb paralysis, infection, gangrene, limb loss, and death.

What causes it

Risk factors for PAD include smoking, aging, inactivity, IV drug use, and family history of vascular disease due to atherosclerosis. A diagnosis of metabolic syndrome (hypertension, obesity, hypercholesterolemia, and insulin resistance), atrial fibrillation, recent MI, and HF are associated with an increased risk of developing CAD and PAD.

These risk factors contribute to the development of plaques (atherosclerosis) and thromboses. Trauma to the arterial vessels can cause an occlusion, rupture, or tearing.

How it happens

In PAD, obstruction or narrowing of the lumen of the aorta, its major branches, and peripheral circulation causes an interruption of blood flow.

Location and timing

Prognosis depends on the location of the occlusion; the development of collateral circulation to counteract reduced blood flow; and in cases of an acute disease, the time elapsed between formation of the occlusion and restoration of adequate blood flow. Intermittent claudication is an indication of PAD. Patients will experience symptomatic pain from decreased blood supply to the affected limb during exercise. The pain is relieved by rest and return of blood flow to the affected limb.

What your patient says

Patients with PAD usually present with symptoms of lower-extremity pain, claudication, numbness, or limb ischemia. However, some patients are asymptomatic. Patients with claudication can complain of buttock, hip, thigh, calf, or foot pain.

There is a relationship between the pain location and the anatomic site of the PAD.

- Buttock and hip pain are associated with aortoiliac disease.
- Thigh pain is associated with aortoiliac or femoral artery disease.

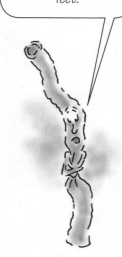

An occluded artery slows blood flow, usually to the legs and feet.

- Upper calf pain is associated with superficial femoral artery disease.
- Lower calf pain is associated with popliteal artery disease.
- Foot pain is associated with tibial or peroneal artery disease. (See *Possible sites of major artery occlusion* and *Types of peripheral arterial disease*, page 247.)

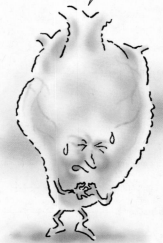

Pain is one of the six classic Ps of arterial occlusion.

Let's not forget the rest

Other signs and symptoms:
- Intermittent claudication with activity or exercise
- Burning pain in the feet (aggravated by elevating the extremity and sometimes relieved by keeping the extremity in a dependent position)
- Pallor on elevation, followed by redness with dependency
- Delayed capillary filling; hair loss; or dry, shiny skin with trophic nail changes

Never forget the classics

Acute arterial occlusion can be caused by a fracture (compartment syndrome) or another trauma that damages the vessels, plaque formation from atherosclerosis, an occluded stent, or emboli. Symptoms are considered as the six classic Ps:
1. Pain
2. Pallor
3. Pulselessness
4. Paresthesia (numbness)
5. Paralysis
6. Poikilothermy (cold).

What to look for

PAD can be suspected if the patient presents with claudication. A physical exam may reveal the following:
- Diminished or absent pulses (may need a Doppler to assess pulses), cool extremities
- Pallor on leg elevation above the heart
- Shiny atrophied skin, nail changes, poor wound healing, hair loss over the anterior lower extremities
- Ulcers located on the bony prominences of the feet which can lead to gangrene
- Calf asymmetry due to muscle atrophy (Bickley, 2020a, 2020b)

  With arterial disease, extremities are cold, numb, and pale. Ulcers occur over the bony areas of the foot and the toes. With venous disease, extremities are reddened, swollen, and warm to touch. Ulcers occur between the medial aspect below the knee and around the ankle.

Possible sites of major artery occlusion

This illustration points out the possible sites of major artery occlusion.

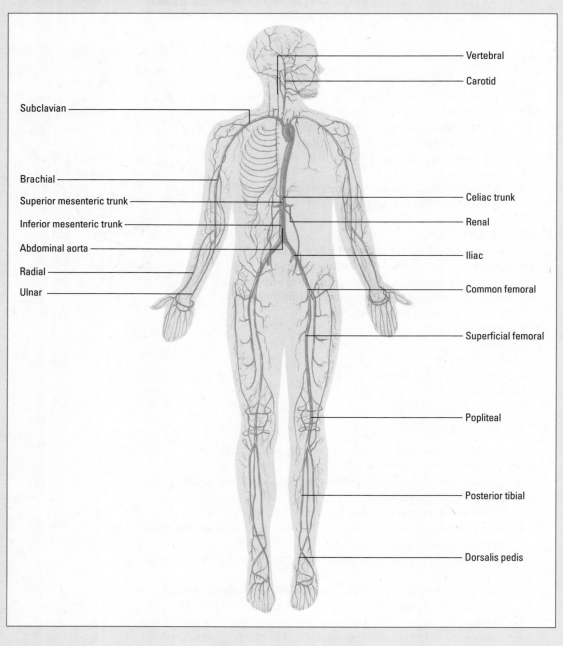

Vertebral

Carotid

Subclavian

Brachial

Superior mesenteric trunk

Inferior mesenteric trunk

Abdominal aorta

Radial

Ulnar

Celiac trunk

Renal

Iliac

Common femoral

Superficial femoral

Popliteal

Posterior tibial

Dorsalis pedis

Types of peripheral arterial disease

The signs and symptoms of PAD depend on the location of the occlusion. Use the *Types of peripheral arterial disease* chart to help determine the site of your patient's occlusion.

Site of occlusion	Signs and symptoms
Carotid arterial system • Internal carotids • External carotids	Neurologic dysfunction: transient ischemic attacks (TIAs) due to reduced cerebral circulation produce unilateral sensory or motor dysfunction (transient monocular blindness, hemiparesis), possible aphasia or dysarthria, confusion, decreased mentation, and, rarely, headache. These recurrent clinical features may last 5–10 minutes but may persist up to 24 hours and may herald a stroke. Decreased pulsation may be palpated or a bruit may be heard over the affected vessels.
Vertebrobasilar system • Vertebral arteries • Basilar arteries	Neurologic dysfunction: TIAs of the brain stem and cerebellum produce binocular visual disturbances, vertigo, dysarthria, and "drop attacks" (falling down without loss of consciousness); less common than carotid territory TIA
Innominate • Brachiocephalic artery	Neurologic dysfunction: signs and symptoms of vertebrobasilar insufficiency; decreased right arm pulses with claudication symptoms; possible bruit over lower right side of neck
Subclavian artery	Subclavian steal syndrome (characterized by reversed blood flow from the brain through the vertebral artery on the same side as the occlusion into the subclavian artery distal to the occlusion); clinical effects of vertebrobasilar insufficiency and exercise-induced arm claudication; rarely, gangrene, usually limited to the digits
Mesenteric artery • Superior (most commonly affected) • Celiac axis • Inferior	Bowel ischemia, infarct necrosis, and gangrene; sudden severe acute abdominal pain; nausea and vomiting; diarrhea; leukocytosis; and shock due to massive intraluminal fluid shifts
Aortic bifurcation (saddle block occlusion; if acute, a medical emergency associated with cardiac embolization)	Sensory and motor deficits (muscle weakness, numbness, paresthesia, paralysis) and signs of ischemia (sudden pain; cold, pale legs with markedly decreased or absent peripheral pulses) and minimal to absent Doppler signals in both legs.
Iliac artery (Leriche's syndrome)	Exercise-induced claudication of lower back, buttocks, and thighs, relieved by rest; absent or reduced femoral or distal pulses; erectile dysfunction in males
Femoral and popliteal artery (may be associated with aneurysm formation)	Intermittent claudication of the calves or thighs on exertion; pain in feet at rest; leg pallor and coolness; blanching of feet on elevation and dependent rubor; gangrene; no palpable pulses in ankles and feet; absent to minimal Doppler signals

What tests tell you

The severity of PAD can be evaluated by calculating the ankle-brachial index (ABI) and by comparing the resting systolic BP at the ankle with the systolic brachial pressure. It is expected to find the pressure in the ankle higher than that in the arm. ABI normal range is 1.00 to 1.09. As the ABI decreases, the pressure in the ankle decreases, and the difference between the ankle arterial pressure and brachial arterial pressure narrows. An ABI of <0.90 is diagnostic for PAD, and that <0.50 is considered severe PAD (Bickley, 2020a, 2020b).

- Ultrasound and duplex imaging provide specific disease location, blood velocity, and grading of extent of disease. Arteriography, which demonstrates the type (thrombus or embolus), location, and degree of obstruction, helps evaluate the collateral circulation. It is particularly useful for diagnosing chronic forms of disease and evaluating candidates for reconstructive surgery.
- Doppler duplex ultrasound and plethysmography show the speed, direction, and pattern of blood flow through the arteries and quantifies the blood flow to extremities.
- CT scanning and magnetic resonance angiography (MRA) are advanced tests, which offer the high-resolution images of disease progression and vascular obstruction.
- Arteriography remains the gold standard for vascular imaging, detection, and treatment angioplasty and stent placement.
- A physical exam may reveal Buerger disease, which is strongly linked to tobacco use. The blood vessels swell, and clots can form and occlude blood flow. This can lead to limb amputation (Bickley, 2020a, 2020b & CDC).

How it's treated

Treatment for PAD depends on the cause, location, and degree of the obstruction.

- Mild chronic disease is treated with supportive measures and risk factor modifications. Smoking cessation is highly recommended along with a supervised exercise regimen to promote walking and reduce symptoms.
- Management of concomitant chronic diseases to halt the progression of PAD such as hypertension, diabetes, and hyperlipidemia.
- Cilostazol, a PHD type 3 inhibitor, causes vasodilation and decreases platelet aggregation. This drug is used to improve claudication symptoms.
- Antiplatelet therapy: aspirin or clopidogrel (if allergic to aspirin) will prevent thromboembolic that can lead to MI or stroke.

Patients with PAD undergoing some surgical interventions for the disease may take both aspirin and clopidogrel together.

- Systemic anticoagulation with heparin or catheter-based thrombolytic therapy may be used to treat acute arterial thrombosis (Gerhard et al., 2017).

Embolectomy, grafting, amputation—oh, my!

Revascularization, percutaneous or surgical, is the best option for patients with advanced PAD. Percutaneous transluminal angioplasty (PTA) is used with or without stenting to relieve symptoms and improve circulation. This is a less invasive alternative to surgery. Appropriate surgical procedures may include embolectomy, thromboendarterectomy, patch arthroplasty, bypass grafting, and lumbar sympathectomy. Bypass grafting surgery is the preferred method because of the long-term lasting benefits of bypass surgery. Amputation becomes necessary with failure of medication therapy and arterial interventions or with the development of nonhealing ulcers, wounds, or untreatable infections.

What to do

- Collaborate care with a skilled team, which may include a vascular surgeon, cardiologist, nutritionist, and physical therapists.
- Assess affected limb for pulses, pain, color, temperature, wound healing, and signs of infection.
- Monitor BP and glucose levels
- Provide a low-cholesterol, DASH diet
- Assess and promote smoking cessation
- Make smoking cessation a priority and strongly advise the patient to stop smoking and refer the patient to a smoking-cessation program, if appropriate.
- Monitor for groin hematoma, pseudoaneurysm, or distal embolization

Pseudoaneurysm

A pseudoaneurysm forms when trauma to the arterial wall causes blood to leak into surrounding tissues, forming a pulsatile hematoma. Pseudoaneurysms are commonly caused by interventional or catheterization procedures in which large catheters and sheaths are used to cannulate arteries. They're also a common complication from vascular surgery. Less commonly, they may be caused by an infection or cancer that damages the arterial wall. Small pseudoaneurysms may spontaneously thrombose and not require treatment.

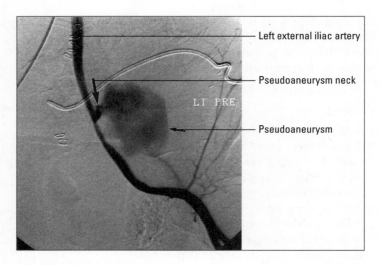

- Left external iliac artery
- Pseudoaneurysm neck

LT PRE

- Pseudoaneurysm

What to look for

- Swelling and pain at the insertion site
- Pulsatile mass
- Bruit
- Palpable thrill
- "To and fro" murmur over mass
- Extensive ecchymosis

What to do

- Evaluate the patient's response to treatment. The patient should be able to increase exercise tolerance without developing pain.
- Teach proper foot care or other appropriate measures, depending on the affected area. Recommend follow-up with a podiatrist.
- Document cardiac and neurovascular status, along with vital signs and wound condition and care, and response to interventions.
- Document teaching provided to the patient and the patient's understanding of instructions.

Patient precautions

- Caution the patient against wearing constrictive clothing or crossing legs while sitting.
- Instruct the patient about signs of recurrence (pain, pallor, numbness, paralysis, absence of pulse) that can result from a graft occlusion or occlusion at another site.
- Teach the patient to palpate pulses and assess skin color and temperature.
- Immediately report any changes to the health-care provider.

RX

Ultrasound-guided
     direct compression
     maneuvers
Thrombin injection
Arterioplasty
Endovascular stent
     placement

- Encourage the patient to follow the prescribed medication regimen closely.
- Advise the patient to avoid temperature extremes.
- Assist the patient in adjusting to lifestyle constraints.

Thrombophlebitis

An acute condition characterized by inflammation and thrombus formation, thrombophlebitis may develop in deep intramuscular veins known as deep vein thrombosis or DVT or superficial (subcutaneous) veins known as superficial vein thrombosis (SVT).

On the surface

SVT is inflammation and clot formation along one or more superficial veins. In the absence of cancer, common types of SVT are varicose veins and infusion thrombophlebitis (IV therapy). The SVT is not dangerous but can increase the risk of a DVT (Goldman, 2017 & DynaMed).

Another form of an SVT is a thrombosed hemorrhoid. This type of hemorrhoid is severely painful, swollen, and bluish in color.

Deep vein, deep trouble

DVT can affect small veins as well as large veins, such as the vena cava and the femoral, iliac, and subclavian veins. DVT is usually progressive and may lead to PE or coronary thrombosis, potentially fatal conditions. Treatment is aimed at treating the symptoms and preventing further complications.

How they happen

Alteration in the epithelial lining causes platelet aggregation and fibrin entrapment of RBCs, white blood cells, and additional platelets. The thrombus initiates a chemical inflammatory process in the vessel epithelium that leads to fibrosis, which may occlude the vessel lumen or embolize.

Even more trouble

Post-thrombotic (or post-phlebitic) syndrome (PTS) is a chronic complication of DVT. This is caused by venous hypertension because the lower-extremity valves are incompetent and cannot push the dependent blood flow back up to the heart. Blood and fluid accumulate in the lower extremities. This syndrome results in an increased risk of future episodes of DVTs. Signs and symptoms are similar to those of chronic venous disease:

- Pitting edema
- Brown hyperpigmented skin

- Telangiectasia particularly around the ankle
- Feeling of heaviness in the extremity
- Pain—leg cramps, paresthesias
- Itchy, thickened skin patches (venous eczema)
- Ulcerations—open or healed

Prevention and treatment for PTS include compression stockings, graduated compression devices, and exercise to promote calf compression (Kahn et al., 2014).

Superficial swell

SVT may produce the following signs and symptoms along the length of the affected vein in a linear pattern.

Varicose veins will present in a clustered appearance:

- Swelling (first sign)
- Pain
- Heat
- Redness

What causes it

SVT may occur due to the following:

- Varicose veins
- Trauma
- Malignancy
- Infection
- IV drug use
- Chemical irritation caused by IV fluid administration
- Systemic inflammatory disorders

What to do

- Apply heat to the area as ordered.
- Give NSAIDs as ordered to decrease inflammation and control the pain.
- Doppler studies may be ordered if the thrombosis is severe or a DVT is suspected.
- Anticoagulants (low-molecular-weight heparin) may be ordered in severe cases.
- In the case of IV fluid administration, discontinue IV fluids and initially apply a cold compress followed by heat to the area. Elevate the arm. Restart the IV access on the opposite arm.
- Assess for signs and symptoms of infection at the IV site such as purulent discharge.
- Assess skin integrity before and after the application of cold and heat.
- Elevate the affected extremity.
- Provide pain management as ordered.
- Watch for signs and symptoms of a dangerous venous thrombosis—severe pain, redness and swelling of the extremity (DVT),

shortness of breath and chest pain (PE), chest pain radiating to left arm, neck or jaw, diaphoresis, shortness of breath (coronary thrombosis).

- Document skin assessment, cardiovascular status of the extremities, vital signs, signs and symptoms of infection and venous thrombosis, and response to pain management (Capriotti, 2021).

Even more trouble

Other complications of thrombophlebitis include respiratory failure, right-sided HF, and postphlebitic syndrome (chronic edema, pain, venous stasis, ulcerations, and recurrent episodes of thrombophlebitis). (See *Understanding thrombophlebitis*.)

Deeper trouble

Although DVT may be idiopathic, it usually results in inflammation and embolism from endothelial damage, infection, accelerated blood clotting, or reduced blood flow.

Certain factors increase the risk of developing DVT. These factors include the following:

- coagulation abnormalities
- endothelial dysfunction
- prolonged immobility (venous stasis)
- IV drug use
- infection
- trauma
- postpartum, usually 1 month after childbirth
- use of estrogen-progestin contraceptives
- estrogen therapy
- abdominal surgery
- major joint replacement surgery.

What to look for

Clinical features vary with the site and length of the affected vein. DVT may produce the following:

- Pain and tenderness
- Swelling of the affected extremity
- Erythema
- Malaise

What tests tell you

- A Doppler duplex ultrasound shows blood flow in a specific area and can reveal the cause of any obstruction to venous blood flow.
- Phlebography (also called venography), which uses dye, is used less frequently and shows filling defects and diverted blood flow.
- CTs and MRIs provide visual images of veins and the presence of thrombus (Woo, 2019).

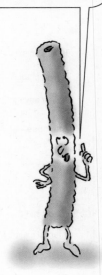

DVT can affect small veins, such as the soleal venous sinuses, and large veins, such as the vena cava.

Understanding thrombophlebitis

Thrombophlebitis can occur in any vein thrombus formation with inflammation. It most commonly occurs at valve sites, as shown below.

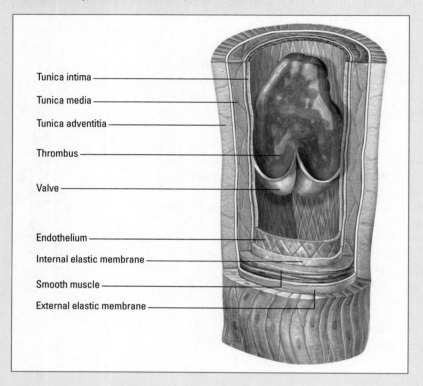

Tunica intima

Tunica media

Tunica adventitia

Thrombus

Valve

Endothelium

Internal elastic membrane

Smooth muscle

External elastic membrane

How it's treated

Treatment aims to control thrombus development, prevent postphlebitic syndrome and other complications, relieve pain, and prevent recurrence. Symptomatic relief measures include bed rest with elevation of the affected arm or leg; warm, moist soaks to the affected area; and analgesics as ordered. Therapy for severe superficial thrombophlebitis may include an anti-inflammatory medication along with antiembolism stockings, elevation of the affected extremity, and anticoagulants for those who are at a higher risk of developing complications. After an acute episode of DVT subsides, the patient may begin to walk while wearing antiembolism stockings (applied before getting out of bed).

Treatment for a DVT includes anticoagulants. The classification of anticoagulants used depends on the setting, cost, and the patient's ability to participate in the plan (given subcutaneous (SC) injections, frequent lab monitoring). Options for pharmacotherapy will include the following:

- IV unfractionated or low-molecular-weight heparin or SC fondaparinux if the patient is hospitalized.
- SC low-molecular-weight heparin or fondaparinux can be started as inpatient or outpatient.
- Oral warfarin, which acts on several different clotting factors or oral direct factor Xa inhibitors, which acts more selectively, will both prolong clotting time. Treatment typically lasts for 3 months.
- Oral antiplatelet drugs like clopidogrel and aspirin are used in the prevention and treatment of recent MI and stroke.

Drugs and surgery

Before any surgical procedure, discontinue anticoagulants and anti-platelet drugs, as ordered, to reduce the risk of bleeding. The timing of the discontinuation depends on the half-life of the prescribed drug. Patients that need to stop their medication preoperatively can take heparin as a "bridge" anticoagulant because the half-life is short, and it can be discontinued closer to the surgery. After some types of surgery, especially major abdominal, knee, or hip replacements, prophylactic doses of anticoagulants may reduce the risk of DVT and PE.

Factor Xa inhibitors and antiplatelet medications are often used for the prevention of thrombosis in at-risk patients when appropriate. These medications are more selective and have less risk of bleeding. Unlike warfarin, they do not require frequent laboratory studies for dose management.

Pardon the interruption

For lysis of acute, extensive DVT, treatment may include thrombolytics (such as streptokinase). In rare cases, DVT may cause complete venous occlusion, which necessitates venous interruption that may be achieved through simple ligation to the vein. An embolectomy may also be performed. Finally, insertion of a vena cava filter may be necessary to prevent PE.

What to do

- Collaborate care with a skilled team, which may include a vascular specialist, surgeon, and physical therapists. A hematological specialist may be consulted if a coagulation disorder is suspected.
- To prevent thrombophlebitis in high-risk patients, perform ROM exercises while the patient is on bed rest.
- Apply antiembolism stockings postoperatively and encourage early ambulation. If the patient is on bed rest for a long period of time, use graduated compression devices as ordered.

- Remain alert for signs of pulmonary emboli, such as chest pain, shortness of breath, crackles hemoptysis, restlessness, and hypotension.
- Closely monitor anticoagulant therapy to prevent serious bleeding complications. Watch for signs of bleeding, such as dark, tarry stools, coffee-ground vomitus, hematuria, and ecchymoses.
- Enforce bed rest, as ordered, and elevate the patient's affected arm or leg. If you plan to use pillows for elevating the leg, place them to support the entire length of the affected extremity and to prevent possible compression of the popliteal space. For the ambulatory patient, encourage walking.
- Apply heat to the affected area as ordered. Assess the skin often.
- Administer analgesics to provide pain relief, as ordered. Monitor for pain relief.
- Measure and record the circumference of the affected extremity daily. Compare this with the unaffected extremity. To ensure accuracy and consistency of serial measurements, always measure the calf 10 cm (about 4 in) below the tibial tuberosity (Bickley, 2020a, 2020b)
- Document neurovascular status and vital signs. Note any respiratory difficulties. Document the patient's response to treatment and pain control. Document teaching provided to the patient and the patient's understanding of the instructions.

After the DVT

- Emphasize the importance of follow-up blood studies to monitor anticoagulant therapy.
- Review any drug or dietary restrictions due to medication interactions.
- Encourage the patient to use an electric razor and a soft toothbrush to avoid trauma to the skin and gums resulting in bleeding
- Caution patient about the increased risk of bleeding and bruising. Apply direct pressure and ice to nosebleeds for 15 minutes before releasing pressure. For wounds, apply direct pressure with a bandage or cloth and reinforce it if the bleeding comes through. If bleeding persists for more than 30 minutes, advise the patient to notify their health-care provider and/or seek urgent care.
- Tell the patient to avoid prolonged sitting or standing to help prevent recurrence. Encourage the patient to walk around at least once an hour when traveling on bus, car, or plane.
- Teach the patient how to apply, remove, and clean antiembolism stockings.
- Review emergency precautions such as signs and symptoms of PE, coronary thrombosis, or DVT.

Suggested references

American Heart Association. (2018a). Aspirin and heart disease. Retrieved from https://www.heart.org/en/health-topics/heart-attack/treatment-of-a-heart-attack/aspirin-and-heart-disease

American Heart Association. (2018b). Treatment of a heart attack: Common heart attack types and treatments. Retrieved fromhttps://www.heart.org/en/health-topics/heart-attack/treatment-of-a-heart-attack

Amsterdam, E. A., Wenger, N. K., Brindis, R. G., Casey, D. E. Jr, Ganiats, T. G., Holmes, D. R. Jr, Jaffe, A. S., Jneid, H., Kelly, R. F., Kontos, M. C., Levine, G. N., Liebson, P. R., Mukherjee, D., Peterson, E. D., Sabatine, M. S., Smalling, R. W., & Zieman, S. J. (2014). 2014 AHA/ACC guideline for the management of patients with non–ST-elevation acute coronary syndromes: A report of the American College of Cardiology/American Heart Association Task force on practice guidelines. *Journal of the American College of Cardiology, 64*(24), e139–e228. https://doi.org/10.1016/j.jacc.2014.09.017

Araújo, C., Laszczyńska, O., Viana, M., Melão, F., Henriques, A., Borges, A., , Severo, M, Maciel, MJ, Moreira, I, Azevedo, A (2018). Sex differences in presenting symptoms of acute coronary syndrome: The EPIHeart cohort study. *BMJ Open, 8*(2), e018798. https://doi.org/10.1136/bmjopen-2017-018798

Bajaj, R., Jain, A., & Knight, C. (2018). Definitions of acute coronary syndromes. *Ischemic Heart Disease, 46*(9), 528–532.

Barish, R. & Hildalgo, K., (2021). Chapter 24 Management of patients with structural, infectious, and inflammatory cardiac disorders. In Hinkle, J. (ed.), *Brunner & Suddarth's Textbook of medical-surgical nursing* (15th ed., pp. 265–272). Wolters Kluwer Health. https://wolterskluwer.vitalsource.com/books/9781975161057

Barstow, C., Rice, M., & McDivitt, J. D. (2017). Acute coronary syndrome: Diagnostic evaluation. *American Family Physician, 95*(3), 170–177.

Bickley, L. S. (2020a). *Chapter 16 cardiovascular system. Bates' guide to physical examination and history taking* (13th ed., pp. 489–560). Wolters Kluwer Health. https://wolterskluwer.vitalsource.com/books/9781975109943

Bickley, L. S. (2020b). *Chapter 17 Peripheral vascular system. Bates' guide to physical examination and history taking* (13th ed., pp. 561–591). Wolters Kluwer Health. https://wolterskluwer.vitalsource.com/books/9781975109943

Capriotti, T. (2021). Chapter 10 fluid and electrolytes. In: Hinkle's, J. (ed.). *Brunner & Suddarth's Textbook of medical-surgical nursing* (15th ed., p. 267). Wolters Kluwer Health. https://wolterskluwer.vitalsource.com/books/9781975161057

Centers for Disease Control. (2022) Smoking and Buerger disease. https://www.cdc.gov/tobacco/campaign/tips/diseases/index.html

Evans, E. (2021). Chapter 27 Assessment and management of patients with hypertension. In: Hinkle, J. (ed.), *Brunner & Suddarth's Textbook of medical-surgical nursing* (15th ed., pp. 865–881). Wolters Kluwer Health. https://wolterskluwer.vitalsource.com/books/9781975161057

Gerhard-Herman, M. D., Gornik, H. L., Barrett, C., Barshes, N. R., Corriere, M. A., Drachman, D. E., Fleisher, L. A., Fowkes, F. G. R., Hamburg, N. M., Kinlay, S., Lookstein, R., Misra, S., Mureebe, L., Olin, J. W., Patel, R. A. G., Regensteiner,

J. G., Schanzer, A., Shishehbor, M. H., Stewart, K. J., ... Walsh, M. E. (2017). 2016 AHA/ACC guideline on the management of patients with lower extremity peripheral artery disease: A report of the American College of Cardiology/American Heart Association Task force on clinical practice guidelines. *Journal of American College of Cardiology, 69*(11), e71–e126. https://doi.org/10.1016/j.jacc.2016.11.007

Geske, J. B., Ommen, S. R., & Gersh, B. J. (2018). Hypertrophic cardiomyopathy: Clinical update. *JACC Heart Failure, 6*(5), 364-375. https://doi.org/10.1016/j.jchf.2018.02.010

Goldman, M.P. (2017). Chapter 2 adverse Sequelae and complications of venous hypertension. In: Goldman, M. P. & Weiss, R. A. (eds.), *Sclerotherapy* (6th ed., pp. 27–54). Elsevier.

Haddad, F., Doyle, R., Murphy, D. J., & Hunt, S. A. (2008). Right ventricular function in cardiovascular disease, part II: Pathophysiology, clinical importance, and management of right ventricular failure. *Circulation, 117*(13), 1717–1731. https://doi.org/10.1161/CIRCULATIONAHA.107.653584

Heidenreich, P. A., Bozkurt, B., Aguilar, D., Allen, L. A., Byun, J. J., Colvin, M. M., Deswal, A., Drazner, M. H., Dunlay, S. M., Evers, L. R., Fang, J. C., Fedson, S. E., Fonarow, G. C., Hayek, S. S., Hernandez, A. F., Khazanie, P., Kittleson, M. M., Lee, C. S., Link, M. S., ... Yancy, CW (2022). 2022 AHA/ACC/HFSA guideline for the management of heart failure: A report of the American College of Cardiology/American Heart Association Joint Committee on clinical practice guidelines. *Circulation, 145*(18), e895–e1032. https://doi.org/10.1161/CIR.0000000000001063

Hubacek, J. A., Stanek, V., Gebauerova, M., Adamkova, V., Lesauskaite, V., Zaliaduonyte-Peksiene, D., , Tamosiunas, A, Supiyev, A, Kossumov, A, Zhumadilova, A, Pitha, J (2017). Traditional risk factors of acute coronary syndrome in four different male populations—total cholesterol value does not seem to be relevant risk factor. *Physiological Research, 66*(Suppl. 1), S121–S128.

Humbert, M., Kovacs, G., Hoeper, M. M., Badagliacca, R., Berger, R. M. F., Brida, M., Carlsen, J., Coats, A. J. S., Escribano-Subias, P., Ferrari, P., Ferreira, D. S., Ghofrani, H. A., Giannakoulas, G., Kiely, D. G., Mayer, E., Meszaros, G., Nagavci, B., Olsson, K. M., Pepke-Zaba, J., ... Rosenkranz, S.; ESC/ERS Scientific Document Group. (2023). 2022 ESC/ERS Guidelines for the diagnosis and treatment of pulmonary hypertension. *European Respiratory Journal, 61*(1), 2200879. https://doi.org/10.1183/13993003.00879-2022

James, P. A., Oparil, S., Carter, B. L., Cushman, W. C., Dennison-Himmelfarb, C., Handler, J., Lackland, D. T., LeFevre, M. L., MacKenzie, T. D., Ogedegbe, O., Smith, S. C. Jr, Svetkey, L. P., Taler, S. J., Townsend, R. R., Wright, J. T. Jr, Narva, A. S., Ortiz, E., Smith, S. C., Jr, & Wright, J. T., Jr. (2014). 2014 evidence-based guideline for the management of high blood pressure in adults: Report from the panel members appointed to the Eighth Joint National Committee (JNC 8). *JAMA: Journal of the American Medical Association, 311*(5), 507–520. https://doi.org/10.1001/jama.2013.284427

Kahn, S. R., Comerota, A. J., Cushman, M., Evans, N. S., Ginsberg, J. S., Goldenberg, N. A., Gupta, D. K., Prandoni, P., Vedantham, S., Walsh, M. E., Weitz, J. I., & American Heart Association Council on Peripheral Vascular Disease Council on Clinical Cardiology and Council on Cardiovascular and Stroke Nursing.

(2014). The postthrombotic syndrome: Evidence-based prevention, diagnosis, and treatment strategies—A scientific statement from the American Heart Association. *Circulation, 130*(18), 1636–1661. https://doi.org/10.1161/CIR.0000000000000130

Keller, K. Sabatino, D. Winland-Brown, J.E., Keller, M., & Porter, B. O. (2022). Chapter 36 dysrhythmias and valvular disorders. In: Dunphy, L. M., Winland-Brown, J. E., Porter, B. O., & Thomas, D. J., (eds.), *Primary care: The art and science of advanced practice nursing -and interprofessional approach* (6th ed.). F. A. Davis Company. https://fadavisreader.vitalsource.com/books/9781719649469

McDonagh, T. A., Metra, M., Adamo, M., Gardner, R. S., Baumbach, A., Böhm, M., Burri, H., Butler, J., Čelutkienė, J., Chioncel, O., Cleland, J. G. F., Coats, A. J. S., Crespo- Leiro, M. G., Farmakis, D., Gilard, M., Heymans, S., Hoes, A. W., Jaarsma, T., Jankowska, E. A., … Kathrine Skibelund, A, ESC Scientific Document Group. (2021). 2021 ESC Guidelines for the diagnosis and treatment of acute and chronic heart failure: Developed by the Task Force for the diagnosis and treatment of acute and chronic heart failure of the European Society of Cardiology (ESC) with the special contribution of the Heart Failure Association (HFA) of the ESC. *European Heart Journal, 42*(36), 3599–3726. https://doi.org/10.1093/eurheartj/ehab368

Monaro, S., & Walsh, M. E. (2021). Chapter 26 Assessment and management of patients with vascular disorders and problems of peripheral circulation. In Hinkle, J. (ed.), *Brunner & Suddarth's Textbook of medical-surgical nursing* (15th ed.). Wolters Kluwer Health. https://wolterskluwer.vitalsource.com/books/9781975161057

Robinson, M. V. (2020). Chapter 29 angina. In: Woo, T. M. & Robinson, M. V. *Pharmacotherapies for advanced practice nurse practitioners* (5th ed.). F. A. Davis Company.

Shim, J. S., Song, W. J., & Morice, A. H. (2020). Drug-induced cough. *Physiological Research, 69*(Suppl. 1), S81–S92. https://doi.org/10.33549/physiolres.934406

Slomski, A. (2017). Redefining acute coronary syndrome therapy. *JAMA, 317*(20), 2054. doi:10.1001/jama.2017.6081

Tong, D. C., Wilson, A. M., & Layland, J. (2016). Novel risk factors for acute coronary syndromes and emerging therapies. *International Journal of Cardiology, 220*, 815–824. https://doi.org/10.1016/j.ijcard.2016.06.148

U.S. Preventive Services Health Task Force. (2019). Abdominal aortic aneurysm: Screening. https://www.uspreventiveservicestaskforce.org/uspstf/recommendation/abdominal-aortic-aneurysm-screening

Whelton, P. K., Carey, R. M., Aronow, W. S., Casey, D. E. Jr, Collins, K. J., Dennison Himmelfarb, C., DePalma, S. M., Gidding, S., Jamerson, K. A., Jones, D. W., MacLaughlin, E. J., Muntner, P., Ovbiagele, B., Smith, S. C. Jr, Spencer, C. C., Stafford, R. S., Taler, S. J., Thomas, R. J., Williams, K. A. Sr, … Wright, J. J. T. (2018). 2017 ACC/AHA/AAPA/ABC/ACPM/AGS/APhA/ASH/ASPC/NMA/PCNA guideline for the prevention, detection, evaluation, and management of high blood pressure in adults: A report of the American College of Cardiology/American Heart Association task force on clinical practice guidelines. *Journal of American College of Cardiology, 71*(19), e127–e248. https://doi.org/10.1016/j.jacc.2017.11.006

Wong, N. D., Budoff, M. J., Ferdinand, K., Graham, I. M., Michos, E. D., Reddy, T., Shapiro, M. D., & Toth, P. P. (2022). Atherosclerotic cardiovascular disease risk assessment: An American Society for Preventive Cardiology clinical practice statement. *American Journal of Preventive Cardiology, 10,* 100335. https://doi.org/10.1016/j.ajpc.2022.100335

Woo, T. M. (2019) Chapter 15 Drugs affecting the hematological system. In Woo, T. M. & Robinson, M. V. (eds.), *Pharmacotherapeutics for advanced practice nurse prescribers* (5th ed.). F. A. Davis Company.

Zychowicz, M. E. (2022). Chapter 78 sports physicals. In: Dunphy, L. M., Winland-Brown, J. E., Porter, B. O., & Thomas, D. J., (eds.), *Primary care: The art and science of advanced Practice nursing—and interprofessional approach* (6th ed.). F. A. Davis Company. https://fadavisreader.vitalsource.com/books/9781719649469

Chapter 8

Emergencies and complications

Just the facts

In this chapter, you'll learn:

♦ cardiac complications that require emergency measures

♦ pathophysiology and treatments related to these complications

♦ diagnostic tests, assessment findings, and nursing interventions for each complication.

A look at cardiac emergencies

Cardiac emergencies, which can result as a complication of another condition, require immediate assessment and treatment. They include cardiac trauma, cardiac tamponade, cardiogenic shock, and hypovolemic shock.

Cardiac trauma

Cardiac trauma, commonly dramatic in presentation, is usually associated with other thoracic injuries; it can occur as a result of blunt or penetrating trauma. Blunt thoracic trauma accounts for 25% of trauma fatalities.

Not always obvious

Although cardiac trauma can be severe, not all injuries are apparent on admission to the emergency department or intensive care unit, especially when the patient exhibits no external signs of chest wall damage. It may be several hours before signs are noticeable and several days before complications are evident. As a result, keen observation and assessment are essential for the early identification of cardiac injuries and potential complications.

The prognosis for a patient with cardiac trauma largely depends on the extent of the cardiac damage and their other injuries. Age and preexisting conditions also affect the prognosis. The population of older people has an increased rate of rib fracture, hospital stay, and mortality. This population may require earlier surgical intervention for survival.

What causes it?

Cardiac trauma is a result of a blunt or penetrating chest injury.

How it happens?

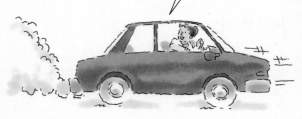

Car accidents are the leading cause of cardiac trauma.

Blunt trauma typically results from vehicular accidents (70% to 80%) or falls from a great height, sport injuries, blast forces, and indirect compression on the abdomen with upward displacement of abdominal viscera. Rapid deceleration may result in shearing forces that tear cardiac structures and cause great vessel disruption. Falls may cause a rapid increase in intra-abdominal and intrathoracic pressures, which can result in myocardial rupture, valvular rupture, or both. Crushing and compression forces may result in contusion or rupture as the heart becomes compressed between the sternum and vertebral column. Blunt trauma commonly results in chest wall injuries (e.g., rib fractures). The pain associated with these injuries can make breathing difficult, and this may compromise ventilation.

Myocardial contusions (or blunt cardiac injury [BCI]) occur when rapid deceleration causes the heart to strike the anterior chest wall and sternum. A cardiac concussion is a less severe form of blunt cardiac trauma. (See *Understanding myocardial contusion*, page 263.)

Penetrating truths

Penetrating trauma to the heart, typically resulting from a knife, gunshots, or foreign bodies in the heart, carries a high risk of mortality and usually requires immediate thoracotomy and surgical repair. This type of cardiac trauma commonly leads to cardiac tamponade. In 94% of cases involving penetrating cardiac trauma, death occurs before the patient reaches the hospital.

What to look for?

Cardiac trauma may initially be overlooked as other life-threatening and more apparent injuries are treated. In addition, signs and symptoms of cardiac injuries, such as myocardial contusion or cardiac tamponade, may not occur for several hours. Therefore, astute assessment skills are needed for early detection and prompt treatment. A common practice involves serial cardiac biomarkers postadmission after a motor vehicle accident.

Accident report

Typically, the patient with cardiac trauma is in pain and feels apprehensive. Attempt to ascertain the following information:

- mechanism of injury (e.g., in an automobile accident, include how the accident occurred, patient location in the vehicle and use of seat belts, and extent of internal car damage; for a fall, include how far the patient fell, onto what type of surface, and how they landed; for a gunshot wound, include the gun caliber (if known) and distance from which the patient was shot; for a stab wound, include the size and type of the weapon)
- history of cardiac or pulmonary problems
- medications the patient is currently taking
- pain location, onset, character, and severity
- presence of dyspnea.

Now I get it!

Understanding myocardial contusion

A myocardial contusion (bruising to the myocardium) is the most common type of injury sustained from blunt trauma. You should suspect it whenever a blow to the chest occurs. The contusion usually results from a fall or from impact with a steering wheel or other object. The right ventricle is the most common site of injury because of its location directly behind the sternum.

Here's what happens:

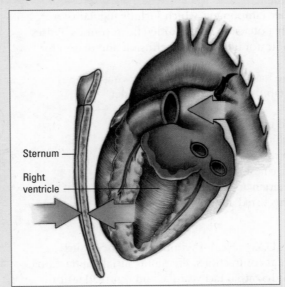

Sternum

Right ventricle

- During deceleration injuries, the myocardium strikes the sternum as the heart and aorta move forward.
- In addition, the aorta may be lacerated by shearing forces.
- Direct force also may be applied to the sternum, causing injury.

Look for more

Other signs and symptoms associated with blunt trauma:

- tachycardia—most common symptom
- precordial chest pain
- bradycardia
- contusion marks on the chest such as steering wheel imprint
- flail chest
- murmurs.

If the patient experienced penetrating trauma, look for the following:

- tachycardia
- shortness of breath with decreased breath sounds
- dullness on percussion
- weakness
- diaphoresis
- acute anxiety
- cool and clammy skin
- upper extremity blood pressure differential or loss of upper or lower extremity pulses
- evidence of an external puncture wound or protrusion of the penetrating instrument
- symptoms of cardiac tamponade, which include jugular vein distention (JVD), hypotension, and muffled heart sounds. Pulses paradoxus is an indicator of pericardial effusion and reason for the tamponade

For the patient who has BCI, look for the following:

- hemodynamic instability, such as severe or sudden hypotension
- arrhythmias caused by ventricular irritability
- heart failure or cardiogenic shock
- pericardial friction rub
- symptoms of cardiac tamponade.

If the patient is experiencing a cardiac concussion, many of the signs and symptoms listed above will be present.

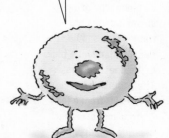

Evidence of cellular injury is absent in cases of cardiac concussion.

What tests tell you?

- Electrocardiogram (ECG) reveals rhythm disturbances, such as premature ventricular contractions, premature atrial contractions, ventricular tachycardia, atrial tachycardia, and ventricular fibrillation along with ischemic changes and nonspecific ST-segment or T-wave changes (with BCI) occurring within 48 hours after the injury.
- Cardiac troponin I shows elevations 24 hours after the injury (suggestive of cardiac injury). If troponin I results are within reference

ranges on admission shortly after trauma, a secondary measurement after 4 to 6 hours is necessary to reliably exclude myocardial injury. Increased troponin I may persist for 4 to 6 days and may aid in evaluating cardiac damage of patients presenting days after the injury.

- Chest X-ray shows widened mediastinum (with cardiac tamponade) and pulmonary edema (with septal defect). Thoracic computed tomography may be an alternative to X-rays and may show associated injury of the great vessels or skeletal or pulmonary structures.
- An echocardiogram (transthoracic echo) shows evidence of cardiac tamponade and valvular abnormalities, abnormal ventricular wall movement, and decreased ejection fraction (with myocardial contusion).
- Transesophageal echocardiogram shows evidence of aortic disruptions, cardiac tamponade, and atrial and septal defects.
- Cardiac enzyme levels show elevated creatine kinase (CK) levels; however, these rise with associated skeletal muscle injury. The usefulness of CK-MB is limited.

How it's treated?

Maintaining hemodynamic stability is crucial to the patient's care. Penetrating trauma may be associated with massive hemorrhage leading to acute hypotension and shock. In addition, cardiac output is affected if the patient develops cardiac tamponade or arrhythmias occurring with BCI. Hemodynamic monitoring is key to evaluating the patient's status and maintaining its adequacy. Intravenous (IV) fluid therapy, including blood component therapy, may be necessary. Continuous ECG monitoring is important to detect possible arrhythmias. Nearly all (81% to 95%) life-threatening ventricular arrhythmias and acute cardiac failures occur within 24 to 48 hours after the trauma. Antiarrhythmics may be used to treat ventricular arrhythmias. Angiotensin-converting enzyme inhibitors may be given for pump failure. Inotropic agents may be used to assist with improving cardiac output and ejection fraction.

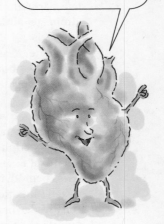

There's a lot to juggle when treating cardiac trauma— but it's all designed to maintain hemodynamic stability.

Look out for the lungs

The patient with cardiac trauma must be monitored closely for signs and symptoms of cardiopulmonary compromise because cardiac trauma is commonly associated with pulmonary trauma. Supplemental oxygen administration and assessment of oxygen saturation are important. If the degree of associated pulmonary trauma is great, endotracheal (ET) intubation and mechanical ventilation may be warranted to maintain adequate oxygenation.

Meds and other measures

Adequate pain management has shown to improve outcomes and should be tailored to the individual patient. Factors such as overall injuries, age, pain level, hydration status, and comorbidities should guide pain control measures. For severe pain, narcotic administration, an epidural anesthetic agent, or a combination drug therapy may be warranted. In addition, corrective surgery may be indicated to correct septal or valvular defects, penetrating injuries, or rupture. Emergency pericardiocentesis is used to treat acute cardiac tamponade.

What to do?

- Collaborate care with a skilled team, which may include emergency medical services personnel, a surgeon, a respiratory therapist, and social services.

Cardiac check-in

Assess the patient's cardiopulmonary status at least every 4 hours—or more frequently, if indicated—to detect signs and symptoms of possible injury. This assessment includes the following:

- Continuous cardiac monitoring for the first 48 to 72 hours to detect arrhythmias or conduction defects. If arrhythmias occur, administer antiarrhythmic agents as ordered and monitor electrolyte levels.
- Auscultate breath sounds and monitor pulse oximeter reading at least every 4 hours (and more frequently as needed), reporting signs of congestion or fluid accumulation, and changes in pulse oximeter.
- Monitor heart rate and rhythm, heart sounds, and blood pressure every hour for changes.
- Evaluate peripheral pulses and capillary refill to detect decreased peripheral tissue perfusion.
- Assess hemodynamic status—which may include mixed venous oxygen saturation, central venous pressure (CVP), pulmonary artery wedge pressure (PAWP), and continuous cardiac output as indicated—at least every 2 hours.

Fluids and other measures

- Administer fluid replacement therapy, including blood component therapy, as prescribed, typically to maintain systolic blood pressure above 90 mm Hg.
- Monitor urine output every hour, notifying the health care provider if output is less than 30 mL/hour.
- Assess the patient's degree of pain and administer analgesic therapy as ordered, monitoring for effectiveness. Position the patient comfortably, usually with the head of the bed elevated 30 to 45°.

- Encourage coughing and deep breathing, splinting the chest as necessary.
- If the patient has undergone surgery, monitor and assess chest tubes for patency, volume and color of drainage, and presence of an air leak.
- Assess vital signs postoperatively, especially temperature.
- Inspect the surgical site for evidence of infection or bleeding at least every 4 hours, noting redness, drainage, warmth, edema, or localized pain at the site.

Preparing for discharge

- Arrange for possible social service consultation depending on the cause of the injury—for example, alcohol-related automobile accident or gang-related gunshot injury.
- Provide brief explanations about the patient's condition and why it's occurring. Inform the patient and their family about how the condition will be treated, being sure to explain new procedures before beginning them.
- Review signs and symptoms of complications and/or a worsening condition, stressing the importance of follow up and alerting the health care provider if any complications occur
- Document vital signs and assessment findings. Document the patient's response to treatment.

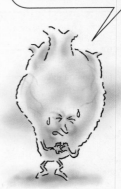

Cardiac tamponade occurs when pressure in the pericardial sac shoots up quickly.

Cardiac tamponade

Cardiac tamponade is a rapid, unchecked increase in pressure within the pericardial sac. This pressure compresses the heart, impairs diastolic filling, and reduces cardiac output.

The increase in pressure usually results from blood or fluid accumulation in the pericardial sac. Even a small amount of fluid (50 to 100 mL) can cause a serious tamponade if it accumulates rapidly.

Quick fill, quick response

If fluid accumulates rapidly, cardiac tamponade requires emergency lifesaving measures to prevent death. A slow accumulation and increase in pressure may not produce immediate symptoms because the fibrous wall of the pericardial sac can gradually stretch to accommodate as much as 1 to 2 L of fluid.

What causes it?

Cardiac tamponade may result from the following:
- idiopathic causes (such as Dressler syndrome)
- effusion (from cancer; bacterial infections; tuberculosis; and rarely, acute rheumatic fever), the most common cause of >50% of all tamponade cases

- hemorrhage caused by trauma (such as gunshot or stab wounds of the chest)
- hemorrhage caused by nontraumatic causes (such as anticoagulant therapy in patients with pericarditis or rupture of the heart or great vessels)
- viral or postirradiation pericarditis
- chronic renal failure requiring dialysis
- drug reaction from procainamide, hydralazine, minoxidil, isoniazid, penicillin, or daunorubicin
- connective tissue disorders (such as rheumatoid arthritis, systemic lupus erythematosus, rheumatic fever, and scleroderma)
- acute myocardial infarction (MI)
- postcardiac procedures such as percutaneous coronary interventions (PCIs), pacemaker, or implantable cardioverter-defibrillator insertion, open-heart surgery, or cardiopulmonary resuscitation.

How it happens?

In a normal heart and pericardium, the pericardial space normally contains 10 to 30 mL of pericardial fluid, which lubricates the layers of the heart and reduces friction when the heart contracts.

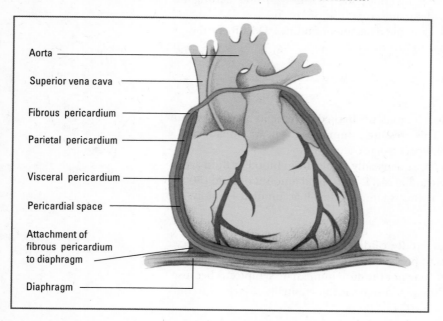

Aorta

Superior vena cava

Fibrous pericardium

Parietal pericardium

Visceral pericardium

Pericardial space

Attachment of fibrous pericardium to diaphragm

Diaphragm

In cardiac tamponade, accumulation of fluid in the pericardial sac causes compression of the heart chambers. This compression obstructs blood flow into the ventricles and reduces the amount of blood that can be pumped out of the heart with each contraction.

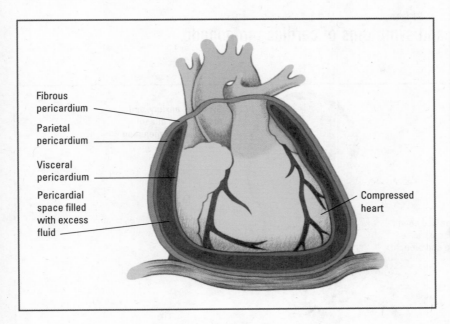

Fibrous pericardium

Parietal pericardium

Visceral pericardium

Pericardial space filled with excess fluid

Compressed heart

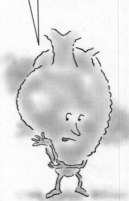

Compression of the heart chambers obstructs blood flow into the ventricles and reduces the amount of blood that can be pumped out of the heart with each contraction.

What to look for?

Cardiac tamponade has three classic features, which are known as *Beck triad*:

1. elevated CVP with JVD
2. muffled heart sounds
3. Hypotension. Pulsus paradoxus (inspiratory drop in systemic blood pressure greater than 10 mm Hg) may be present indicating pericardial effusion is present.

That's not all

Other signs include the following:

- tachycardia (first compensatory sign)
- narrowed pulse pressure
- tachypnea
- orthopnea
- diaphoresis
- anxiety or confusion
- restlessness
- cyanosis
- weak, rapid peripheral pulse.

Understanding signs and symptoms of cardiac tamponade.

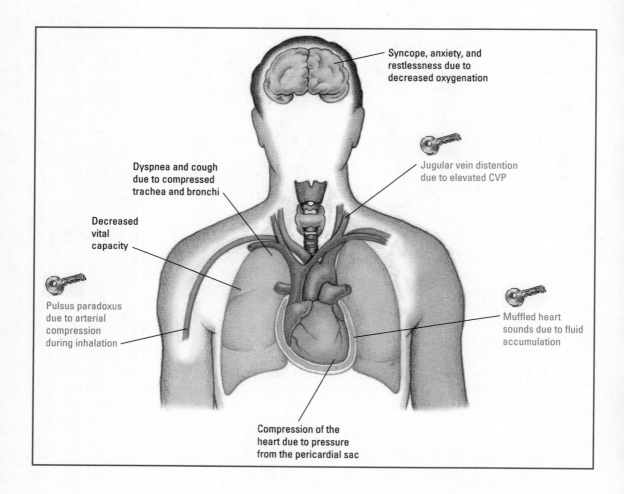

Syncope, anxiety, and restlessness due to decreased oxygenation

Jugular vein distention due to elevated CVP

Dyspnea and cough due to compressed trachea and bronchi

Decreased vital capacity

Pulsus paradoxus due to arterial compression during inhalation

Muffled heart sounds due to fluid accumulation

Compression of the heart due to pressure from the pericardial sac

What tests tell you?

- Chest X-ray shows a slightly widened mediastinum and cardiomegaly.
- ECG commonly shows sinus tachycardia. On rare occasions, the ECG may show a low-amplitude QRS complex and electrical alternans, an alternating beat-to-beat change in amplitude of the P wave, QRS complex, and T wave. Generalized ST-segment elevation is noted in all leads. An ECG is used to rule out other cardiac disorders; it may reveal changes produced by acute pericarditis.

- Echocardiography may reveal pericardial effusion with signs of right ventricular and atrial compression. This is the gold standard to determine cardiac tamponade.
- Computed tomography scanning or magnetic resonance imaging can be used to identify pericardial effusions or pericardial thickening caused by constrictive pericarditis.

How it's treated?
The goal of treatment is to relieve intrapericardial pressure and cardiac compression by removing accumulated blood or fluid. This removal can be done in three different ways:
- pericardiocentesis (needle aspiration of the pericardial cavity) done with guidance by echocardiography
- surgical creation of an opening, called a pericardial window
- insertion of a drain into the pericardial sac to drain the effusion.

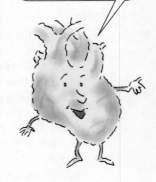

The goals of treatment for cardiac tamponade are to drain fluid and relieve pressure.

When pressure is low

If the patient is hypotensive, two large bore IVs should be initiated, and trial volume loading with crystalloids, such as normal saline solution, may be used to maintain systolic blood pressure. Inotropic drugs may be necessary to improve myocardial contractility until fluid in the pericardial sac can be removed. The use of a vasopressor drug may increase the mean arterial pressure (MAP) without causing additional strain to the heart.

More to do

Additional treatment may be necessary, depending on the cause. Examples of such causes and treatments follow:
- traumatic injury—blood transfusion or a thoracotomy to drain reaccumulating fluid or to repair bleeding sites
- heparin-induced tamponade—administration of the heparin antagonist protamine sulfate
- warfarin-induced tamponade (rare)—vitamin K administration.
  In some cases, early tamponade has been shown to resolve with steroids/nonsteroidal anti-inflammatory drugs, making early recognition a key element.

What to do?
- Collaborate care with a skilled team, which may include emergency medical personnel, a cardiovascular surgeon, and critical care personnel. Echocardiography is the most useful diagnostic tool for evaluating patients with cardiac tamponade. It should be performed without delay on patients where tamponade is suspected.

- Monitor the patient's cardiovascular status frequently, at least every hour, noting the extent of JVD, the quality of heart sounds, and blood pressure.
- Assess hemodynamic status, including CVP, right atrial pressure, and pulmonary artery pressure (PAP), and determine cardiac output.

It's a paradox

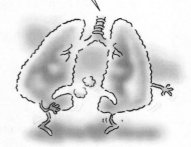

Don't forget me! Be sure to monitor for signs of respiratory distress.

- Monitor for pulsus paradoxus (pulse that rapidly decreases during inspiration).
- Be alert for ST-segment and T-wave changes on ECG. Note rate and rhythm and report evidence of any arrhythmias.
- Watch closely for signs of increasing tamponade or dyspnea and report them immediately.
- Infuse IV solutions and inotropic drugs, such as dopamine, as ordered to maintain the patient's blood pressure.
- Administer oxygen therapy as needed and assess oxygen saturation levels. Monitor the patient's respiratory status for signs of respiratory distress, such as severe tachypnea and changes in the patient's level of consciousness. Anticipate the need for ET intubation and mechanical ventilation if the patient's respiratory status deteriorates.
- Prepare the patient for pericardiocentesis or thoracotomy.
- If the patient has trauma-induced tamponade, assess for other signs of trauma and institute appropriate care, including the use of colloids, crystalloids, and blood component therapy under pressure or by rapid volume infuser, if massive fluid replacement is needed; administration of protamine sulfate for heparin-induced tamponade; and vitamin K administration for warfarin-induced tamponade.
- Assess renal function status closely, monitoring urine output every hour and notifying the health care provider if output is less than 30 mL/hour.
- Monitor capillary refill time, level of consciousness, peripheral pulses, and skin temperature for evidence of diminished tissue perfusion.
- Explain the patient's condition and why it's occurring. Inform the patient and their family how the condition will be treated, being sure to explain new procedures before beginning them.
- Review signs and symptoms of a worsening condition, stressing the importance of alerting the health care provider if such signs occur.
- Document the patient's vital signs, cardiac and respiratory status, and response to treatment.

Cardiogenic shock

Cardiogenic shock is a condition of diminished cardiac output that severely impairs tissue perfusion. It's sometimes called *pump failure*. Cardiogenic shock is defined as a systolic blood pressure of less than 90 mm Hg for at least 30 minutes. The cardiac index and the pulmonary capillary wedge pressure are usually less than 2.2 L/min/m^2 and greater than 15 mm Hg, respectively. Lactate levels of >2 mmol/L are noted and indicative of diminished perfusion to the end organs.

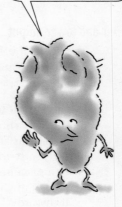

Did I hear that right? Cardiogenic shock occurs in 7% to 10% of patients with acute MI.

Shocking stats

Cardiogenic shock is a serious complication in 7% to 10% of all patients hospitalized with acute MI. It typically affects patients whose area of infarction involves 40% or more of left ventricular (LV) muscle mass; in such patients, the overall in-hospital mortality rate is 35% to 50%.

What causes it?

Cardiogenic shock can result from any condition that causes significant LV dysfunction with reduced cardiac output, such as follows:

- MI (most common)
- myocardial ischemia
- papillary muscle dysfunction
- end-stage cardiomyopathy
- myocardial free wall rupture.

Other offenders

Other causes include myocarditis, pericarditis, and depression of myocardial contractility after cardiac arrest and prolonged cardiac surgery. Mechanical abnormalities of the ventricle, such as acute mitral or aortic insufficiency or an acutely acquired ventricular septal defect or ventricular aneurysm, may also result in cardiogenic shock.

Patients at risk:

- Diabetics
- Older people
- Females
- Those with prior history of LV injury

How it happens?

Regardless of the cause, here's what happens:

- LV dysfunction initiates a series of compensatory mechanisms that attempt to increase cardiac output and, in turn, maintain vital organ function.
- If cardiogenic shock results from an acute MI, a systemic inflammatory response syndrome may occur, possibly resulting in delayed pumping recovery (stunned myocardium).

- As cardiac output falls, baroreceptors in the aorta and carotid arteries initiate responses in the sympathetic nervous system. These responses, in turn, increase heart rate, LV filling pressure, and peripheral resistance to flow to enhance venous return to the heart.
- These compensatory responses initially stabilize the patient but later cause the patient to deteriorate as the oxygen demands of the already compromised heart increase.

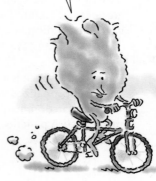

Cardiogenic shock begins a cycle that increasingly lowers cardiac output.

Lower and lower output

The events involved in cardiogenic shock comprise a vicious cycle of low cardiac output, sympathetic compensation, myocardial ischemia, and even lower cardiac output.

What to look for?

Cardiogenic shock produces signs of poor tissue perfusion:

- cold, pale, and clammy skin
- drop in systolic blood pressure to 30 mm Hg below baseline or a sustained reading below 90 mm Hg that isn't attributable to medication
- tachycardia
- rapid, shallow respirations
- oliguria (urine output less than 20 mL/hour)
- restlessness and anxiety
- confusion
- narrowing pulse pressure
- cyanosis
- gallop murmur (S3), faint heart sounds, and possibly, a holosystolic murmur.

INCREASED

- Heart rate
- Respiratory rate
- PAP and PAWP
- B-type natriuretic peptide
- Lactate

DECREASED

- Systolic pressure (<80 mm Hg)
- Urine output (<20 mL/hour)
- Pulse pressure
- Cardiac index
- Oxygen saturation

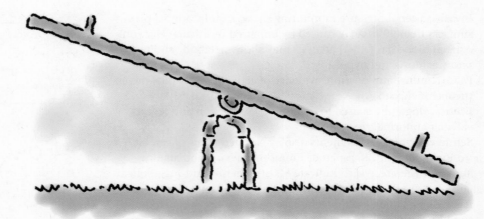

What tests tell you?

- Hemodynamic pressure monitoring reveals increased PAP, PAWP, and right ventricular end-diastolic volume index reflecting an increase in LV end-diastolic pressure (preload) and heightened resistance to LV emptying (afterload) caused by ineffective pumping and increased peripheral vascular resistance. Thermodilution catheterization reveals a reduced cardiac index. (See *Interpreting hemodynamic parameters in cardiogenic shock.*)

Interpreting hemodynamic parameters in cardiogenic shock

Interpreting hemodynamic parameters in cardiogenic shock can help you quickly determine hemodynamic parameters associated with cardiogenic shock.

Parameter	Values associated with cardiogenic shock
Right atrial pressure	6–10 mm Hg
Right ventricular pressure	40–50/6 to 15 mm Hg
Pulmonary artery pressure	50/25–30 mm Hg
Pulmonary artery wedge pressure	25–40 mm Hg
Systemic vascular resistance	>1,200 dynes/second/cm^5
Mixed venous oxygen saturation	50%
Cardiac output	<4 L/minute
Cardiac index	<1.5 L/minute/m^2

- Invasive arterial pressure monitoring shows systolic arterial pressure less than 90 mm Hg caused by impaired ventricular ejection.
- Arterial blood gas (ABG) analysis may show metabolic and respiratory acidosis and hypoxemia.
- ECG demonstrates possible evidence of acute MI, ischemia, or ventricular aneurysm.
- Echocardiography is used to determine LV function and reveals valvular abnormalities.
- Serum enzyme measurements display elevated levels of cardiac troponin I and T, CK, aspartate aminotransferase, and alanine aminotransferase, which indicate MI or ischemia and suggest heart failure or shock. Troponins confirm acute MI. An increased brain natriuretic peptide level may indicate heart failure and help predict survival. Lactate should be monitored to assess perfusion to end organs.
- Cardiac catheterization and echocardiography may reveal other conditions that can lead to pump dysfunction and failure, such as cardiac tamponade, papillary muscle infarct or rupture, ventricular septal rupture, pulmonary emboli, venous pooling (associated with vasodilators and continuous or intermittent positive-pressure breathing), and hypovolemia.

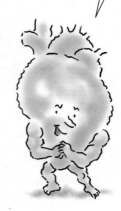

A combo of cardio drugs and mechanical assistance gets me pumped up again.

How it's treated?

The goal of treatment is to enhance cardiovascular status by increasing cardiac output, improving myocardial perfusion, and decreasing cardiac workload. Treatment consists of administering a combination of cardiovascular drugs, revascularization of the culprit coronary artery causing MI via PCI, and mechanical-assist techniques.

Treatment ABCs

Treatment begins with these measures:
- maintaining a patent airway, including preparing for intubation and mechanical ventilation if the patient develops respiratory distress
- administering supplemental oxygen to increase oxygenation
- continuous cardiac monitoring to detect changes in heart rate and rhythm and administration of antiarrhythmics as necessary
- initiating and maintaining at least two IV lines with large bore needles for fluid and drug administration
- administering IV fluids, crystalloids, colloids, or blood products, as necessary, to maintain intravascular volume

memory board

To help you recall the treatment protocol for cardiogenic shock, remember your **ABC**s (plus a **D** and an **E**).

Airway control with possible mechanical assistance

Breathing with high-flow rate oxygen therapy

Circulation monitoring and maintenance of large-bore IV lines

Drugs to increase cardiac output and stabilize the patient hemodynamically

Emergency intra-aortic balloon pump (IABP), ventricular assist device, or surgery

    ○   MI patients in cardiac arrest should be transported by emergency medical services to a facility that performs PCI to improve patient outcomes.

Increase flow

Drug therapy commonly used may include IV medication adjuncts such as vasopressors and inotropes. Vasopressors, such as dopamine, phenylephrine (Neo-Synephrine), or norepinephrine (Levophed), work to increase blood pressure and blood flow to the kidneys. Inotropic agents, such as inamrinone (Inocor) or dobutamine, work to increase myocardial contractility and cardiac output.

Decrease resistance and pressure

A vasodilator—nitroglycerin or nitroprusside (Nitropress)—may be used with a vasopressor to further improve cardiac output by decreasing peripheral vascular resistance (afterload) and reducing LV end-diastolic pressure (preload). However, the patient's blood pressure must be adequate to support nitroprusside therapy and must be monitored closely. Diuretics also may be used to reduce preload in patients with fluid volume overload.

Bring in the hardware

Extracorporeal membrane oxygenation is becoming a more common intervention used in patients with poor prognosis. When attached to an extracorporeal membrane oxygenation machine, the patient's blood is pumped out of the body through the machine, which then removes carbon dioxide and oxygenates the blood. The blood is then pumped back into the patient's body.

Treatment may also include mechanical assistance by the IABP to improve coronary artery perfusion and decrease cardiac workload. The IABP is inserted through the femoral artery into the descending thoracic aorta. The balloon inflates during diastole to increase coronary artery perfusion pressure and deflates before systole (before the aortic valve opens) to reduce resistance to ejection (afterload) and therefore reduce cardiac workload.

Improved ventricular ejection, as a result of the mechanical assistance of the IABP, significantly improves cardiac output. Subsequent vasodilation in the peripheral vessels leads to lower preload volume and reduced workload of the left ventricle because of decreasing systemic vascular resistance.

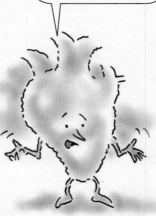

Heart transplantation is the last resort for treatment of cardiogenic shock.

End–stage effort

When the above therapies fail, a ventricular assist device may be inserted to assist the pumping action of the heart. When this intervention fails, heart transplantation may be considered.

Even more

Additional treatment measures for cardiogenic shock may include the following:

- thrombolytic therapy or coronary artery revascularization to restore coronary artery blood flow, if cardiogenic shock is due to acute MI
- emergency surgery to repair papillary muscle rupture or ventricular septal defect if either is the cause of cardiogenic shock.

RX

- Vasopressor agents, such as dopamine (Intropin), phenylephrine (Neo-Synephrine), or norepinephrine (Levophed)
- Inotropic agents, such as inamrinone (Amrinone) or dobutamine (Dobutrex)
- Nitrates, such as nitroglycerin (Tridil)
- IABP or LV assist device
- Thrombolytic therapy or coronary artery revascularization
- Emergency surgery, if applicable

What to do?

- Collaborate care with a skilled team, which may include emergency medical personnel, a cardiologist, a nutritional therapist, and a cardiac interventional team.
- Begin IV infusions of normal saline solution or lactated Ringer's solution using a large-bore (16G to 18G) catheter, which allows easier administration of fluids, medications, and possible blood transfusions.
- Administer oxygen via the appropriate adjunct to ensure adequate oxygenation of tissues. Adjust the oxygen flow rate to a higher or lower level, as ABG measurements indicate. Many patients need mechanical ventilation to ensure proper oxygenation and may need positive end-expiratory pressure or continuous positive airway pressure.
- Document vital signs, hemodynamic parameters, and assessment findings. Document the patient's response to treatment and patient and family wishes associated with patient care.

Monitor, record, and then monitor more

- Monitor and record blood pressure, pulse, respiratory rate, and peripheral pulses every 1 to 5 minutes until the patient's condition stabilizes. Monitor cardiac rhythm continuously. Systolic blood pressure less than 90 mm Hg usually results in inadequate coronary artery blood flow, cardiac ischemia, arrhythmias, and further complications of low cardiac output.

- Using a thermodilution catheter, closely monitor CVP, PAP, PAWP, and cardiac output. High PAWP indicates heart failure, increased systemic vascular resistance, decreased cardiac output, and decreased cardiac index and should be reported immediately.
- Determine how much fluid to give by checking blood pressure, urine output, CVP, or PAWP. (To increase accuracy, measure CVP at the level of the right atrium, using the same reference point on the chest each time.) Whenever the fluid infusion rate is increased, watch for signs of fluid overload, such as an increase in PAWP. If the patient is hypovolemic, preload may need to be increased; this is typically accomplished with IV fluids. However, IV fluids must be given cautiously, increasing them gradually while hemodynamic parameters are closely monitored. In this situation, diuretics aren't given.
- Insert an indwelling urinary catheter to measure hourly urine output. If output is less than 30 mL/hour in adults, increase the fluid infusion rate but watch for signs of fluid overload such as an increase in PAWP. Notify the health care provider if urine output doesn't improve.
- Administer a diuretic, such as furosemide (Lasix) or bumetanide (Bumex), as ordered, to decrease preload and improve stroke volume and cardiac output.
- Monitor ABG values, complete blood count, and lactate and electrolyte levels. Monitor and treat acidosis when noted. Administer electrolyte replacement therapy as ordered.
- During therapy, assess skin color and temperature and note any changes. Cold and clammy skin may be a sign of continuing peripheral vascular constriction, indicating progressive shock.

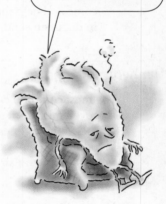

Report high PAWP readings, which may indicate complications such as heart failure and fluid overload.

Minimize movement

- During use of the IABP, move the patient as little as possible. Never flex the "ballooned" leg at the hip because this may displace or kink the catheter. Never place the patient in a sitting position for any reason (including chest X-rays) while the balloon is inflated because the balloon will tear through the aorta and result in immediate death.
- Also, during use of the IABP, assess leg pulses and skin temperature and color to ensure adequate peripheral circulation. Check the dressing over the insertion site frequently for bleeding and change it according to facility protocol. Also check the site for hematoma or signs of infection and culture any drainage.

- If the patient becomes hemodynamically stable, gradually reduce the frequency of balloon inflation to wean them from the IABP as ordered.
- When weaning the patient from the IABP, watch for ECG changes, chest pain, decreased cardiac output, and other signs of recurring cardiac ischemia as well as for shock.
- Prepare the patient for possible emergency cardiac catheterization to determine eligibility for PCI or coronary artery bypass grafting to restore blood flow to areas with reversible injury patterns.

Provide regular rest and support

- To ease emotional stress, plan care measures to allow frequent rest periods and provide as much privacy as possible. Allow family members to visit and comfort the patient as much as possible.
- Because the patient and their family may be anxious about the intensive care unit and about the IABP and other devices, offer explanations and reassurance.
- Prepare the patient and their family for a possible fatal outcome and help them find effective coping strategies. Assist in discussing end-of-life issues.

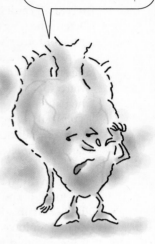

When weaning the patient from IABP, watch for signs of cardiac ischemia and shock.

Hypovolemic shock

The most common cause of hypovolemic shock is traumatic injury. Hypovolemic shock results from acute blood loss (about 25% to 30% of total volume) or extracellular fluid volume loss. Without sufficient blood or fluid replacement, hypovolemic shock may lead to irreversible damage to organs and systems.

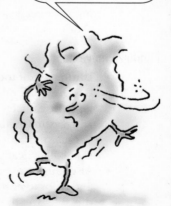

Acute blood loss can lead to hypovolemic shock.

What causes it?

Massive volume loss may result from the following:

- gastrointestinal (GI) bleeding, internal or external hemorrhage, or any condition that reduces circulating intravascular volume or other body fluids
- extensive burns or interruption of skin barrier
- intestinal obstruction
- peritonitis
- acute pancreatitis
- ascites
- dehydration from excessive perspiration, severe diarrhea or protracted vomiting, diabetes insipidus, diuresis, or inadequate fluid intake.

How it happens?

Potentially life threatening, hypovolemic shock stems from reduced intravascular blood volume, which leads to decreased cardiac output and inadequate tissue perfusion. The subsequent tissue anoxia prompts a shift in cellular metabolism from aerobic to anaerobic pathways. This results in an accumulation of lactic acid, which produces metabolic acidosis.

The road to shockville

When compensatory mechanisms fail, hypovolemic shock occurs in this sequence:

1. decreased intravascular fluid volume
2. diminished venous return, which reduces preload and decreases stroke volume
3. reduced cardiac output
4. decreased MAP
5. impaired tissue perfusion
6. decreased oxygen and nutrient delivery to cells
7. multiple organ dysfunction syndrome.

Between a rock and a hard space

Third-space fluid shift can also cause hypovolemic shock. It can occur in the abdominal cavity (ascites), pleural cavity, or pericardial sac. Third spacing of fluid may occur in conditions, such as intestinal obstruction, peritonitis, acute pancreatitis, and burns.

Hydrostatic pressure forces me out of the intravascular space.

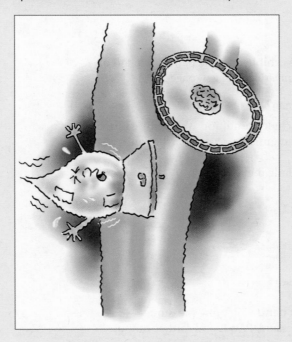

(Continued)

Between a rock and a hard space *(continued)*

But increased capillary permeability or decreased plasma colloid osmotic pressure traps me in the third, or interstitial, space.

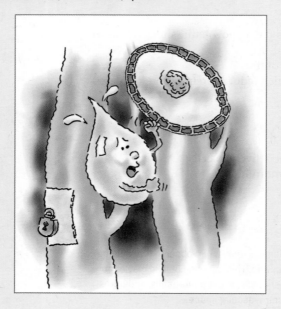

What to look for?

The specific signs and symptoms exhibited by the patient depend on the amount of fluid loss. (See *Estimating fluid loss,* page 283.)

Where, oh where, has the blood volume gone?

Typically, the patient's history includes conditions that reduce blood volume, such as GI hemorrhage, trauma, or severe diarrhea and vomiting.

Assessment findings may include the following:
- pale skin
- dry mucous membranes
- decreased skin turgor
- decreased sensorium
- rapid, shallow respirations
- urine output below 25 mL/hour
- rapid, thready peripheral pulses
- cold, clammy skin
- MAP below 60 mm Hg and a narrowing pulse pressure
- decreased CVP, right atrial pressure, PAWP, and cardiac output.

Estimating fluid loss

Use the following assessment parameters to determine the severity of fluid loss.

Minimal fluid loss
Signs and symptoms of minimal fluid loss include the following:
- slight tachycardia
- normal supine blood pressure
- positive postural vital signs, including a decrease in systolic blood pressure >10 mm Hg or an increase in pulse rate >20 beats/minute

- increased capillary refill time >3 seconds
- urine output >30 mL/hour
- cool, pale skin on arms and legs
- anxiety.

Moderate fluid loss
Signs and symptoms of moderate fluid loss include the following:
- rapid, thready pulse
- supine hypotension
- cool, truncal skin
- urine output of 10 to 30 mL/hour

- severe thirst
- restlessness, confusion, or irritability.

Severe fluid loss
Signs and symptoms of severe fluid loss include the following:
- marked tachycardia
- marked hypotension
- weak or absent peripheral pulses
- cold, mottled, or cyanotic skin
- urine output <10 mL/hour
- unconsciousness.

What tests tell you?

No single diagnostic test confirms hypovolemic shock, but these test results help to support the diagnosis:
- Decreased hemoglobin and hematocrit levels, but also both, may exhibit as elevated because of fluid loss and hemoconcentration of the blood
- decreased red blood cell and platelet counts
- coagulation studies for coagulopathy from disseminated intravascular coagulation (late stage)
- lactate levels elevated secondary to anaerobic metabolism
- elevated serum potassium, sodium, creatinine, and blood urea nitrogen levels
- increased urine-specific gravity (greater than 1.020) and urine osmolality
- urine sodium levels less than 50 mEq/L
- decreased pH and partial pressure of arterial oxygen and increased partial pressure of arterial carbon dioxide
- gastroscopy, X-rays, aspiration of gastric contents through a nasogastric tube, and tests for fecal occult blood.

How it's treated?

Emergency treatment relies on prompt and adequate fluid and blood replacement to restore intravascular volume and to raise blood pressure and maintain it above 90 mm Hg.

Stop the bleed! If hypovolemic shock is due to bleeding—stop the bleed by applying pressure or tourniquet. In hemorrhagic hypovolemic shock, blood replacement is critical. Trauma centers follow massive transfusion protocols to assist in getting blood to the patient rapidly (using O-negative uncrossmatched blood until a type and crossmatch is done).

If hypovolemic shock is due to fluid volume loss, rapid infusion of normal saline or lactated Ringer's solution may expand volume adequately. (See *When blood pressure drops.*)

When blood pressure drops

A drop below 90 mm Hg in systolic blood pressure usually signals inadequate cardiac output from reduced intravascular volume. Such a drop usually results in inadequate coronary artery blood flow, cardiac ischemia, arrhythmias, and other complications of low cardiac output.

Increase flow and go

If systolic blood pressure drops below 90 mm Hg and the patient's pulse is thready, increase the oxygen flow rate and notify the health care provider immediately.

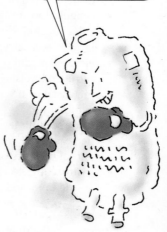

Fluid and blood replacement is the first step in treating hypovolemic shock.

Fashion forward

Three goals that exist in the emergency treatment of the patient with hypovolemic shock are as follows: (1) control further blood loss; (2) maximize oxygen delivery—completed by ensuring adequacy of ventilation, and administration of oxygen to increase oxygen saturation in the blood; and (3) fluid resuscitation. Treatment may also include the use of inotropic drugs to support blood pressure and surgery, if appropriate.

What to do?

- Collaborate care with a skilled team, which may include emergency medical personnel, a health care provider, blood bank personnel, and surgical team.
- Assess the patient for the extent of fluid loss and begin fluid replacement as ordered. Obtain a type and crossmatch for blood component therapy.

ABCs of Care

- Assess ABCs. If the patient experiences cardiac or respiratory arrest, start cardiopulmonary resuscitation.
- Administer supplemental oxygen as ordered. Monitor oxygen saturation and ABG studies for evidence of hypoxemia and anticipate the need for ET intubation and mechanical ventilation should the patient's respiratory status deteriorate.
- Monitor vital signs, neurologic status, and cardiac rhythm continuously for such changes as cardiac arrhythmias or myocardial ischemia. Observe skin color and check capillary refill. Notify the health care provider if capillary refill is greater than 2 seconds.
- Monitor hemodynamic parameters, including CVP, PAWP, and cardiac output, frequently—as often as every 15 minutes—to evaluate the patient's status and response to treatment.
- Monitor intake and output closely. Insert an indwelling urinary catheter and assess urine output hourly. If urine output falls below 30 mL/hour in an adult, expect to increase the IV fluid infusion rate, but watch for signs of fluid overload, such as elevated PAWP. Notify the health care provider if urine output doesn't increase. If bleeding from the GI tract is the suspected cause, check all stools, emesis, and gastric drainage for occult blood.
- Administer blood component therapy as ordered; monitor serial hemoglobin and hematocrit values to evaluate the effects of treatment.
- Administer inotropes or vasopressors as ordered, to increase cardiac contractility and renal perfusion.

Positioning for shock

For years, patients in hypovolemic shock were placed in Trendelenburg position. However, research now shows that only the legs should be elevated to avoid affecting gas exchange in the lungs or increasing intracranial pressure.

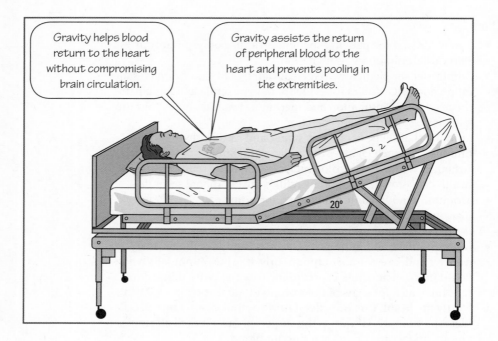

RX

- Supplemental oxygen or mechanical ventilation to maintain oxygenation
- Legs-up position
- Bleeding control
- Fluid and blood replacement

Clot concerns

- Watch for signs of impending coagulopathy (such as petechiae, bruising, and bleeding or oozing from the gums or venipuncture sites) and report them immediately.
- Provide emotional support and reassurance appropriately in the wake of massive fluid losses.
- Prepare the patient for surgery as indicated. Explain the treatment needed as well as expectations for the patient's condition after surgery.
- Document vital signs and assessment findings. Note the patient's response to treatment.

Suggested references

Bellone, A., Bossi, I., Etteri, M., Cantaluppi, F., Pina, P., Guanziroli, M., Bianchi, A., & Casazza, G. (2016). Factors associated with ICU admission following blunt chest trauma. *Canadian Respiratory Journal, 2016*, 3257846. https://doi.org/10.1155/2016/3257846

Bergman Schieman, K., Pattison, K., & Early, C. (2017). Caring for trauma patients with coexisting heart failure. *Journal of Trauma Nursing, 24*(5), 312–316. https://doi.org/10.1097/JTN.0000000000000316

Chrysou, K., Halat, G., Hoksch, B., Schmid, R., & Kocher, G. (2017). Lessons from a large trauma center: Impact of blunt chest trauma in polytrauma patients—still a relevant problem? *Scandinavian Journal of Trauma Resuscitation and Emergency Medicine, 25*(1), 42. https://doi.org/10.1186/s13049-017-0384-y

Hanschen, M., Kanz, K. G., Kirchhoff, C., Khalil, P. N., Wierer, M., van Griensven, M., Laugwitz, KL, Biberthaler, P, Lefering, R, Huber-Wagner, S; TraumaRegister DGU. (2015). Blunt cardiac injury in the severely injured—a retrospective multicentre study. *PloS One, 10*(7), e0131362. https://doi.org/10.1371/journal.pone.0131362

Kosaraju, A, Pendela, V.S., & Hai, O. (2023, April 7). *Cardiogenic shock. StatPearls.* [Internet]. StatPearls Publishing. https://www.ncbi.nlm.nih.gov/books/NBK482255/

Kragholm, K., Malta Hansen, C., Dupre, M. E., Xian, Y., Strauss, B., Tyson, C., Monk, L., Corbett, C., Fordyce, C. B., Pearson, D. A., Fosbøl, E. L., Jollis, J. G., Abella, B. S., McNally, B., & Granger, C. B. (2017). Direct transport to a percutaneous cardiac intervention center and outcomes in patients with out-of-hospital cardiac arrest. *Circulation: Cardiovascular Quality and Outcomes, 10*(6), e003414. https://doi.org/10.1161/CIRCOUTCOMES.116.003414

Kyriazidis, I. P., Jakob, D. A., Vargas, J. A., Franco, O. H., Degiannis, E., Dorn, P., Pouwels, S., Patel, B., Johnson, I., Houdlen, C. J., Whiteley, G. S., Head, M., Lala, A., Mumtaz, H., Soler, J. A., Mellor, K., Rawaf, D., Ahmed, A.R., Ahmad, S. J., & Exadaktylos, A. (2023). Accuracy of diagnostic tests in cardiac injury after blunt chest trauma: A systematic review and meta-analysis. *World Journal of Emergency Surgery, 18*(1), 36. https://doi.org/10.1186/s13017-023-00504-9

Makdisi, G., & Wang, I. W. (2015). Extra corporeal membrane oxygenation (ECMO) review of a lifesaving technology. *Journal of Thoracic Disease, 7*(7), 166–176. https://doi.org/10.3978/j.issn.2072-1439.2015.07.17

Odor, P., & Bailey, A. (2013, March 13). *Cardiac Tamponade. Anesthesia tutorial of the week – 283.* World Federation of Societies of Anaesthes.

Patil, V., & Shetmahajan, M. (2014). Massive transfusion and massive transfusion protocol. *Indian Journal of Anaesthesia, 58*(5), 590–595. https://doi.org/10.4103/0019-5049.144662

Singh, S., Heard, M., Pester, J., & Angus, L. D. (2022, October 28). *Blunt cardiac injury. StatPearls.* StatPearls Publishing. https://www.ncbi.nlm.nih.gov/books/NBK532267/

Stashko, E., & Meer, J. M., (2023, August 7). *Cardiac tamponade. StatPearls.* (Internet). StatPearls Publishing. https://www.ncbi.nlm.nih.gov/books/NBK431090/

Taghavi, S., & Askari, R. (2018). *Hypovolemic shock.* Retrieved from https://www.ncbi.nlm.nih.gov/books/NBK513297/.

Taghavi, S., Nassar, A. K., & Askari, R. (2023, June 5). *Hypovolemic shock. StatPearls.* (Internet). StatPearls Publishing. https://www.ncbi.nlm.nih.gov/books/ NBK513297/

Tehrani, B. N., Truesdell, A. G., Psotka, M. A., Rosner, C., Singh, R., Sinha, S. S., Damluji, A. A., & Batchelor, W. B. (2020). A standardized and comprehensive approach to the management of cardiogenic shock. *JACC Heart Failure, 8*(11), 879–891. https://doi.org/10.1016/j.jchf.2020.09.005

Tien, Y. T., Chen, W. J., Huang, C. H., Wang, C. H., Chen, W. T., Hung, C. S., Lin, J. J., Huang, C. C., Chang, W. T., & Tsai, M. S. (2022). The CSP (cardiogenic shock prognosis) score: A tool for risk stratification of cardiogenic shock. *Frontiers in Cardiovascular Medicine, 9*, 842056. https://doi.org/10.3389/ fcvm.2022.842056

Vahdatpour, C., Collins, D., & Goldberg, S. (2019). Cardiogenic shock. *Journal of American Heart Association, 8*(8), e011991. https://doi.org/10.1161/ JAHA.119.011991

Chapter 9

Treatments

Just the facts

In this chapter, you will learn:

◆ treatments for cardiovascular disorders

◆ patient preparation for specific types of cardiovascular treatments

◆ monitoring and home care techniques for the patient after discharge.

A look at treatments for cardiovascular disorders

Many treatments are available for patients with cardiovascular disorders; the dramatic ones, such as heart transplantation and artificial heart insertion, have received a lot of publicity. However, some more commonly used treatment measures include drug therapy, surgery, balloon catheter treatments, defibrillation, synchronized cardioversion, and pacemaker insertion.

Drug therapy

Several types of medications are critical to the treatment of cardiovascular disorders. These drugs include the following:

- Antiarrhythmics
- Inotropics
- Antianginals
- Antihypertensives
- Antilipemics
- Anticoagulants
- Antiplatelets
- Thrombolytics

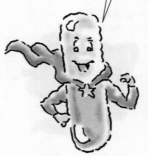

Looks like we are on!

Many drug types play critical roles in the treatment of cardiovascular disorders.

Antiarrhythmics

Antiarrhythmic drugs work to decrease abnormal heart rhythms otherwise known as dysrhythmias. They work in many different ways and are grouped in one of four classes.

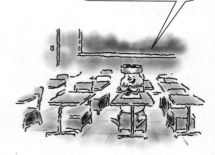

As far as class I antiarrhythmics go, I am a class act, but I am also in a class of my own.

Class	Features	Rhythms treated	Examples
I Sodium channel blockers	• Largest class • Three subdivisions plus adenosine • Decrease automaticity, conduction velocity, and membrane responsiveness	• IA: atrial and ventricular arrhythmias • IB: acute ventricular arrhythmias • IC: severe refractory ventricular arrhythmias • Adenosine: paroxysmal supraventricular tachycardia	• IA: disopyramide (Norpace) • IB: lidocaine (Xylocaine) • IC: flecainide (Tambocor)
II Beta-adrenergic blockers	• Slow automaticity of sinoatrial node • Reduce conduction of atrioventricular node and pacer cells • Decrease strength of contraction	• Atrial flutter and fibrillation • Paroxysmal atrial tachycardia	• Atenolol (Tenormin) • Metoprolol (Lopressor) • Propranolol (Inderal) • Carvedilol (Coreg) • Nebivolol (Bystolic)
III Diverse group	• Mechanism of action poorly understood • May slow repolarization • May prolong refractory period	• Ventricular arrhythmias	• Amiodarone (Cordarone) • Dofetilide (Tikosyn) • Sotalol (Betapace) • Ibutilide (Corvert)
IV Calcium channel blockers	• Decrease cardiac contractility and oxygen demand • Dilate coronary arteries and arterioles	• Supraventricular arrhythmias with rapid ventricular response	• Diltiazem (Cardizem) • Nifedipine (Procardia) • Verapamil (Calan)

Ionotropics

These drugs increase the force of the heart's contractions. There are two types:

- digoxin (Lanoxin)—which slows the heart rate and electrical impulse conduction through the sinoatrial and atrioventricular (AV) nodes

- phosphodiesterase inhibitors, which provide short-term management of heart failure or long-term management in patients awaiting heart transplant surgery. Two examples of phosphodiesterase inhibitors are inamrinone and milrinone.

Antianginals

Antianginal drugs relieve chest pain (angina) by reducing myocardial oxygen demand, increasing the supply of oxygen to the heart, or both. There are three main types:
- nitrates, used primarily to treat acute angina
- beta-adrenergic blockers, prescribed for long-term prevention of angina
- ranolazine (Ranexa), prescribed for patients with ischemic stable heart disease, if unable to tolerate acceptable doses of beta-blockers
- calcium channel blockers (used when other drugs fail to prevent angina).

How antianginal drugs work?

When the coronary arteries cannot supply enough oxygen to the myocardium, angina occurs. This forces the heart to work harder, increasing heart rate, preload, afterload, and the force of myocardial contractility. Antianginal drugs relieve angina by decreasing one or more of these four factors.

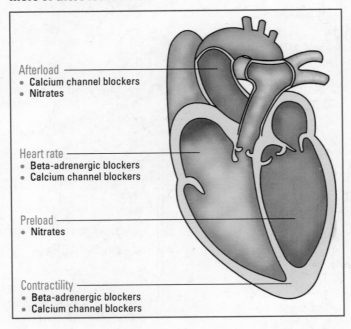

Afterload
- Calcium channel blockers
- Nitrates

Heart rate
- Beta-adrenergic blockers
- Calcium channel blockers

Preload
- Nitrates

Contractility
- Beta-adrenergic blockers
- Calcium channel blockers

Antihypertensives

Treatment for hypertension begins with modifying diet, encouraging exercise, and, if indicated, counseling about weight loss. If these measures are not enough, drugs can help.

There are many different kinds of antihypertensives. Some of the categories are listed below.

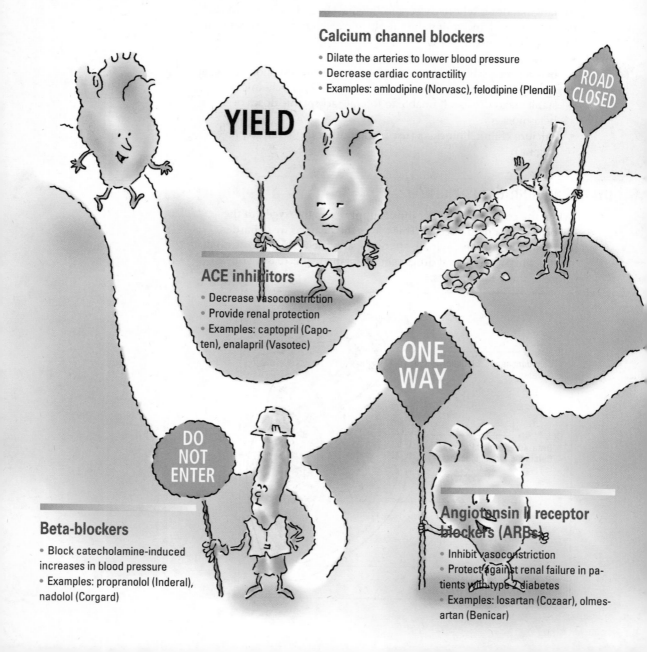

Calcium channel blockers

- Dilate the arteries to lower blood pressure
- Decrease cardiac contractility
- Examples: amlodipine (Norvasc), felodipine (Plendil)

ACE inhibitors

- Decrease vasoconstriction
- Provide renal protection
- Examples: captopril (Capoten), enalapril (Vasotec)

Beta-blockers

- Block catecholamine-induced increases in blood pressure
- Examples: propranolol (Inderal), nadolol (Corgard)

Angiotensin II receptor blockers (ARBs)

- Inhibit vasoconstriction
- Protect against renal failure in patients with type 2 diabetes
- Examples: losartan (Cozaar), olmesartan (Benicar)

Sympatholytics

- Decrease peripheral vascular resistance by inhibiting the sympathetic nervous system
- Examples: clonidine (Catapres), doxazosin (Cardura), carvedilol (Coreg)

Direct renin inhibitors

- Block renin and help blood vessels relax
- Example: aliskiren (Tekturna)

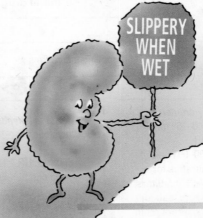

Diuretics

- Help kidneys excrete water and electrolytes, which lowers blood pressure
- Thiazide example: hydrochlorothiazide (HydroDIURIL)
- Loop example: furosemide (Lasix)
- Potassium sparing, example: triamterene (spironolactone) and Dyrenium (Aldactone) (http://www.mayoclinic.org/diseases-conditions/high-blood-pressure/in-depth/diuretics/art-20048129)

Selective aldosterone receptor antagonists

- Used as a second-line treatment when other drugs fail
- Eplerenone (Inspra), spironolactone (Aldactone) (https://www.drugs.com/drug-class/aldosterone-receptor-antagonists.html)

Vasodilators

- Relax arteries, veins, or both
- Oral example: hydralazine

For hypertensive crisis

- Example: I.V. nitroprusside (Nitropress)

Treating hypertension

Lifestyle modifications

↓

Not at goal blood pressure (<140/90 mm Hg)
(<130/80 mm Hg for patients with diabetes or chronic kidney disease)

↓

Initial drug choices

↓ (Without compelling indications)　　　　　　　↓ (With compelling indications)

Without compelling indications　　　　　**With compelling indications**

Stage 1 hypertension
(systolic BP 140–159 mm Hg
OR
diastolic BP 90–99 mm Hg)
Thiazide-type diuretics for
most. Consider ACE inhibitors,
ARBs, beta-blockers, calcium
channel blockers, direct renin
inhibitors, or combination.

Stage 2 hypertension
(systolic BP ≥ 160 mm Hg
OR
diastolic BP ≥ 100 mm Hg)
Two-drug combination for most
(usually thiazide-type diuretic and
ACE inhibitor, ARB, beta-blocker,
or calcium channel blocker).

- Drug(s) for compelling indications.
(See prescriber.)
- Other antihypertensive drugs
(diuretics, ACE inhibitors, ARBs, beta-
blockers, calcium channel blockers)
as needed.

↓

Not at goal blood pressure

↓

- Optimize dosages or add additional drugs until goal blood pressure is achieved.
- Consider consultation with hypertension specialist.
- Consider consultation with a nephrologist (https://www.uptodate.com/contents/
treatment-of-resistant-hypertension)

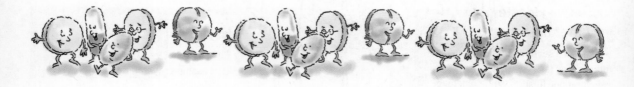

Antihypertensives and the renin–angiotensin–aldosterone system

The renin-angiotensin-aldosterone system (RAAS) regulates the body's sodium and water levels and blood pressure.

1. Juxtaglomerular cells near the glomeruli in each kidney secrete the enzyme renin into the blood.

2. Renin circulates throughout the body and converts angiotensinogen, made in the liver, to angiotensin I.

3. In the lungs, angiotensin I is converted by hydrolysis to angiotensin II.

4. Angiotensin II acts on the adrenal cortex to stimulate production of the hormone aldosterone. Aldosterone acts on the juxtaglomerular cells to increase sodium and water retention and to stimulate or depress further renin secretion, completing the feedback system that automatically readjusts homeostasis.

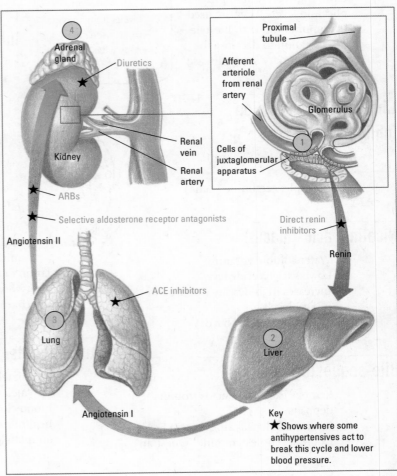

Adverse reactions of antihypertensive drugs

All	Angiotensin-converting enzyme inhibitors	Angiotensin II receptor blockers	Direct renin inhibitors
• Headache • Fatigue • Angioedema • Gastrointestinal reactions • Electrolyte imbalance (specific to drug used)	• Altered renal function when used with nonsteroidal anti-inflammatory drugs • Dry, nonproductive, and persistent cough	• Transient elevations of blood urea nitrogen and serum creatinine levels • Cough • Tickling in throat	• Dizziness • Fainting • Diarrhea

Antilipemics

Antilipemics lower cholesterol, triglyceride, and phospholipid levels. They are used in combination with lifestyle modification to decrease the risk of coronary artery disease.

Cholesterol absorption inhibitors

- Lower total cholesterol levels
- Example: ezetimibe (Zetia)

Nicotinic acid (niacin)

- Water-soluble vitamin
- Lowers triglyceride levels
- Increases high-density lipoprotein (HDL) levels
- Example: niacin (Niacor)

Bile-sequestering drugs

- Remove excess bile acids from fat deposits
- Lower low-density lipoprotein levels
- Example: cholestyramine (Questran)

Fibric acid derivatives

- Lower triglyceride levels
- Minimally increase HDL levels
- Examples: fenofibrate (Tricor) and gemfibrozil (Lopid)

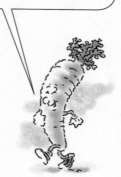

To lower cholesterol levels, combine pharmacologic therapy with lifestyle modification.

3-Hydroxy-3-methyl-glutaryl-coenzyme A reductase reductase inhibitors

- Also known as *statins*
- Lower total cholesterol and low-density lipoprotein levels
- Minimally increase HDL levels
- Examples: atorvastatin (Lipitor), simvastatin (Zocor), and rosuvastatin (Crestor)

Anticoagulants

Anticoagulants reduce the blood's ability to clot. They are prescribed for mitral insufficiency or atrial fibrillation or to dissolve clots that block an artery. Some anticoagulants are listed in the chart that follows.

Antiplatelets

Antiplatelets interfere with the binding of platelets or the process preceding the blood clotting process (https://www.healthline.com/health/anticoagulant-and-antiplatelet-drugs#what-they-do).

Category	Features	Examples
Heparins	• Used in patients with unstable angina, myocardial infarction, and deep vein thrombosis • Acts immediately when given intravenously (IV) • Available in regular and low molecular weight forms	• Heparin (Liquaemin) *low molecular weight* • Dalteparin (Fragmin) • Enoxaparin (Lovenox)
Coumarin derivative	• Antagonizes production of vitamin K–dependent clotting factors • Prevents deep vein thrombosis • Used in patients who have undergone prosthetic heart valve surgery and those with diseased valves • Given orally and takes days to reach effect	• Warfarin (Coumadin)
Antiplatelet drugs	• Prevent thromboembolism	• Brilinta (Ticagrelor) • Clopidogrel (Plavix)
Direct thrombin inhibitors (IIa)	• Treat heparin-induced thrombocytopenia • Used when heparin cannot be prophylactically used before angioplasty and stent placement • Available IV	• Argatroban • Bivalirudin (Angiomax) • Lepirudin (Refludan)
Glycoprotein IIb/IIIa inhibitors	• Used in patients with unstable angina and before and during angioplasty • Prevent platelets from binding together • Available IV	• Abciximab (ReoPro) • Eptifibatide (Integrilin) • Tirofiban (Aggrastat)

Thrombolytics

Thrombolytics can dissolve a preexisting clot or thrombus in acute myocardial infarction (MI), ischemic stroke, or peripheral artery occlusion. They also can dissolve thrombi and reestablish blood flow in arteriovenous cannulas and IV catheters. In an acute situation or an emergent situation, they must be administered within 3 to 6 hours after the onset of symptoms. Thrombolytics include alteplase (Activase), reteplase (Retavase), urokinase (Abbokinase), and tenecteplase (TNKase).

How thrombolytics help restore circulation?

When a thrombus forms in an artery, it obstructs the blood supply, causing ischemia and necrosis. Thrombolytics can dissolve thrombi in the coronary and pulmonary arteries, restoring the blood supply to the area beyond the blockage.

Obstructed artery

A thrombus blocks blood flow through the artery, causing distal ischemia.

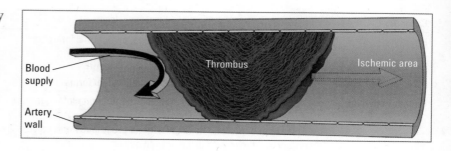

Blood supply

Thrombus

Ischemic area

Artery wall

Inside the thrombus

The thrombolytic enters the thrombus and binds to the fibrin–plasminogen complex, converting inactive plasminogen into active plasmin. Active plasmin digests fibrin, dissolving the thrombus. As the thrombus dissolves, blood flow resumes.

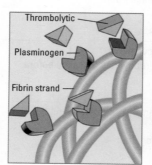

Thrombolytic

Plasminogen

Fibrin strand

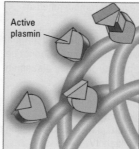

Active plasmin

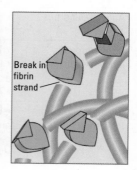

Break in fibrin strand

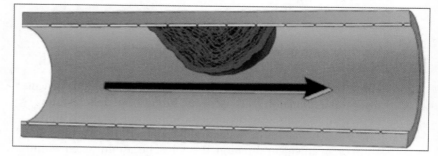

Surgery

Despite successful advances, such as single- and multiple-organ transplants, improved immunosuppressants, and improved ventricular assist devices (VADs), far more patients undergo conventional surgeries. Surgeries for the treatment of disorders of the cardiovascular system include coronary artery bypass grafting (CABG), minimally invasive direct coronary artery bypass (MIDCAB), totally endoscopic coronary artery bypass (TECAB), off-pump CABG, heart transplantation, vascular repair, valve surgery, and VAD insertion.

Coronary artery bypass grafting

A CABG circumvents an occluded coronary artery with an autogenous graft (usually a segment of the saphenous vein or internal mammary artery) to restore blood flow to the myocardium. CABG techniques vary according to the patient's condition and the number of arteries needing bypass.

Construction ahead

The most common procedure, aortocoronary bypass, involves suturing one end of the autogenous graft to the ascending aorta and the other end to a coronary artery distal to the occlusion. (See *Bypassing coronary occlusions*, page 301.)

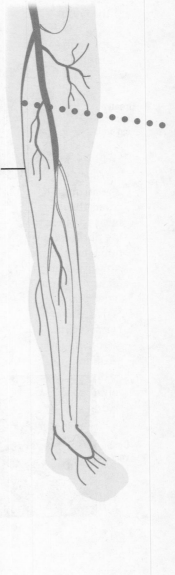

Greater saphenous vein (donor vein)

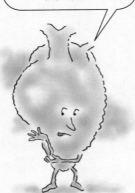

CABG circumvents an occluded coronary artery by using a segment of the saphenous vein, radial artery, or internal mammary artery to restore blood flow to the heart.

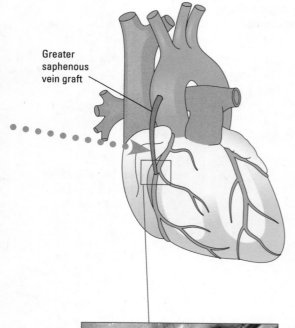

Greater
saphenous
vein graft

Performing CABG surgery

CABG surgery is performed either "on pump" (the traditional method) or "off pump" (also called the "beating heart method" or OPCAB). A technician monitors the heart–lung machine (cardiopulmonary bypass pump), shown below.

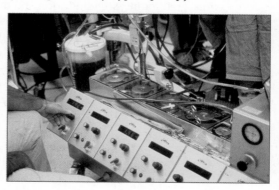

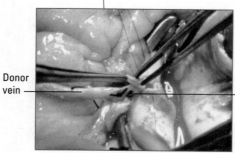

Donor vein

Sutures

Bypassing coronary occlusions

After the patient receives general anesthesia and is placed on mechanical ventilation, aortocoronary bypass surgery begins with graft harvesting. The surgeon makes a series of incisions in the patient's thigh or calf and removes a saphenous vein segment for grafting. Most surgeons prefer to use a segment of the internal mammary artery.

Exposing the heart

Once the autografts are obtained, the surgeon performs a median sternotomy to expose the heart and then initiates cardiopulmonary bypass. Sometimes, small multiple incisions are made when a sternotomy is not the traditional approach.

To reduce myocardial oxygen demands during surgery and to protect the heart, the surgeon induces cardiac hypothermia and standstill by injecting a cold cardioplegic solution (potassium-enriched saline solution) into the aortic root.

One fine sewing lesson

After the patient is prepared, the surgeon sutures one end of the venous graft to the ascending aorta and the other end to a patent coronary artery that is distal to the occlusion. The graft is sutured in a reversed position to promote proper blood flow. The surgeon repeats this procedure for each occlusion to be bypassed.

In the example depicted below, saphenous vein segments bypass occlusions in three sections of the coronary artery.

Finishing up

When the grafts are in place, the surgeon flushes the cardioplegic solution from the heart and discontinues cardiopulmonary bypass. The surgeon then implants epicardial pacing electrodes, inserts a chest tube, closes the incision, and applies a sterile dressing.

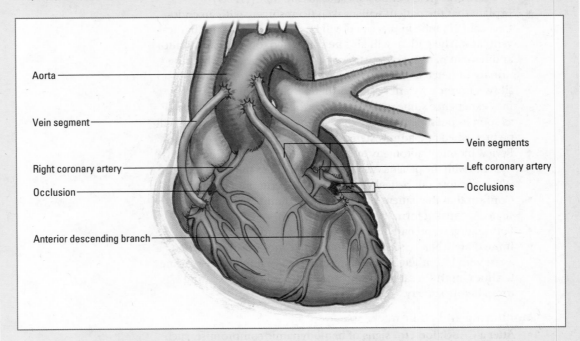

Aorta

Vein segment

Right coronary artery

Occlusion

Anterior descending branch

Vein segments

Left coronary artery

Occlusions

CABG candidates

More than 200,000 Americans (most of them male) undergo CABG each year, making it one of the most common cardiac surgeries. Prime candidates include patients with severe angina from atherosclerosis and others with coronary artery disease that have a high risk of MI. Successful CABG can relieve anginal pain, improve cardiac function, and, possibly, enhance the patient's quality of life and resumption to normal life.

CABG caveat

Although the surgery relieves pain in about 90% of patients, its long-term effectiveness is unclear. In addition, such problems as graft closure and development of atherosclerosis in other coronary arteries may make repeat surgery necessary. In addition, because CABG does not resolve the underlying disease associated with arterial blockage, CABG may not reduce the risk of MI recurrence.

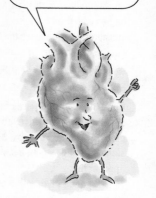

The most common bypass builds a new road from the aorta to a coronary artery.

Patient preparation

- Reinforce the health care provider's explanation of the surgery.
- Explain the complex equipment and procedures used in the intensive care unit (ICU) or postanesthesia care unit (PACU).
- Explain that the patient will awaken from surgery with an endotracheal (ET) tube in place and will be connected to a mechanical ventilator. The patient will also be connected to a cardiac monitor and have in place a nasogastric tube, a chest tube, an indwelling urinary catheter, arterial lines, epicardial pacing wires, and, possibly, a pulmonary artery (PA) catheter. Tell the patient that they may experience some discomfort, but the equipment is removed as soon as possible. Reassure the patient that pain medication will be prescribed and administered.
- Review incentive spirometry techniques and range of motion (ROM) exercises with the patient. Also teach the patient to splint the incision. When possible, this patient teaching should occur prior to surgery.
- Confirm that the patient or a responsible family member has signed a consent form.
- Before surgery, prepare the patient's skin as ordered.
- Immediately before surgery, begin cardiac monitoring and then assist with PA catheterization and insertion of arterial lines. Some facilities insert PA catheters and arterial lines in the operating room before surgery.

Monitoring and aftercare

- After a CABG, look for signs of hemodynamic compromise, such as severe hypotension, decreased cardiac output, and shock.
- Begin warming procedures according to your facility's policy.
- Check and record vital signs and hemodynamic parameters every 5 to 15 minutes until the patient's condition stabilizes. Administer

medications as ordered and titrate according to the patient's response.

- Monitor electrocardiograms (ECGs) continuously for disturbances in heart rate and rhythm. If you detect serious abnormalities, notify the health care provider and be prepared to assist with epicardial pacing or, if necessary, cardioversion or defibrillation.

Reading the map

- To ensure adequate myocardial perfusion, keep arterial pressure within the limits set by the health care provider. Usually, mean arterial pressure (MAP) less than 70 mm Hg results in inadequate tissue perfusion; pressure greater than 110 mm Hg can cause hemorrhage and graft rupture. Monitor pulmonary artery pressure (PAP), central venous pressure (CVP), left atrial pressure, and cardiac output as ordered.
- Frequently evaluate the patient's peripheral pulses, capillary refill time, skin temperature, and color and auscultate for heart sounds; report any abnormalities.
- Evaluate tissue oxygenation by assessing breath sounds, chest excursion, and symmetry of chest expansion. Check arterial blood gas (ABG) results upon arrival in ICU. Collaborate with respiratory therapy to extubate the patient as soon as possible per order/policy.
- Maintain chest tube drainage at the ordered negative pressure (usually −10 to −40 cm H_2O) and assess regularly for hemorrhage, excessive drainage (greater than 200 mL/hour), and sudden decrease or cessation of drainage.

In and out

- Monitor the patient's intake and output and assess for electrolyte imbalance, especially hypokalemia and hypomagnesemia. Assess urine output at least hourly during the immediate postoperative period and then less frequently as the patient's condition stabilizes.
- As the patient's incisional pain increases, give an analgesic or other drugs as ordered.
- Throughout the recovery period and postoperative course, assess for signs and symptoms of stroke, pulmonary embolism, pneumonia, and impaired renal perfusion.
- After weaning the patient from the ventilator and removing the ET tube, provide chest physiotherapy. Start with incentive spirometry and encourage the patient to splint the incision, cough, turn frequently, and deep breathe. Assist with ROM exercises, as ordered, to enhance peripheral circulation and prevent thrombus formation.
- Monitor blood sugar and administer insulin per postoperative protocol. Blood sugar results can fluctuate greatly after surgery. This is important for patients with and without a history of diabetes.

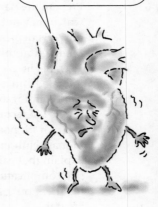

After a CABG, be on the lookout for severe hypotension, decreased cardiac output, and shock. These signs indicate hemodynamic compromise.

Postperi problems

- Explain that postpericardiotomy syndrome commonly develops after open-heart surgery. Instruct the patient about signs and symptoms, such as fever, muscle and joint pain, weakness, and chest discomfort. Keep in mind that a mild transient temperature elevation may be a normal physiological response after surgery; however, temperature should be monitored closely and reported promptly if the patient does not respond to temperature-reducing medications.
- Prepare the patient for the possibility of postoperative depression, which may not develop until weeks after discharge. Reassure them that this depression is normal and should pass quickly.
- Maintain nothing-by-mouth status until bowel sounds return. Then begin the patient on clear liquids and advance the diet as tolerated and as ordered. Tell the patient to expect sodium and cholesterol restrictions and explain that this diet can help reduce the risk of recurrent arterial occlusion.
- Monitor for postoperative complications, such as stroke, pulmonary embolism, pneumonia, and impaired renal perfusion.
- Explain that early mobility is important to prevent postoperative complications. Inform the patient that staff will be assisting them out of bed to the chair and ambulating when they are stable.
- Gradually allow the patient to increase activities as ordered. (See *Using cardiac rehabilitation*.)
- Monitor the incision site for signs of infection or drainage.
- Provide support to the patient and their family to help them cope with recovery and lifestyle changes. (See *Teaching the patient after CABG*, page 305.)
- Monitor ECG tracings, assessing for arrhythmias, such as atrial fibrillation, or torsades de pointes because of hypomagnesemia and premature ventricular contractions because of hypokalemia.

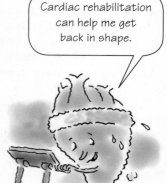

Cardiac rehabilitation can help me get back in shape.

Using cardiac rehabilitation

Cardiac rehabilitation is an exercise program to monitor and improve cardiovascular status and help the patient learn how to manage heart disease.

Elements of cardiac rehabilitation include the following:
- individualized exercise program
- diet, nutrition, and weight control
- stress management
- reduction of risk factors
- lipid and cholesterol control.

Sessions are held weekly, based on patient's needs and tolerance. Heart rate, blood pressure, and symptoms are continuously monitored during the session. Education is provided based on the patient's individual needs.

Teaching the patient after CABG

Before discharge from the hospital, instruct the patient on the following:

• watch for and immediately notify the health care provider of any signs of infection (redness, swelling, or drainage from the leg or chest incisions; fever; or sore throat) or possible arterial reocclusion (angina, dizziness, dyspnea, rapid or irregular pulse, or prolonged recovery time from exercise)

• check weight daily (at the same time every day and preferably in the morning)

• call the health care provider in the case of weight gain greater than 3 lb (1.4 kg) in 1 week; the patient may be developing congestive heart failure

• follow their prescribed diet, especially sodium and cholesterol restrictions

• maintain a balance between activity and rest by trying to sleep at least 8 hours each night, scheduling a short rest period each afternoon, and resting frequently when engaging in tiring physical activity

• participate in an exercise program or cardiac rehabilitation, if prescribed

• follow lifestyle modifications (no smoking, improved diet, and regular exercise) to reduce atherosclerotic progression

• contact a local chapter of the Mended Hearts and the American Heart Association for information and support

• understand the dose, frequency of administration, and possible adverse effects of prescribed medications; discuss pain medications and pain management

• follow up with cardiology, the surgeon, and the primary care physician.

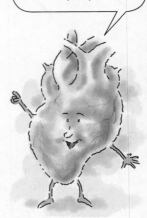

Wow! MIDCAB and TECAB can be performed while I pump.

Minimally invasive direct coronary artery bypass and totally endoscopic coronary artery bypass

Originally, cardiac surgery required stopping the heart and using cardiopulmonary bypass to oxygenate and circulate blood. MIDCAB and TECAB can be performed on a pumping heart through small thoracotomies. The patient may receive only right lung ventilation along with drugs, such as beta-adrenergic blockers, to slow the heart rate and reduce heart movement during surgery. MIDCAB is more widely available than TECAB.

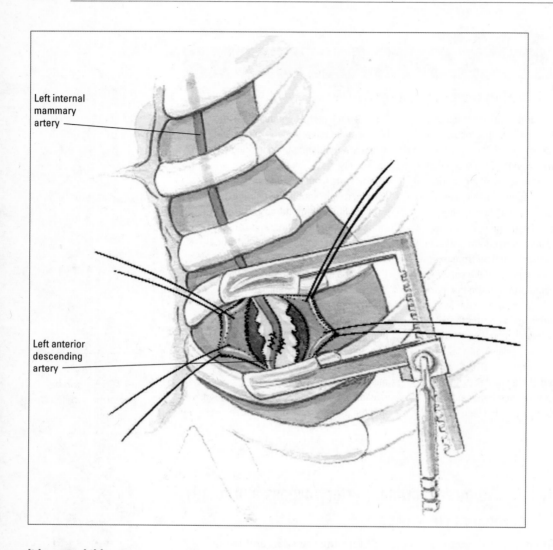

Left internal mammary artery

Left anterior descending artery

It is a good thing

Advantages of MIDCAB and TECAB include shorter hospital stays, use of short-acting anesthetic agents, fewer postoperative complications (such as infection), earlier extubation, reduced cost, smaller incisions, and earlier return to work. Patients eligible for MIDCAB and TECAB include those with proximal left anterior descending lesions and some lesions of the right coronary and circumflex arteries.

Patient preparation

- Review the procedure with the patient and answer their questions. Tell the patient that they will be extubated in the operating room or within 2 to 4 hours after surgery.

- Teach the patient to splint their incision, cough and breathe deeply, and use an incentive spirometer.
- Explain the use of pain medications after surgery as well as non-pharmacologic methods to control pain.
- Let the patient know that they should be able to walk with assistance the first postoperative day and be discharged within 48 hours.

Comparing types of CABG

Features	On-pump CABG	OPCAB	MIDCAB
Access site	• Breastbone severed for heart access	• Breastbone severed for heart access	• Incisions made between ribs for anterior heart access, no bones cut
Indications	• Suitable for multivessel disease, any coronary artery	• Suitable for multivessel disease, any coronary artery	• Only used for one-vessel diseases in anterior portions of the heart, such as left anterior descending artery, or some portions of the right coronary and circumflex arteries
Graft types	• Combination of artery and vein grafts	• Combination of artery and vein grafts	• Arterial grafts (better long-term results)
Complications	• Highest risk of postoperative complications	• Reduced blood usage, fewer rhythm problems, less kidney dysfunction than on-pump CABG	• Reduced blood usage, fewest complications, fastest recovery
Intubation	• Up to 24 hours	• Up to 24 hours	• Usually for 2–4 hours
Incisions	• Leg incisions for vein grafting, possibly arm incision for radial artery grafting	• Leg incisions for vein grafting, possibly arm incision for radial artery grafting	• No leg incisions, possibly arm incision for radial artery grafting
Heart and lung function	• Heart and lung circulation bypassed mechanically, affecting blood cells	• Drugs and special equipment used to slow heart and immobilize it; cardiopulmonary and systemic circulation still function	• Drugs used to slow heart; cardiopulmonary and systemic circulation still function

Monitoring and aftercare

- After a MIDCAB or TECAB, look for signs of hemodynamic compromise, such as severe hypotension, decreased cardiac output, and shock.
- Check and record vital signs and hemodynamic parameters every 5 to 15 minutes until the patient's condition stabilizes. Administer medications as ordered and titrate according to the patient's response.

- Monitor ECGs continuously for disturbances in heart rate and rhythm. If you detect serious abnormalities, notify the health care provider and be prepared to assist with epicardial pacing or, if necessary, cardioversion or defibrillation because the most common arrhythmia is atrial fibrillation.
- To ensure adequate myocardial perfusion, keep arterial pressure within the limits set by the health care provider. Usually, an MAP less than 70 mm Hg results in inadequate tissue perfusion; pressure greater than 110 mm Hg can cause hemorrhage and graft rupture. Monitor hemodynamic parameters such as CVP as ordered. If PA catheter is inserted, monitor PAP and cardiac output as ordered.
- Frequently evaluate the patient's peripheral pulses, capillary refill time, skin temperature and color, and auscultate for heart sounds; report any abnormalities.
- Evaluate tissue oxygenation by assessing breath sounds, chest excursion, and symmetry of chest expansion.
- Monitor the patient's intake and output and assess for electrolyte imbalance, especially hypokalemia and hypomagnesemia. Assess urine output at least hourly during the immediate postoperative period and then less frequently as the patient's condition stabilizes.
- Provide analgesia or encourage the use of patient-controlled analgesia, if appropriate.
- Throughout the recovery period, assess for symptoms of stroke, pulmonary embolism, and impaired renal perfusion.
- Provide incentive spirometry and encourage the patient to splint their incision, cough, turn frequently, and deep breathe. Assist with ROM exercises, as ordered, to enhance peripheral circulation and prevent thrombus formation.
- Explain that postpericardiotomy syndrome commonly develops after open-heart surgery. Instruct the patient about signs and symptoms, such as fever, muscle and joint pain, weakness, and chest discomfort.
- Prepare the patient for the possibility of postoperative depression, which may not develop until weeks after discharge. Reassure the patient that this depression is normal and should pass quickly.
- Maintain nothing-by-mouth status until bowel sounds return. Then begin the patient on clear liquids and advance the diet as tolerated and as ordered. Tell the patient to expect sodium and cholesterol restrictions and explain that this diet can help reduce the risk of recurrent arterial occlusion.
- Gradually allow the patient to increase activities as ordered.
- Monitor the incision site for signs of infection or drainage.
- Provide support to the patient and their family to help them cope with recovery and lifestyle changes. (See *Teaching the patient after MIDCAB or TECAB.*)

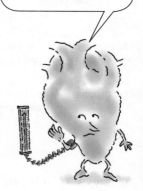

After a MIDCAB or TECAB, check and record vital signs and hemodynamic parameters every 5 to 15 minutes until the patient's condition stabilizes.

Teaching the patient after MIDCAB or TECAB

Before discharge from the hospital following MIDCAB or TECAB, instruct the patient to:
• continue with the progressive exercise started in the facility
• perform coughing and deep-breathing exercises (while splinting the incision with a pillow to reduce pain) and use the incentive spirometer to reduce pulmonary complications
• avoid lifting objects that weigh more than 10 lb (4.5 kg) for the next 4 to 6 weeks
• wait 2 to 4 weeks before resuming sexual activity

• check the incision site daily and immediately notify the health care provider of signs of infection (redness, foul-smelling drainage, or swelling) or possible graft occlusion (slow, rapid, or irregular pulse; angina; dizziness; or dyspnea)
• perform necessary incisional care
• follow lifestyle modifications
• take medications as prescribed and report adverse effects to the health care provider
• consider participation in a cardiac rehabilitation program.

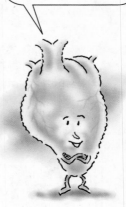

Coughing is encouraged following cardiac procedures such as MIDCAB and TECAB.

Heart transplantation

Heart transplantation involves the replacement of a person's heart with a donor heart. It is the treatment of choice for patients with end-stage cardiac disease that have a poor prognosis, estimated survival of 6 to 12 months, and poor quality of life. A heart transplant candidate typically has uncontrolled symptoms and no other surgical options. Transplantation does not guarantee a cure. Serious postoperative complications include infection and tissue rejection. Most patients experience one, or both, of these complications postoperatively.

Heart to heart

The donor's heart

The donor's heart is removed after the surgeon cuts along these dissection lines.

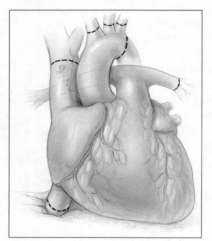

Anterior view

The transplanted heart

The transplanted heart is sutured.

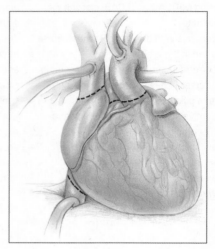

The recipient's heart

Before it can be removed, the recipient's heart is resected along these lines.

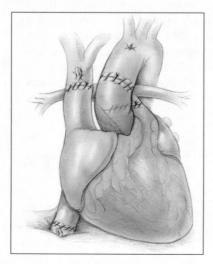

Rejection and infection

Rejection typically occurs in the first 6 weeks after surgery, but it may still occur after this time (up to 1 year following transplantation). The patient is treated with monoclonal antibodies and potent immunosuppressants. The resulting immunosuppression places the patient at risk for life-threatening infection.

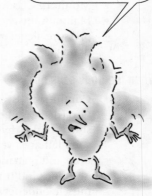

Most patients experience infection, tissue rejection, or both after heart transplantation.

Patient preparation

- Reinforce the health care provider's explanation of the surgery.
- Explain the complex equipment and procedures used in ICU and PACU.
- Explain that the patient will awaken from surgery with an ET tube in place and will be connected to a mechanical ventilator. They will also be connected to a cardiac monitor and have in place a nasogastric tube, a chest tube, an indwelling urinary catheter, arterial lines, epicardial pacing wires, and, possibly, a PA catheter. Tell the patient that if they experience discomfort and pain, medication will be available. The equipment will be removed as soon as possible.
- Review incentive spirometry techniques and ROM exercises with the patient.
- Confirm that the patient or a responsible family member has signed an informed consent form.
- Before surgery, prepare the patient's skin as ordered.
- Immediately before surgery, begin cardiac monitoring and then assist with PA catheterization and insertion of arterial lines. Some facilities insert PA catheters and arterial lines in the operating room before surgery.

Monitoring and aftercare

- Provide emotional support to the patient and their family. Begin to address their fears by discussing the procedure, possible complications, and the impact of transplantation and a prolonged recovery period on the patient's life.
- After surgery, maintain protective (reverse) isolation.
- Administer immunosuppressants and monitor the patient closely for signs of infection. Transplant recipients may exhibit only subtle signs because immunosuppressants mask obvious signs. Prophylactic regimens are sometimes recommended for recipients. These may include sulfamethoxazole and trimethoprim to prevent *Pneumocystis carinii*. CMV hyperimmune globulin and ganciclovir are also given to CMV-seronegative recipients of a seropositive donor organ (Abbott, 2019).
- Monitor vital signs every 15 minutes until stabilized and assess the patient for signs of hemodynamic compromise, such as hypotension, decreased cardiac output, and shock.
- If necessary, administer nitroprusside (Nipride) during the first 24 to 48 hours to control blood pressure. An infusion of dopamine can improve contractility.

- Volume replacement with normal saline, plasma expanders, or blood products may be necessary to maintain CVP. Monitor the patient for signs and symptoms of fluid overload, such as edema, jugular vein distention, and increased PAPs.
- Patients with an elevated PAP may receive prostaglandin E to produce pulmonary vasodilation and reduced right ventricular afterload.
- Monitor ECGs for rhythm disturbances.
- Maintain the chest tube drainage system at the prescribed negative pressure. Regularly assess for hemorrhage or sudden cessation of drainage.

When the body says no

- Continually assess the patient for signs of tissue rejection (decreased electrical activity on the ECG, right-axis shift, atrial arrhythmias, conduction defects, weight gain, lethargy, ventricular failure, jugular vein distention, and increased T-cell count).
- Keep in mind that the effects of denervated heart muscle or denervation (in which the vagus nerve is cut during heart transplant surgery) makes drugs such as edrophonium (Tensilon) and anticholinergics (such as atropine) ineffective. (See *Teaching the patient after heart transplantation.*)

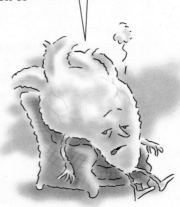

Since my surgery, I have experienced such problems as atrial arrhythmias, conduction defects, and jugular vein distention.

No place like home

Teaching the patient after heart transplantation

Before discharge from the hospital, instruct the patient to:
- continue with the progressive exercise started in the facility
- perform coughing and deep-breathing exercises (while splinting the incision with a pillow to reduce pain) and use the incentive spirometer to reduce pulmonary complications
- avoid lifting objects that weigh more than 10 lb (4.5 kg) for the next 4 to 6 weeks
- wait 2 to 4 weeks before resuming sexual activity
- check the incision site daily and immediately notify the health care provider of any signs of infection (such as redness,

foul-smelling drainage, swelling, fever, or excessive pain)
- perform incisional care as directed
- follow lifestyle modifications
- take medications (**which will be lifelong**), as prescribed, and report adverse effects to the health care provider
- consider participation in a cardiac rehabilitation program, as advised
- immediately report any episodes of chest pain or shortness of breath
- avoid crowds and anyone with an infectious illness
- comply with follow-up visits, as instructed
- get any recommended seasonal vaccine (flu, COVID, and pneumonia)
- perform regular handwashing.

Vascular repair

Vascular repair includes aneurysm resection, aneurysm exclusion, grafting, embolectomy, vena cava filtering, endarterectomy, vein stripping, and vein ablation. The specific surgery used depends on the type, location, and extent of vascular occlusion or damage. (See *Types of vascular repair*, page 313.) Vascular surgery can be performed as traditional open surgery or as a less invasive endovascular surgery.

Types of vascular repair

Several procedures exist to repair damaged or diseased vessels. These options include aortic aneurysm repair, vena cava filter insertion, embolectomy, and bypass grafting.

Aortic aneurysm repair

Open abdominal surgery: Aortic aneurysm repair involves removing or excluding an aneurysmal segment of the aorta. The surgeon first makes an incision to expose the aneurysm site. If necessary, the patient is placed on a cardiopulmonary bypass machine. Next, the surgeon clamps the aorta, resects the aneurysm, and repairs the damaged portion of the aorta. A synthetic bypass graft may be used.

Endovascular aneurysm repair involves an incision in the femoral artery. A catheter (and the graft) is threaded through the vessel to the site of the aneurysm. The graft is expanded into place.

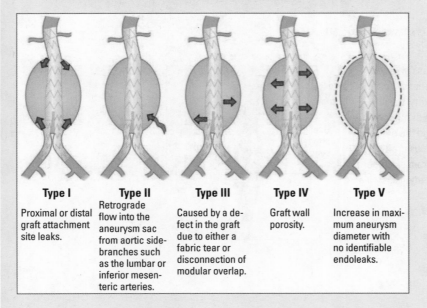

Type I	Type II	Type III	Type IV	Type V
Proximal or distal graft attachment site leaks.	Retrograde flow into the aneurysm sac from aortic side-branches such as the lumbar or inferior mesenteric arteries.	Caused by a defect in the graft due to either a fabric tear or disconnection of modular overlap.	Graft wall porosity.	Increase in maximum aneurysm diameter with no identifiable endoleaks.

Types of vascular repair *(continued)*

Vena cava filter insertion

A vena cava filter traps emboli in the vena cava, preventing them from reaching the pulmonary vessels. Inserted percutaneously by catheter, the vena cava filter, or *umbrella*, traps emboli but allows venous blood flow.

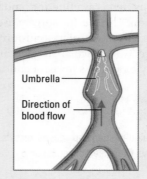

Umbrella

Direction of blood flow

Embolectomy

To remove an embolism from an artery, a surgeon may perform an embolectomy. In this procedure, the surgeon inserts a balloon-tipped indwelling catheter in the artery and passes it through the thrombus (as shown below left). The surgeon then inflates the balloon and withdraws the catheter to remove the thrombus (as shown above right).

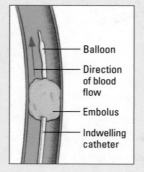

Balloon

Direction of blood flow

Embolus

Indwelling catheter

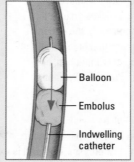

Balloon

Embolus

Indwelling catheter

Bypass grafting

Bypass grafting serves to bypass an arterial obstruction resulting from arteriosclerosis. After exposing the affected artery, the surgeon anastomoses a synthetic or autogenous graft to divert blood flow around the occluded arterial segment. The autogenous graft may be a vein or artery harvested from elsewhere in the patient's body. The illustration shows a femoropopliteal bypass.

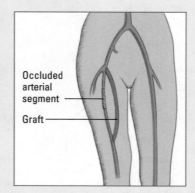

Occluded arterial segment

Graft

Life and limb

Vascular repair can be used to treat the following:
- vessels damaged by arteriosclerotic or thromboembolic disorders (such as aortic aneurysm or arterial occlusive disease), trauma, infections, or congenital defects
- vascular obstructions that severely compromise blood flow
- vascular disease that does not respond to drug therapy or nonsurgical treatments such as balloon catheterization
- life-threatening dissecting or ruptured aortic aneurysms
- limb-threatening acute arterial occlusion.

Repair despairs

All vascular surgeries have the potential for vessel trauma, emboli, hemorrhage, infection, and other complications. Grafting carries added risks because the graft may occlude, narrow, dilate, or rupture.

Patient preparation

- Make sure the patient and their family understand the health care provider's explanation of the surgery and its possible complications.
- Ensure a patient consent is signed.
- Tell the patient that they will receive a general anesthetic and will awaken from the anesthetic in the ICU or PACU. Explain that they will have an IV line in place, ECG electrodes for continuous cardiac monitoring, and, possibly, an arterial line or a PA catheter to provide continuous pressure monitoring. The patient may also have a urinary catheter in place to allow accurate output measurement. If appropriate, explain that they will be intubated and placed on mechanical ventilation.

Flow check

- Before surgery, perform a complete vascular assessment and document it. Take vital signs to provide a baseline. Evaluate the strength and sound of the blood flow and the symmetry of the pulses and note bruits. Record the temperature of the extremities; their sensitivity to motor and sensory stimuli; and pallor, cyanosis, or redness. Rate peripheral pulse volume and strength on a scale of 0 (pulse absent) to 4 (bounding pulse) and check capillary refill time by blanching the fingernail or toenail; normal refill time is less than 3 seconds.
- Instruct the patient that they may be ordered to restrict food/fluid for a period of time preoperatively. Failure to adhere to these directions may cause the surgery to be postponed.

Keep your guard

- If the patient is awaiting surgery for aortic aneurysm repair, be on guard for signs and symptoms of acute dissection or rupture. Especially note sudden, severe, tearing pain in the chest, abdomen, or lower back; severe weakness; diaphoresis; tachycardia; or a precipitous drop in blood pressure. If any of these signs or symptoms occurs, notify the health care provider immediately.

Monitoring and aftercare

- Check and record the patient's vital signs every 15 minutes until their condition stabilizes, then every 30 minutes for 1 hour, and hourly thereafter for 2 to 4 hours. Report hypotension and hypertension immediately.
- Auscultate heart, breath, and bowel sounds and report abnormal findings. Monitor the ECG for abnormalities in heart rate or rhythm. Also monitor other pressure readings and carefully record intake and output.
- Check the patient's dressing regularly for excessive bleeding.
- Assess the patient's neurologic and renal function and report abnormalities.
- Provide analgesics, as ordered, for incisional pain.
- Frequently assess peripheral pulses, using a handheld Doppler if palpation is difficult. Mark on the skin the location of the Doppler signals. Check all extremities bilaterally for muscle strength and movement, color, temperature, and capillary refill time.
- Change dressings and provide incision care as ordered. Position the patient to avoid pressure on grafts and to reduce edema. Administer antithrombotics, as ordered, and monitor appropriate laboratory values to evaluate effectiveness.
- Assess for complications and immediately report relevant signs and symptoms. (See *Vascular repair complications*.)

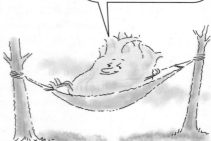

After vascular repair, position the patient to avoid pressure on grafts and to reduce edema.

Vascular repair complications

After a patient has undergone vascular repair surgery, monitor for these potential complications.

Complication	Signs and symptoms
Pulmonary infection	• Fever • Cough • Congestion • Dyspnea • Abnormal lung sounds • Fatigue • Malaise

(Continued)

Vascular repair complications *(continued)*

Complication	Signs and symptoms
Infection	• Redness • Warmth • Drainage • Pain • Fever • Increased heart rate • Hypertension or hypotension • Malaise • Microalbuminuria
Renal dysfunction	• Low urine output • Elevated blood urea nitrogen and serum creatinine levels
Occlusion	• Reduced or absent peripheral pulses • Paresthesia • Severe pain • Cyanosis • Loss of Doppler signal in bypass graft
Hemorrhage	• Hypotension • Tachycardia • Restlessness and confusion • Shallow respirations • Abdominal pain • Increased abdominal girth • Lethargy

- As the patient's condition improves, take steps to wean them from the ventilator, if appropriate. To promote good pulmonary hygiene, encourage the patient to cough, turn, and deep breathe frequently.
- Assist the patient with ROM exercises, as ordered, to prevent thrombus formation. Assist with early ambulation to prevent complications of immobility.
- Provide support to the patient and their family to help them cope with recovery and lifestyle changes. (See *Teaching the patient after vascular repair.*)

Teaching the patient after vascular repair

Before discharge from the hospital, instruct the patient to:

- check their pulse (or have a family member do it) in the affected extremity before rising from bed each morning and to notify the health care provider if the patient cannot palpate their pulse or if they develop coldness, pallor, numbness, tingling, weakness, or pain in their extremities
- continue with the progressive exercise started in the facility
- perform coughing and deep-breathing exercises (if open abdominal surgical approach was conducted, splint the incision with a pillow to reduce pain) and use the incentive spirometer to reduce pulmonary complications
- avoid lifting objects that weigh more than 10 lb (4.5 kg) for the next 4 to 6 weeks
- check the incision site daily and immediately notify the health care provider of any signs and symptoms of infection
- take medications as prescribed and report adverse effects to the health care provider
- comply with the laboratory schedule for monitoring international normalized ratio (INR), if the patient is receiving warfarin (Coumadin).

Valve surgery

Types of valve surgery include valvuloplasty (valvular repair), commissurotomy (separation of the adherent thickened leaflets of the mitral valve), and valve replacement (with a mechanical or tissue valve). Historically, repair and replacement of these valves required open surgeries. Increasingly, minimally invasive valve surgery called transcatheter aortic valve replacement or transcatheter aortic valve implantation is available.

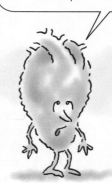

Because they are under the most pressure, the mitral and aortic valves are the most likely to need repair.

Valve replacement

In valve replacement, the natural heart valve is excised and a prosthetic valve is sutured in place.

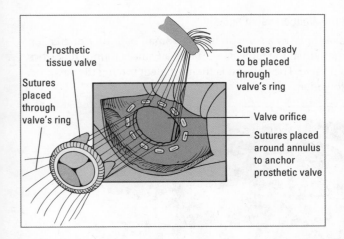

Prosthetic
tissue valve

Sutures
placed
through
valve's ring

Sutures ready
to be placed
through
valve's ring

Valve orifice

Sutures placed
around annulus
to anchor
prosthetic valve

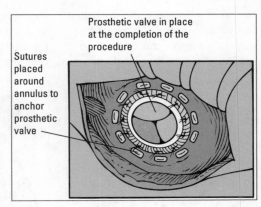

Prosthetic valve in place
at the completion of the
procedure

Sutures
placed
around
annulus to
anchor
prosthetic
valve

Types of replacement valves

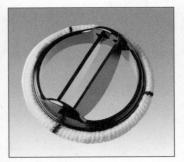

**Bileaflet valve
(St. Jude, mechanical)**

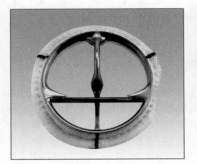

**Tilting-disk valve
(Medtronic-Hall, mechanical)**

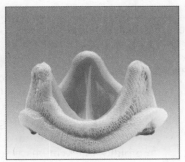

**Porcine heterograft valve
(Carpentier-Edwards, tissue)**

Valve leaflet resection and repair

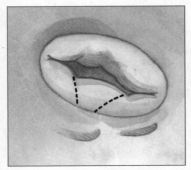

**The section between the dashed
lines is excised.**

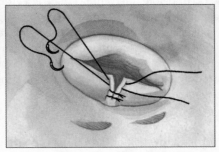

The edges are approximated and sutured.

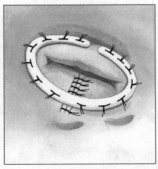

**The repair is finished off with
an annuloplasty ring.**

Commissurotomy

In commissurotomy, the thickened leaflets are surgically separated. The surgeon removes scar tissues and calcium deposits from leaflets.

Percutaneous balloon valvuloplasty

During valvuloplasty, a surgeon inserts a small balloon catheter through the skin at the femoral vein and advances it until it reaches the affected valve. The balloon is then inflated, forcing the valve opening to widen.

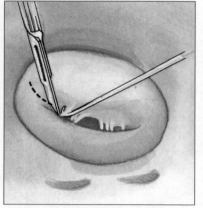

Commissurotomy of mitral valve

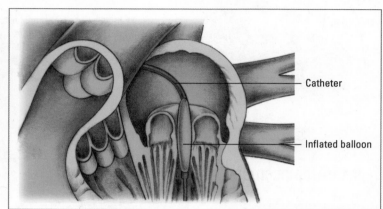

Catheter

Inflated balloon

Attention to prevention

Valve surgery is typically used to prevent heart failure in a patient with valvular stenosis (too tight of a valve) or insufficiency (a too loose or leaking valve). Many factors go into deciding the timing of surgery. Since the advent of newer minimally invasive procedures with a decreased morbidity, interventions are often performed earlier than in the past.

Pressure points

Because of the high pressure generated by the left ventricle during contraction, stenosis and insufficiency most commonly affect the mitral and aortic valves. Other indications for valve surgery depend on the patient's symptoms and on the affected valve. In general, most cardiologists do not wait for symptoms to occur before intervening. There is a growing emphasis on cardiac imaging such as magnetic resonance imaging and advanced echocardiogram techniques looking for decreased left ventricular ejection fraction and increased left ventricular end diastolic dimension and serial biomarkers such as brain natriuretic peptide to determine timing for surgical intervention. It is generally thought that waiting until symptoms occur is no longer the best practice.

It gets complicated

Although valve surgery carries a low risk of mortality, it can cause serious complications. Hemorrhage, for instance, may result from unligated vessels, anticoagulant therapy, or coagulopathy resulting from cardiopulmonary bypass during surgery. Stroke may result from thrombus formation caused by turbulent blood flow through the prosthetic valve or from poor cerebral perfusion during cardiopulmonary bypass. In valve replacement, bacterial endocarditis can develop within days of implantation or months later. Valve dysfunction or failure may occur as the prosthetic device wears out.

Patient preparation

- As necessary, reinforce and supplement the health care provider's explanation of the procedure.
- Confirm that the patient consent is signed.
- Tell the patient that they will awaken from surgery in an ICU or a PACU. Mention that they will be connected to a cardiac monitor and have IV lines, an arterial line, and, possibly, a PA or left atrial catheter in place. There will also be epicardial pacer wires in place.
- Explain that they will breathe through an ET tube connected to a mechanical ventilator; this will be removed as soon as they are breathing on their own after surgery and they may or may not remember it. Assure them that they will be given medication for pain and anxiety.
- They will have at least one and possibly two chest tubes in place after surgery, and these will remain in place for a few days.

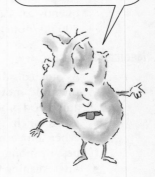

Distant heart sounds or new murmurs may indicate prosthetic valve failure.

Monitoring and aftercare

- Closely monitor the patient's hemodynamic status for signs of compromise. Watch especially for severe hypotension, decreased cardiac output, and shock. Check and record vital signs every 15 minutes until their condition stabilizes. Frequently assess heart sounds; report distant heart sounds or new murmurs, which may indicate prosthetic valve failure.
- Monitor the ECG continuously for disturbances in heart rate and rhythm, such as bradycardia, ventricular tachycardia, and heart block. Such disturbances may signal injury of the conduction system, which may occur during valve replacement from proximity of the atrial and mitral valves to the AV node. Arrhythmias may also result from myocardial irritability or ischemia, fluid and electrolyte imbalance, hypoxemia, or hypothermia. If you detect serious abnormalities, notify the health care provider and be prepared to assist with temporary epicardial pacing.

Blood check

- Take steps to maintain the patient's MAP between 70 and 100 mm Hg. Also, monitor PA and left atrial pressure as ordered.
- Frequently assess the patient's peripheral pulses, capillary refill time, and skin temperature and color and auscultate for heart sounds. Evaluate tissue oxygenation by assessing breath sounds, chest excursion, and symmetry of chest expansion. Report any abnormalities.

Breathing check

- Check ABG values upon arrival in ICU. Collaborate with respiratory therapy to extubate the patient as soon as possible per order/policy and have the ventilator settings adjusted as needed.
- Maintain chest tube drainage at the prescribed negative pressure (usually −10 to −40 cm H_2O for adults). Assess chest tubes frequently for signs of hemorrhage, excessive drainage (greater than 200 mL/hour), and a sudden decrease or cessation of drainage.

Medication check

- As ordered, administer analgesic, anticoagulant, antibiotic, antiarrhythmic, inotropic, and pressor medications as well as IV fluids and blood products. Monitor intake and output and assess for electrolyte imbalances, especially hypokalemia. When anticoagulant therapy begins, evaluate its effectiveness by monitoring prothrombin time and INR daily.
- After weaning from the ventilator and removing the ET tube, promote chest physiotherapy. Start the patient on incentive spirometry and encourage them to splint the incision, cough, turn frequently, and deep breathe.
- Throughout the patient's recovery period, observe them carefully for complications. (See *Teaching the patient after valve surgery.*)

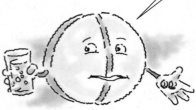

The effectiveness of anticoagulant therapy can be evaluated by monitoring prothrombin time and INR daily.

No place like home

Teaching the patient after valve surgery

Before discharge from the hospital, instruct the patient to:
- immediately report chest pain, fever, redness, swelling, or drainage at the incision site
- immediately notify the health care provider if signs or symptoms of heart failure (weight gain, dyspnea, or edema) develop
- notify the health care provider if signs or symptoms of postpericardiotomy syndrome (fever, muscle and joint pain, weakness, or chest discomfort) develop
- follow the prescribed medication regimen and report adverse effects
- follow their prescribed diet, especially sodium and fat restrictions
- maintain a balance between activity and rest
- follow their exercise or rehabilitation program, if prescribed
- inform their dentist and other health care providers of their prosthetic valve before undergoing surgery or dental work and to take prophylactic antibiotics as directed before such procedures
- follow up with the cardiologist, surgeon, and primary care physician.

VAD insertion

A VAD is a device that is implanted to support a failing heart. A VAD consists of a blood pump, cannulas, and a pneumatic or electrical drive console.

More output, less work

VADs are designed to decrease the heart's workload and increase cardiac output in patients with ventricular failure.

A temporary diversion

A VAD is commonly used as a "bridge to destination therapy" while a patient waits for a heart transplant. Increasingly, VAD can be used as a "destination therapy." This means the patient receives a VAD as a palliative treatment for heart failure. In a surgical procedure, blood is diverted from a ventricle to an artificial pump. This pump, which is synchronized to the patient's ECG, then functions as the ventricle. (See *VAD: Help for a failing heart.*)

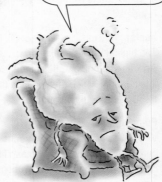

A closer look at VADs

There are three types of VADs.

1

A right VAD (RVAD) provides pulmonary support by diverting blood from the failing right ventricle to the VAD, which then pumps the blood to the pulmonary circulation via the VAD connection to the left PA.

2

With a left VAD (LVAD), blood flows from the left ventricle to the VAD, which then pumps blood back to the body via the VAD connection to the aorta.

3

When RVAD and LVAD are used, it is referred to as a *biventricular VAD*.

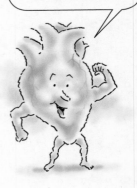

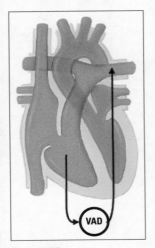

Right VAD

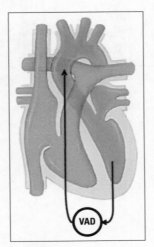

Left VAD

VAD: Help for a failing heart

A VAD is a mechanical pump that relieves the workload of the ventricle as the heart heals or until a donor heart is located.

Implantable

The typical VAD is implanted in the upper abdominal wall. An inflow cannula drains blood from the left ventricle into a pump, which then pushes the blood into the aorta through the outflow cannula.

Pump options

VADs are available as continuous flow or pulsatile pumps. A continuous flow pump fills continuously and returns blood to the aorta at a constant rate. A pulsatile pump may work in one of two ways: It may fill during systole and pump blood into the aorta during diastole, or it may pump irrespective of the patient's cardiac cycle.

Many types of VAD systems are available. This illustration shows a VAD implanted in the left abdominal wall and connected to an external battery pack by a percutaneous lead.

Potential complications

Despite the use of anticoagulants, the VAD may cause thrombi formation, leading to pulmonary embolism or stroke. Other complications may include heart failure, bleeding, cardiac tamponade, or infection.

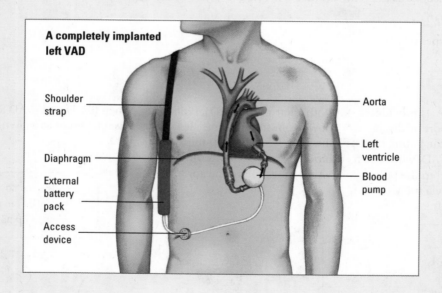

A completely implanted left VAD

Shoulder strap

Diaphragm

External battery pack

Access device

Aorta

Left ventricle

Blood pump

Right or left or both?

A VAD is used to provide systemic or pulmonary support, or both:

- An RVAD provides pulmonary support by diverting blood from the failing right ventricle to the VAD, which then pumps the blood to the pulmonary circulation by way of the VAD connection to the PA.
- With an LVAD, blood flows from the left ventricle to the VAD, which then pumps blood back to the body by way of the VAD connection to the aorta.
- When biventricular support is needed, both may be used.

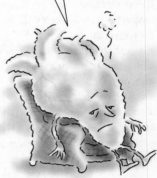

A VAD can help when the patient is waiting for a heart transplant.

Patient preparation

- Prepare the patient and their family for VAD insertion; be sure to explain how the device works, what its purpose is, and what to expect after insertion.
- Confirm that informed consent is obtained.
- Continue close patient monitoring, including continuous ECG monitoring, PA and hemodynamic status monitoring, and intake and output monitoring.

Monitoring and aftercare

- Assess the patient's cardiovascular status at least every 15 minutes until stable and then hourly. Monitor blood pressure and hemodynamic parameters, including cardiac output and cardiac index, ECG, and peripheral pulses.
- Inspect the incision and dressing at least every hour initially and then every 2 to 4 hours as indicated by the patient's condition.
- Monitor urine output hourly and maintain IV fluid therapy as ordered. Watch for signs of fluid overload or decreasing urine output.
- Assess chest tube drainage and function frequently. Notify the health care provider if drainage is greater than 150 mL over 2 hours. Auscultate lungs for evidence of abnormal breath sounds. Evaluate oxygen saturation or mixed venous oxygen saturation levels and administer oxygen as needed and as ordered.
- Obtain hemoglobin levels, hematocrit, and coagulation studies as ordered. Administer blood component therapy as indicated and as ordered.
- Assess for signs and symptoms of bleeding.
- Turn the patient every 2 hours and begin ROM exercises when they are stable.
- Administer antibiotics prophylactically if ordered. (See *Teaching the patient after VAD insertion*, page 326.)

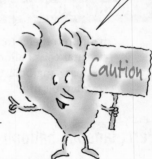

Notify the health care provider if chest tube drainage is greater than 150 mL over 2 hours.

Caution

Teaching the patient after VAD insertion

Before discharge from the hospital following the insertion of a VAD, instruct the patient to:
- immediately report redness, swelling, or drainage at the incision site; chest pain; or fever
- immediately notify the health care provider if signs or symptoms of heart failure (weight gain, dyspnea, or edema) develop
- follow the prescribed medication regimen and report adverse effects
- follow their prescribed diet, especially sodium and fat restrictions
- maintain a balance between activity and rest
- follow their exercise or rehabilitation program (if prescribed)
- comply with the laboratory schedule for monitoring international normalized ratio if the patient is receiving warfarin (Coumadin)
- be always connected to a source of electricity: battery pack or outlet
- be familiar with the particular VAD device and follow manufacturer's instructions for use, programming, and care
- know who to call in an emergency and keep the number with them
- charge battery per manufacturer guidelines
- perform insertion site/drive line care.

Balloon catheter treatments

Balloon catheter treatments for cardiovascular disorders include percutaneous balloon valvuloplasty, percutaneous transluminal coronary angioplasty (PTCA), and intra-aortic balloon pump (IABP) counterpulsation.

Percutaneous balloon valvuloplasty

Percutaneous balloon valvuloplasty may be performed in the cardiac catheterization laboratory. It is intended to improve valvular function by enlarging the orifice of a stenotic heart valve caused by congenital defect, calcification, rheumatic fever, or aging. A small balloon valvuloplasty catheter is introduced through the skin at the femoral vein.

Although valve surgery remains the treatment of choice for valvular heart disease, percutaneous balloon valvuloplasty offers an alternative for individuals who are considered poor candidates for surgery.

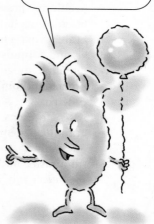

Percutaneous balloon valvuloplasty enlarges the orifice of a stenotic heart valve. That is my kind of inflation!

Balloon bungles

Unfortunately, elderly patients with aortic disease commonly experience restenosis 1 to 2 years after undergoing balloon valvuloplasty. In addition, despite decreasing the risks associated with more invasive procedures, balloon valvuloplasty can lead to complications, including:

- worsening valvular insufficiency (a valve leak) by misshaping the valve so that it does not close completely
- pieces breaking off of the calcified valve, which may travel to the brain or lungs and cause embolism (rare)
- severely damaging delicate valve leaflets, requiring immediate surgery to replace the valve (rare)
- bleeding and hematoma at the arterial puncture site
- MI (rare), arrhythmias, myocardial ischemia, and circulatory defects distal to the catheter entry site.

Patient preparation

- Describe the procedure to the patient and their family and tell them that it takes 1 to 4 hours to complete.
- Explain that a catheter will be inserted into an artery or a vein in the patient's groin and that they may feel pressure as the catheter moves along the vessel.
- Reassure the patient that although they will be awake during the procedure, they will be given a sedative. Instruct them to report any angina during the procedure.
- Check the patient's history for allergies; if they have had allergic reactions to shellfish, iodine, or contrast media, notify the health care provider.
- Confirm that the patient has signed an informed consent form.
- Restrict food and fluids before the procedure as directed by the surgeon or anesthesia team. Advise the patient that they will be instructed whether to take their medications.
- Make sure that the results of coagulation studies, complete blood count, serum electrolyte studies, blood typing and crossmatching, blood urea nitrogen, and serum creatinine are available.
- Obtain baseline vital signs and assess peripheral pulses.
- Apply ECG electrodes and insert an IV line if not already in place.
- Administer oxygen through a nasal cannula.
- Perform skin preparation according to your facility's policy.
- Give the patient a sedative as ordered.

Monitoring and aftercare

- Assess the patient's vital signs and oxygen saturation every 15 minutes for the first hour and then every 30 minutes for 4 hours, unless the patient's condition warrants more frequent checking.
- Monitor IV infusions, such as heparin or nitroglycerin, as indicated.
- Assess peripheral pulses distal to the catheter insertion site as well as the color, sensation, temperature, movement, and capillary refill time of the affected extremity.

- Monitor cardiac rhythm continuously and assess hemodynamic parameters closely for changes.
- Instruct the patient to remain in bed for 8 hours and to keep the affected extremity straight. Apply pressure to catheter site per hospital policy. Elevate the head of the bed 15 to 30°. If a hemostatic device was used to close the catheter insertion site, anticipate that the patient may be allowed out of bed in only a few hours.
- Assess the catheter site for hematoma, ecchymosis, and hemorrhage. If bleeding occurs, locate the artery and apply manual pressure and then notify the health care provider.
- Administer IV fluids as ordered (usually 100 mL/hour) to promote excretion of the contrast medium. Be sure to assess for signs of fluid overload.
- Document the patient's tolerance of the procedure and status after it, including vital signs, hemodynamic parameters, appearance of the catheter site, ECG findings, condition of the extremity distal to the insertion site, complications, and necessary interventions. (See *Teaching the patient after percutaneous balloon valvuloplasty.*)

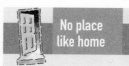

No place like home

Teaching the patient after percutaneous balloon valvuloplasty

Before discharge from the hospital, instruct the patient to:
- resume normal activity
- notify the health care provider if they experience bleeding or increased bruising at the puncture site or recurrence of symptoms of valvular insufficiency, such as breathlessness or decreased exercise tolerance
- comply with regular follow-up visits.

Percutaneous transluminal coronary angioplasty

PTCA offers a nonsurgical alternative to coronary artery bypass surgery. The health care provider uses a balloon-tipped catheter to dilate a coronary artery that has become narrowed because of atherosclerotic plaque. (See *Looking at PTCA.*)

Shorter stay, shorter return to activity

Performed in the cardiac catheterization laboratory under local anesthesia, PTCA does not involve a thoracotomy, so it is less costly and requires shorter hospitalization. Patients can usually walk the same day and return to work in 2 weeks.

Best working conditions

PTCA works best when lesions are readily accessible, noncalcified, less than 10 mm, concentric, discrete, and smoothly tapered. Patients with a history of less than 1 year of disabling angina make good candidates because their lesions tend to be softer and more compressible.

Harrowing narrowing

Complications of PTCA are acute vessel closure and late restenosis. To prevent restenosis, such procedures as stenting, atherectomy, and laser angioplasty may be performed. Also, vascular brachytherapy and drug-eluting stents may decrease the incidence of restenosis. (See *Preventing restenosis,* page 330.)

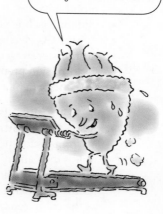

Although they may not be ready for the treadmill, patients can usually walk the day of the PTCA.

Looking at PTCA

PTCA can open an occluded coronary artery without opening the chest. This procedure is outlined in the steps below.

1. First, the health care provider must thread the catheter into the artery. The illustration below shows the entrance of a guide catheter into the coronary artery.

2. When angiography shows the guide catheter positioned at the occlusion site, the health care provider carefully inserts a smaller double-lumen balloon catheter through the guide catheter and directs the balloon through the occlusion.

3. The health care provider then inflates the balloon, causing arterial stretching and plaque fracture, as shown below. The balloon may need to be inflated or deflated several times until successful arterial dilation occurs.

4. After the artery is dilated, a balloon catheter with a stent is inserted. The balloon is inflated, and the stent is wedged against the vessel wall. The stent remains in the vessel to prevent reocclusion.

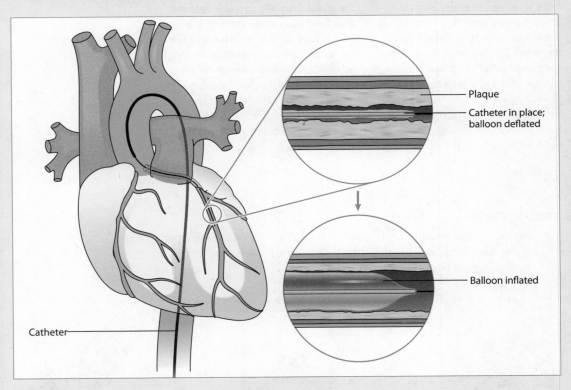

Plaque

Catheter in place; balloon deflated

Balloon inflated

Catheter

Preventing restenosis

Standard angioplasty is performed to remove the plaque blockage in the coronary artery. However, restenosis of the vessel is a frequent complication that occurs from scar tissue formation rather than plaque buildup.

Vascular brachytherapy

Vascular brachytherapy is the use of radiation in the coronary vessels to inhibit the development of this scar tissue, thus preventing restenosis of the vessel. The procedure involves a specialized radiation catheter that is inserted after angioplasty to direct beta radiation to the treated area for a few minutes. The radiation and catheter are then removed, with no radiation source being left in the body. This therapy is not commonly used anymore. It is usually only done if the patient is resistant to anticoagulation or drug-eluting stents.

Coronary drug-eluting stents

Stents are used to open arteries that feed the heart, thereby improving circulation to myocardial tissue. One complication of stents is restenosis of the vessel. Drug-eluting stents open the artery and also release a drug to the implantation site that helps reduce restenosis. The medication works by blocking proliferation of smooth muscle cells.

Placement of drug-eluting stents during a cardiac catheterization or angioplasty procedure is the same as for regular stents. Postprocedural care is also the same.

Intravascular stents

An intravascular stent may be used to hold the walls of a vessel open. Some stents are coated with a drug that is slowly released to inhibit further aggregation of fibrin or clots.

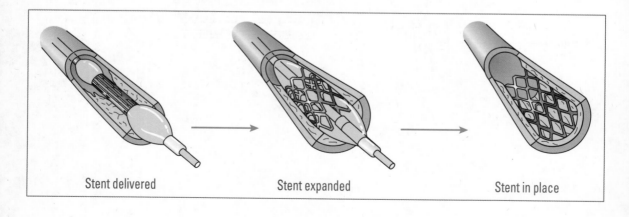

Stent delivered   Stent expanded   Stent in place

Patient preparation

- Describe the procedure to the patient and their family and tell them that it takes 1 to 4 hours to complete.
- Explain that a catheter will be inserted into an artery or a vein in the patient's groin and that they may feel pressure as the catheter moves along the vessel.
- Reassure the patient that although they will be awake during the procedure, they will be given a sedative. Instruct them to report any angina during the procedure.
- Explain that the health care provider will inject a contrast medium to outline the lesion's location. Warn the patient that they may feel a hot and flushing sensation or transient nausea during the injection.
- Check the patient's history for allergies; if they have had allergic reactions to shellfish, iodine, or contrast media, notify the health care provider.
- Give 650 mg of aspirin the evening before the procedure, if ordered, to prevent platelet aggregation.
- Confirm that the patient has signed an informed consent form.
- Restrict food and fluids for at least 6 hours before the procedure.
- Make sure that the results of coagulation studies, complete blood count, serum electrolyte studies, blood typing and crossmatching, blood urea nitrogen, and serum creatinine are available.
- Obtain baseline vital signs and assess peripheral pulses.
- Apply ECG electrodes and insert an IV line if not already in place.
- Administer oxygen through a nasal cannula.
- Perform skin preparation according to your facility's policy.
- Give the patient a sedative as ordered.

Monitoring and aftercare

- Assess the patient's vital signs and oxygen saturation every 15 minutes for the first hour and then every 30 minutes for 4 hours, unless the patient's condition warrants more frequent checking.
- Monitor IV infusions, such as heparin or nitroglycerin, as indicated.
- Assess peripheral pulses distal to the catheter insertion site as well as the color, sensation, temperature, movement, and capillary refill time of the affected extremity.
- Monitor cardiac rhythm continuously and assess hemodynamic parameters closely for changes. Respond to monitor alarms promptly.
- Instruct the patient to remain in bed for 8 hours and to keep the affected extremity straight. Apply pressure to catheter site per hospital policy. Elevate the head of the bed 15° to 30°. If a hemostatic device was used to close the catheter insertion site, anticipate that the patient may be allowed out of bed in only a few hours.

- Administer IV fluids as ordered (usually 100 mL/hour) to promote excretion of the contrast medium. Be sure to assess for signs of fluid overload.
- Assess the catheter site for hematoma, ecchymosis, and hemorrhage. If bleeding occurs, locate the artery and apply manual pressure and then notify the health care provider.
- After the health care provider removes the catheter, apply direct pressure for at least 10 minutes and assess the site often.
- Document the patient's tolerance of the procedure and status afterward, including vital signs, hemodynamic parameters, appearance of the catheter site, ECG findings, condition of the extremity distal to the insertion site, complications, and necessary interventions. (See *Teaching the patient after PTCA*.)

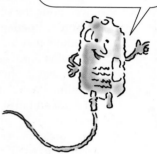

Administer IV fluids to promote excretion of the contrast medium.

IABP counterpulsation

IABP counterpulsation temporarily reduces left ventricular workload and improves coronary perfusion. (See *Understanding a balloon pump*.)

What for?

IABP counterpulsation may benefit patients with the following:
- cardiogenic shock because of acute MI
- septic shock
- intractable angina before surgery
- intractable ventricular arrhythmias
- ventricular septal or papillary muscle ruptures.

It is also used for patients who suffer pump failure before or after cardiac surgery.

No place like home

Teaching the patient after PTCA

If the patient does not experience complications from PTCA, they may go home in 6 to 12 hours. Before discharge from the hospital, instruct the patient to do the following:
- call their health care provider if they experience any bleeding or bruising at the arterial puncture site

- return for a stress thallium imaging test and follow-up angiography, as recommended by their health care provider
- report chest pain to the health care provider because restenosis can occur after PTCA.

Now I get it!

Understanding a balloon pump

An IABP consists of a polyurethane balloon attached to an external pump console by means of a large-lumen catheter. It is inserted percutaneously through the femoral artery and positioned in the descending aorta just distal to the left subclavian artery and above the renal arteries.

Push...

This external pump works in precise counterpoint to the left ventricle, inflating the balloon with helium early in diastole and deflating it just before systole. As the balloon inflates, it forces blood toward the aortic valve, thereby raising pressure in the aortic root and augmenting diastolic pressure to improve coronary perfusion. It also improves peripheral circulation by forcing blood through the brachiocephalic, common carotid, and subclavian arteries arising from the aortic trunk.

...and pull

The balloon deflates rapidly at the end of diastole, creating a vacuum in the aorta. This vacuum action reduces aortic volume and pressure, thereby decreasing the resistance to left ventricular ejection (afterload). This decreased workload, in turn, reduces the heart's oxygen requirements and, combined with the improved myocardial perfusion, helps prevent or diminish myocardial ischemia.

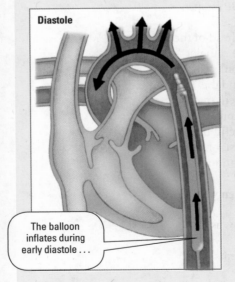

Diastole

The balloon inflates during early diastole . . .

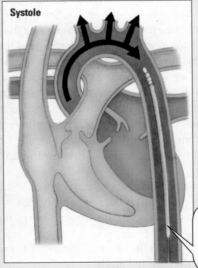

Systole

. . . and deflates just before systole.

How so?

The health care provider may perform balloon catheter insertion at the patient's bedside as an emergency procedure or in the operating room.

Patient preparation

- Explain to the patient that the health care provider is going to place a catheter in the aorta to help their heart pump more easily. Tell them that while the catheter is in place, they cannot sit up, bend their knee, or flex their hip more than 30°.
- Confirm that a signed patient consent was obtained.
- Attach the patient to a continuous ECG monitor and make sure they have an arterial line, a central line, and a peripheral IV line in place.
- Gather a surgical tray for percutaneous catheter insertion, heparin, normal saline solution, the IABP catheter, and the pump console. Connect the ECG monitor to the pump console. Then prepare the femoral site.

Monitoring and aftercare

- After the IABP catheter is inserted, select either the ECG or the arterial waveform to regulate inflation and deflation of the balloon. With the ECG waveform, the pump inflates the balloon in the middle of the T wave (diastole) and deflates with the R wave (before systole). With the arterial waveform, the upstroke of the arterial wave triggers balloon inflation. (See *Timing IABP counterpulsation*, page 335.)
- Frequently assess the insertion site. Do not elevate the head of the bed more than 30° to prevent upward migration of the catheter and occlusion of the left subclavian artery. If the balloon occludes the artery, you may see a diminished left radial pulse and the patient may report dizziness. Incorrect balloon placement may also cause flank pain or a sudden decrease in urine output.
- Assess distal pulses, color, temperature, and capillary refill time of the patient's extremities every 15 minutes for the first 4 hours after insertion. After 4 hours, assess hourly for the duration of IABP therapy.
- Watch for signs of thrombus formation, such as a sudden weakening of pedal pulses, pain, and motor or sensory loss.
- Apply antiembolism stockings or antithrombotic pumps as ordered.
- Encourage active ROM exercises every 2 hours for the arms, the unaffected leg, and the affected ankle.
- Maintain adequate hydration to help prevent thrombus formation.
- If bleeding occurs at the catheter insertion site, apply direct pressure and notify the health care provider.

Now I get it!

Timing IABP counterpulsation

IABP counterpulsation is synchronized with either the ECG or the arterial waveform. Ideally, balloon inflation should begin when the aortic valve closes—at the dicrotic notch on the arterial waveform. Deflation should occur just before systole.

Proper timing is crucial

Early inflation can damage the aortic valve by forcing it closed, whereas late inflation permits most of the blood emerging from the ventricle to flow past the balloon, reducing pump effectiveness.

Late deflation increases the resistance against which the left ventricle must pump, possibly causing cardiac arrest.

At the peak
The illustration below depicts how IABP counterpulsation boosts peak diastolic pressure and lowers peak systolic and end-diastolic pressures.

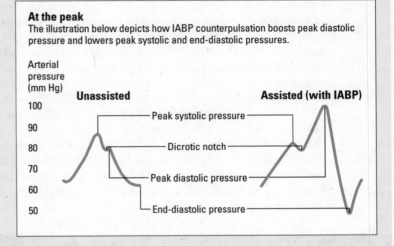

How timing affects waveforms
The arterial waveforms below show correctly and incorrectly timed balloon inflation and deflation.

Inflation

Early Normal Late

Deflation

Early Normal Late

Quick response required
- An alarm on the console may indicate a gas leak from a damaged catheter or a ruptured balloon. If the alarm sounds or you see blood in the catheter, shut down the pump console and immediately place the patient in Trendelenburg position to prevent an embolus from reaching the brain. Then notify the health care provider.

Weaning ways

- After the patient's signs and symptoms of left-sided heart failure diminish, only minimal drug support is required and the health care provider begins weaning the patient from IABP counterpulsation by reducing the frequency of pumping or decreasing the balloon volume. A minimum volume or pumping ratio must be maintained to prevent thrombus formation. Most consoles have a flutter function that moves the balloon to prevent clot formation. Use the flutter function when the patient has been weaned from counterpulsation but the catheter has not yet been removed.
- To discontinue the IABP, the health care provider deflates the balloon, clips the sutures, removes the catheter, and allows the site to bleed for 5 seconds to expel clots.
- After the health care provider discontinues the IABP, apply direct pressure for 30 minutes and then apply a pressure dressing. Evaluate the site for bleeding and hematoma formation hourly for the next 4 hours. (See *Teaching the patient after IABP treatment.*)

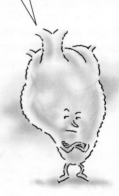

IABP counterpulsation patients should be watched for signs of thrombus formation, such as sudden weakening of pedal pulses, pain, and motor or sensory loss.

Cardiovascular resynchronization techniques

When the electrical conduction of the heart is disrupted, cardiac output is diminished and perfusion of blood and oxygen to all body tissues is affected. Treatment to restore the heart's conduction needs to begin quickly. Such treatments include defibrillation, an implantable cardioverter-defibrillator (ICD), synchronized cardioversion, and pacemaker insertion.

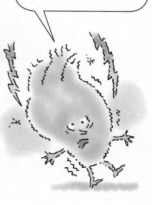

Shock it to me! In defibrillation, an electric current is directed through the heart.

No place like home

Teaching the patient after IABP treatment

Before discharge from the hospital, instruct the patient to:
- call their health care provider if they experience bleeding, bruising, or a pulsatile mass at the insertion site
- return for follow-up testing as recommended by the health care provider
- report chest pain promptly.

Defibrillation

In defibrillation, electrode paddles or hands-free pads are used to direct an electric current through the patient's heart. The current causes the myocardium to depolarize, which in turn encourages the SA node to resume control of the heart's electrical activity.

The electrode paddles delivering the current may be placed on the patient's chest or, during cardiac surgery, directly on the myocardium. (See *Biphasic versus monophasic: what is the difference?*)

Act early and quickly

Because some arrhythmias, such as ventricular fibrillation, can cause death if not corrected, the success of defibrillation depends on early recognition and quick treatment.

In addition to treating ventricular fibrillation, defibrillation may also be used to treat ventricular tachycardia without a pulse.

Automated external defibrillators

An automated external defibrillator (AED) has a cardiac rhythm analysis system. The AED interprets the patient's cardiac rhythm and gives the operator step-by-step directions on how to proceed if

Biphasic versus monophasic: what is the difference?

There are two types of defibrillators: monophasic and biphasic.

• Monophasic defibrillators were developed before biphasic defibrillators. A monophasic defibrillator delivers a single current traveling in one direction, between the two pads or paddles on the patient's chest, which requires a large amount of electrical energy.

• Biphasic defibrillators are more common. A biphasic defibrillator delivers a current that in a positive direction for a specified duration and then reverses and flows in a negative direction for the remaining time of the electrical discharge.

Most automated external defibrillators are biphasic, and many manufacturers are discontinuing monophasic defibrillators. Hands-free pads or paddle placement is the same with both types.

Advantages of Biphasic defibrillators

• **Energy efficient**—The biphasic defibrillator delivers two currents of electricity and lowers the defibrillation threshold of the heart muscle, making it possible to successfully defibrillate ventricular fibrillation with smaller amounts of energy. Instead of using 200 joules, an initial shock of 150 joules is usually effective.

• **Adjustable**—The biphasic defibrillator is able to adjust for differences in impedance (the resistance of the current through the chest). This functionality reduces the number of shocks needed to terminate ventricular fibrillation.

• **Less damage to the myocardium**—Because the biphasic defibrillator requires lower energy levels and fewer shocks, damage to the myocardial muscle is reduced. Biphasic defibrillators used at the clinically appropriate energy level may be used for defibrillation and, in the synchronized mode, for synchronized cardioversion.

defibrillation is indicated. AEDs are commonly found in public areas throughout the United States. They are designed so that a lay person can use them if necessary.

Come equipped

The defibrillator

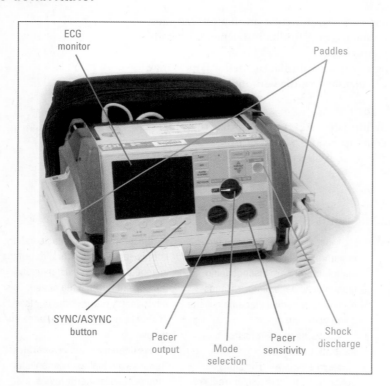

Who is in charge here?

The AED is equipped with a microcomputer that analyzes a patient's heart rhythm at the push of a button. It then audibly or visually prompts you to deliver a shock.

Patient preparation

- Assess the patient to determine if they lack a pulse. Call for help and perform cardiopulmonary resuscitation (CPR) until the defibrillator and other emergency equipment arrive.
- Connect the monitoring leads of the defibrillator to the patient and assess their cardiac rhythm in two leads.

- Expose the patient's chest and apply conductive pads at the paddle placement positions. (See *Defibrillator paddle placement*, page 339.)

Monitoring and aftercare

- Turn on the defibrillator. If performing manual external defibrillation, set the energy level at 120 to 200 joules (based on biphasic defibrillator manufacturer recommendation) or 360 joules (for a monophasic defibrillator).
- Charge the paddles by pressing the CHARGE buttons, which are located on either the machine or the paddles.

Ready

- Place the paddles over the conductive pads and press firmly against the patient's chest, using 25 lb (11.3 kg) of pressure. Sometimes, hands-free pads (such as with an AED) are used in place of paddles.
- Reassess the patient's cardiac rhythm in two leads.

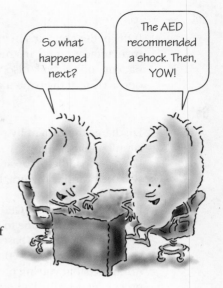

So what happened next?

The AED recommended a shock. Then, YOW!

Peak technique

Defibrillator paddle placement

Here is a guide to correct paddle placement for defibrillation.

Anterolateral placement
For anterolateral placement, place one paddle to the right of the upper sternum, just below the right clavicle, and the other over the fifth or sixth intercostal space at the left anterior axillary line.

Anteroposterior placement
For anteroposterior placement, place the anterior paddle directly over the heart at the precordium to the left of the lower sternal border. Place the flat posterior paddle under the patient's body beneath the heart and immediately below the scapulae.

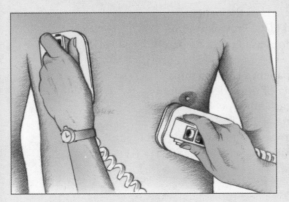

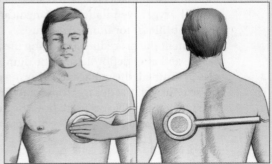

Set

- If the patient remains in ventricular fibrillation or pulseless ventricular tachycardia, instruct all personnel to stand clear of the patient and the bed. Also, make a visual check to make sure everyone is clear of the patient and the bed.

Go!

- Discharge the current by pressing both paddle DISCHARGE buttons simultaneously.
- Leave the paddles in position on the patient's chest while you reassess their cardiac rhythm; have someone else assess the patient's pulse.
- If necessary, continue CPR and prepare to defibrillate a second time. Instruct someone to reset the energy level on the defibrillator to 120 to 200 joules (based on biphasic defibrillator manufacturer recommendation) or 360 joules (for a monophasic defibrillator). Announce that you are preparing to defibrillate and follow the procedure described above.

One more time

- Reassess the patient. If defibrillation is again necessary, follow the same procedure as before.
- Perform the three countershocks in rapid succession, reassessing the patient's rhythm before each attempt.
- If the patient still has no pulse after three initial defibrillations, resume CPR, give supplemental oxygen, and follow advanced cardiac life support guidelines. Also, consider possible causes for failure of the patient's rhythm to convert, such as acidosis and hypoxia.

It worked!

- If defibrillation restores a normal rhythm, assess the patient. Obtain baseline ABG levels and a 12-lead ECG. Provide supplemental oxygen, ventilation, and medications as needed. Prepare the defibrillator for immediate reuse.
- Document the procedure, including the patient's ECG rhythms before and after defibrillation; the number of times defibrillation was performed; the voltage used during each attempt; whether a pulse returned; the dosage, route, and time of any drugs administered; whether CPR was used; how the airway was maintained; and the patient's outcome. (See *Teaching the patient after defibrillation.*)

No place like home

Teaching the patient after defibrillation

Before discharge from the hospital, instruct the patient to:
- report episodes of chest pain to the health care provider
- encourage the family to learn cardiopulmonary resuscitation as well as how to use an automated external defibrillator (AED)
- consider an ICD, if recommended by the health care provider.

Implantable cardioverter-defibrillator

An ICD has a programmable pulse generator and lead system that monitors the heart's activity, detects ventricular bradyarrhythmias and tachyarrhythmias, and responds with appropriate therapies. It is used for antitachycardia and bradycardia pacing, cardioversion, and defibrillation. Some ICDs also have the ability to pace the atrium and the ventricle.

Power station nearby

To implant an ICD, the cardiologist positions the lead (or leads) transvenously in the endocardium of the right ventricle (and the right atrium, if both chambers require pacing). The lead connects to a generator box, which is implanted in the right or left upper chest near the clavicle. (See *Location of an ICD*.)

Patient preparation
- Reinforce the cardiologist's instructions to the patient and their family, answering any questions they may have.
- Confirm that a patient consent is signed.
- Be sure to emphasize the need for the device, the potential complications, and ICD terminology.
- Restrict food and fluids as directed by the anesthesia team.
- If ordered, provide a sedative on the morning of the procedure, to help the patient relax. If a sedative is given, remember to make sure the consent is signed PRIOR to administration of the medication, siderails are up, and the bed is in the lowest position. Make sure the call bell is in reach and patient knows to ask for help getting up.

Location of an ICD

To insert an ICD, the cardiologist makes a small incision near the collarbone and accesses the subclavian vein. The lead wires are inserted through the subclavian vein, threaded into the heart, and placed in contact with the endocardium.

Pocket placement
The leads are connected to the pulse generator, which is placed under the skin in a specially prepared pocket in the right or left upper chest. (Placement is similar to that used for a pacemaker.) The cardiologist then closes the incision and programs the device.

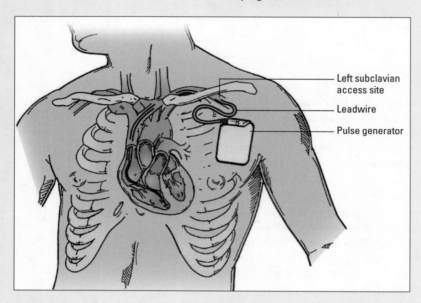

Left subclavian access site

Leadwire

Pulse generator

Monitoring and aftercare

- The patient will be monitored on a telemetry unit.
- Monitor for arrhythmias and proper device functioning.
- Gradually allow the patient to increase activities as ordered.
- Monitor the incision site for signs of infection or drainage.
- Provide support to the patient and their family to help them cope with recovery and lifestyle changes.
- Encourage family members to learn CPR. (See *Teaching the patient after ICD implantation.*)

Teaching the patient after ICD implantation

Before discharge from the hospital, instruct the patient to:

• avoid placing excessive pressure over the insertion site or moving or jerking the area until the postoperative visit

• check the incision site daily and immediately notify the health care provider of signs and symptoms of infection

• wear medical alert identification and carry information regarding their ICD at all times

• increase exercise and sexual activity as allowed by the health care provider

• take medications as prescribed and report adverse effects to the health care provider.

Encourage family members to learn CPR. Provide resources for finding classes.

Synchronized cardioversion

Cardioversion (synchronized countershock) is an elective or emergency procedure used to correct tachyarrhythmias (such as atrial tachycardia, atrial flutter, atrial fibrillation, and symptomatic ventricular tachycardia). It is also the treatment of choice for patients with arrhythmias who do not respond to drug therapy.

Small shock

In synchronized cardioversion, an electric current is delivered to the heart to correct an arrhythmia. Compared with defibrillation, it uses much lower energy levels and is synchronized to deliver an electric charge to the myocardium at the peak R wave.

Back in control

The procedure causes immediate depolarization, interrupting reentry circuits (abnormal impulse conduction that occurs when cardiac tissue is activated two or more times, causing reentry arrhythmias) and allowing the sinoatrial node to resume control.

Synchronizing the electrical charge with the R wave ensures that the current would not be delivered on the vulnerable T wave and disrupt repolarization. Thus, it reduces the risk that the current will strike during the relative refractory period of a cardiac cycle and induce ventricular fibrillation.

Patient preparation

- Describe this elective procedure to the patient and make sure an informed consent is obtained.
- Withhold all food and fluids for 6 to 12 hours, or as directed, before the procedure. If cardioversion is urgent, withhold food beginning as soon as possible.
- Obtain a baseline 12-lead ECG.
- Connect the patient to a pulse oximeter and blood pressure cuff.
- If the patient is awake, administer a sedative as ordered and wait for positive effects of the medication.
- Place the leads on the patient's chest and assess their cardiac rhythm.
- Apply conductive gel to the paddles or attach defibrillation pads to the chest wall; position the pads so that one pad is to the right of the sternum, just below the clavicle, and the other is at the fifth or sixth intercostal space in the left anterior axillary line.

Monitoring and aftercare

- Turn on the defibrillator and select the ordered energy level, usually between 50 and 100 joules. (See *Choosing the correct cardioversion energy level.*)
- Activate the synchronized mode by depressing the synchronizer switch.

Advice from the experts

Choosing the correct cardioversion energy level

When choosing an energy level for cardioversion, try the lowest energy level first. If the arrhythmia is not corrected, repeat the procedure using the next energy level.

Try, try again

Repeat this procedure until the arrhythmia is corrected or until the highest energy level is reached. The monophasic energy doses (or clinically equivalent biphasic energy dose) used for cardioversion are:

- 100, 200, 300, and 360 joules for unstable ventricular tachycardia with a pulse
- 50, 100, 200, 300, and 360 joules for unstable paroxysmal supraventricular tachycardia
- 100, 200, 300, and 360 joules for unstable atrial fibrillation with a rapid ventricular response
- 50, 100, 200, 300, and 360 joules for unstable atrial flutter with a rapid ventricular response.
- The numbers above are correct when using a monophasic cardioverter-defibrillator. Most machines are biphasic now. It is important to refer to the recommended energy levels of your specific device in order to maximize first shock success.

- Check that the machine is sensing the R wave correctly.
- Place the paddles on the chest and apply firm pressure.
- Charge the paddles.
- Instruct other personnel to stand clear of the patient and the bed to avoid the risk of an electric shock.
- Discharge the current by pushing both paddles' discharge buttons simultaneously.
- If cardioversion is unsuccessful, repeat the procedure two or three times, as ordered, gradually increasing the energy with each additional countershock.
- If normal rhythm is restored, continue to monitor the patient and provide supplemental ventilation as long as needed.
- If the patient's cardiac rhythm changes to ventricular fibrillation, switch the mode from SYNCHRONIZED to DEFIBRILLATE and defibrillate the patient immediately after charging the machine.

Use your hands

- When using handheld paddles, continue to hold the paddles on the patient's chest until the energy is delivered.
- Remember to reset the SYNC MODE on the defibrillator after each synchronized cardioversion. Resetting this switch is necessary because most defibrillators automatically reset to an unsynchronized mode.

Write it down

- Document the use of synchronized cardioversion, the rhythm before and after cardioversion, the amperage used, and how the patient tolerated the procedure. (See *Teaching the patient after synchronized cardioversion*, page 345.)

No place like home

Teaching the patient after synchronized cardioversion

Before discharge from the hospital, instruct the patient to:
- report chest pain or palpitations to the health care provider
- encourage family members to learn cardiopulmonary resuscitation and use of an automated external defibrillator
- take medication and attend follow-up visits with the health care provider, as recommended.

Permanent pacemaker insertion

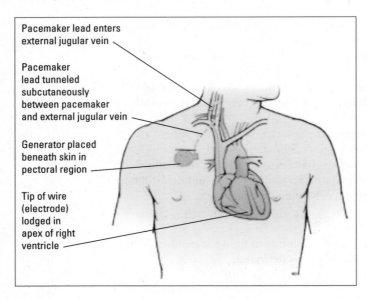

Pacemaker lead enters external jugular vein

Pacemaker lead tunneled subcutaneously between pacemaker and external jugular vein

Generator placed beneath skin in pectoral region

Tip of wire (electrode) lodged in apex of right ventricle

A permanent pacemaker is a self-contained device that is surgically implanted in a pocket under the patient's skin. This implantation is usually performed in an operating room or a cardiac catheterization laboratory.

Permanent pacemakers function in the DEMAND mode, allowing the patient's heart to beat on its own but preventing it from falling below a preset rate.

And the nominees for insertion are...

Permanent pacemakers are indicated for patients with the following:
- persistent bradyarrhythmia
- complete heart block
- congenital or degenerative heart disease
- Stokes–Adams syndrome
- Wolff–Parkinson–White syndrome
- sick sinus syndrome.

Setting the pace

Pacing electrodes can be placed in the atria, the ventricles, or both chambers (AV sequential or dual chamber). Biventricular pacemakers are also available for cardiac resynchronization therapy in some patients with heart failure. (See *Understanding pacemaker codes*.)

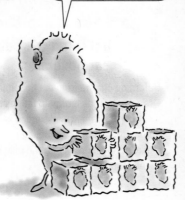

Complete heart block is just one reason I might need a pacemaker.

Now I get it!

Understanding pacemaker codes

The capabilities of pacemakers are described by a five-letter coding system, although typically, only the first three letters are used.

First letter

The first letter identifies which heart chambers are paced. Here are the letters used to signify these options:
- V = ventricle
- A = atrium
- D = dual (ventricle and atrium)
- O = none.

Second letter

The second letter signifies the heart chamber where the pacemaker senses the intrinsic activity:
- V = ventricle
- A = atrium
- D = dual
- O = none.

Third letter

The third letter shows the pacemaker's response to the intrinsic electrical activity it senses in the atrium or the ventricle:
- T = triggers pacing
- I = inhibits pacing
- D = dual; can be triggered or inhibited depending on the mode and where intrinsic activity occurs
- O = none; the pacemaker does not change its mode in response to sensed activity.

Fourth letter

The fourth letter denotes the pacemaker's programmability; it tells whether the pacemaker can be modified by an external programming device:
- P = basic functions programmable
- M = multiprogrammable parameters
- C = communicating functions such as telemetry
- R = rate responsiveness (rate adjusts to fit the patient's metabolic needs and achieve normal hemodynamic status)
- O = none.

Fifth letter

The fifth letter denotes the pacemaker's response to a tachyarrhythmia:
- P = pacing ability—pacemaker's rapid burst paces the heart at a rate above its intrinsic rate to override the tachycardia source
- S = shock—an ICD identifies ventricular tachycardia and delivers a shock to stop the arrhythmia
- D = dual ability to shock and pace
- O = none.

Understanding pacemaker codes

A   S   P

First letter

Identifies heart chambers that are paced:
V = ventricle
A = atrium
D = dual (ventricle and atrium)
O = none

> ### memory board
>
> The letters of the pacemaker code help you to understand what the pacemaker is doing. To remember this important **ASP**ect of pacemaker coding, think of Cleopatra's **ASP**:
>
> **A**ssisted heart chamber
>
> **S**ensed heart chamber
>
> **P**acemaker response to intrinsic activity it sensed.

Second letter

Signifies the heart chamber where the pacemaker senses the intrinsic activity:
V = ventricle
A = atrium
D = dual
O = none

Third letter

Shows the pacemaker's response to the intrinsic electrical activity it senses in the atrium or ventricle:
T = triggers pacing
I = inhibits pacing
D = dual (can be triggered or inhibited depending on the mode and where intrinsic activity occurs)
O = none (the pacemaker does not change its mode in response to sensed activity)

Pacemaker spikes

Pacemaker impulses—the stimuli that travel from the pacemaker to the heart—are visible on the patient's ECG tracing as spikes. Large or small pacemaker spikes appear above or below the isoelectric line. This example shows an atrial and a ventricular pacemaker spike.

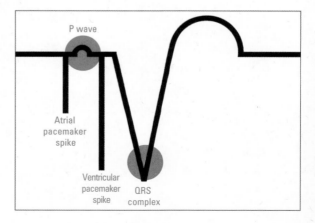

The most common pacing codes are VVI for single-chamber pacing and DDD for dual-chamber pacing. To keep the patient healthy and active, newer pacemakers are designed to increase the heart rate with exercise. (See *Biventricular pacemaker*, page 349.)

Patient preparation

- Explain the procedure to the patient.
- Confirm that a patient consent has been signed.
- Before pacemaker insertion, follow the institutions protocol for skin preparation and hair removal. This may include clipping the hair, using a depilatory or just a skin prep on the chest from the axilla to the midline and from the clavicle to the nipple line on the side selected by the health care provider.
- Establish an IV line.
- Obtain baseline vital signs and a baseline ECG.
- Provide sedation as ordered.

Now I get it!

Biventricular pacemaker

A biventricular pacemaker is a type of pacemaker that is currently being used to treat heart failure.

All together now
It works by sending tiny electrical signals to the left and right ventricles at the same time, ultimately causing the walls of the left ventricle to pump

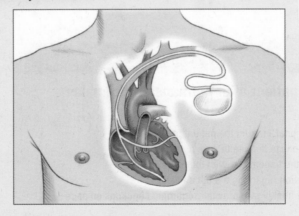

together. The result is more efficient pumping of the heart, improved circulation, and decreased fluid backup in the heart muscle and lungs.

Another lead
Insertion is similar to a regular pacemaker. However, in addition to the two leads that are used in most pacemakers, a third lead is placed into a cardiac vein and paces the left ventricle.

Monitoring and aftercare
- Monitor the patient's ECG to check for arrhythmias and to ensure correct pacemaker functioning.
- Check the dressing for signs of bleeding and infection.
- Change the dressing according to your facility's policy.
- Check vital signs and level of consciousness every 15 minutes for the first hour, every hour for the next 4 hours, and then every 4 hours unless the patient's condition warrants more frequent checking.
- Provide the patient with an identification card that lists the pacemaker type and manufacturer, serial number, pacemaker rate setting, date implanted, and the health care provider's name. (See *Teaching the patient after permanent pacemaker insertion.*)

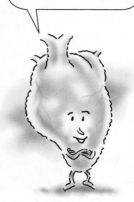

When you have enough time, a transvenous pacemaker is the more comfortable—and more reliable—choice.

Temporary pacemaker insertion

A temporary pacemaker is typically used in an emergency. The device consists of an external battery-powered pulse generator and a lead or electrode system.

Temporary pacemakers usually come in three types:
- transcutaneous
- transvenous
- epicardial.

No place like home

Teaching the patient after permanent pacemaker insertion

Before discharge from the hospital, instruct the patient to:
- report chest pain or palpitations to the health care provider
- carry information regarding the pacemaker with them at all times
- wear medical alert identification regarding the pacemaker
- follow instructions from their health care provider regarding checkups on pacemaker function.

Dire straits

In a life-threatening situation, a transcutaneous pacemaker is the best choice. This device works by sending an electrical impulse from the pulse generator to the patient's heart by way of two electrodes, which are placed on the front and back of the patient's chest.

Transcutaneous pacing is quick and effective, but it is used only until the health care provider can institute transvenous or permanent pacing.

When you have more time

In addition to being more comfortable for the patient, a transvenous pacemaker is more reliable than a transcutaneous pacemaker.

Transvenous pacing involves threading an electrode catheter through a vein into the patient's right atrium or right ventricle. The electrode is attached to an external pulse generator that can provide an electrical stimulus directly to the endocardium.

Come equipped

Transvenous pulse generator

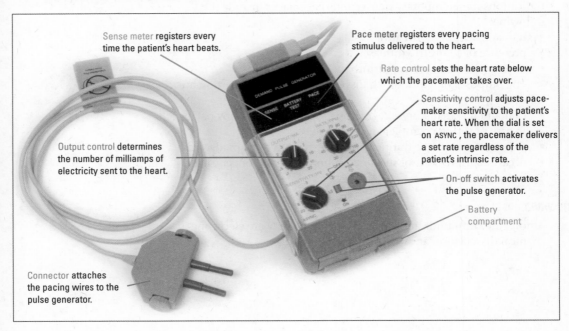

Sense meter **registers every time the patient's heart beats.**

Pace meter **registers every pacing stimulus delivered to the heart.**

Rate control **sets the heart rate below which the pacemaker takes over.**

Sensitivity control **adjusts pace-maker sensitivity to the patient's heart rate. When the dial is set on** ASYNC **, the pacemaker delivers a set rate regardless of the patient's intrinsic rate.**

Output control **determines the number of milliamps of electricity sent to the heart.**

On-off switch **activates the pulse generator.**

Battery compartment

Connector **attaches the pacing wires to the pulse generator.**

Temporary transvenous pacemaker

Transvenous pacing provides a more reliable pacing beat. This type of pacing is more comfortable for the patient because the pacing wire is inserted in the heart via a major vein.

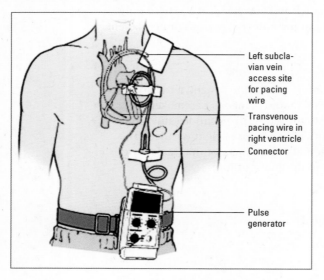

Left subcla-
vian vein
access site
for pacing
wire

Transvenous
pacing wire in
right ventricle

Connector

Pulse
generator

When to use...

Indications for a temporary transvenous pacemaker include the following:

- management of bradycardia
- presence of tachyarrhythmias
- other conduction system disturbances.

The purposes of temporary transvenous pacemaker insertion are as follows:

- to maintain circulatory integrity by providing for standby pacing in case of sudden complete heart block
- to increase heart rate during periods of symptomatic bradycardia
- occasionally, to control sustained supraventricular or ventricular tachycardia.

...and when not to

Among the contraindications to pacemaker therapy are electromechanical dissociation and ventricular fibrillation.

Suited for surgery

Epicardial pacing is used during cardiac surgery, when the surgeon may insert electrodes through the epicardium of the right ventricle and, if they want to institute AV sequential pacing, the right atrium. From there, the electrodes pass through the chest wall, where they remain available if temporary pacing becomes necessary.

Patient preparation

- Teach measures to prevent microshock; warn the patient not to use any electrical equipment that is not grounded.
- When using a transcutaneous pacemaker, do not place the electrodes over a bony area because bone conducts current poorly. With a female patient, place the anterior electrode under the patient's breast but not over their diaphragm.
- If the health care provider inserts the transvenous pacer wire through the brachial or femoral vein, immobilize the patient's arm or leg to avoid putting stress on the pacing wires.

Monitoring and aftercare

- After instituting use of any temporary pacemaker, assess the patient's vital signs, skin color, level of consciousness, and peripheral pulses to determine the effectiveness of the paced rhythm. Perform a 12-lead ECG to serve as a baseline and then perform additional ECGs daily or with clinical changes. Also, if possible, obtain a rhythm strip before, during, and after pacemaker placement; anytime the pacemaker settings are changed; and whenever the patient receives treatment because of a complication due to the pacemaker.
- Continuously monitor the ECG reading, noting capture, sensing, rate, intrinsic beats, and competition of paced and intrinsic rhythms. If the pacemaker is sensing correctly, the sense indicator on the pulse generator should flash with each beat.
- Record the date and time of pacemaker insertion, the type of pacemaker, the reason for insertion, and the patient's response. Record the pacemaker settings. Document any complications and the measures taken to resolve them.
- If the patient has epicardial pacing wires in place, clean the insertion site and change the dressing daily. At the same time, monitor the site for signs of infection. Always keep the pulse generator nearby in case pacing becomes necessary.
- Prepare the patient for permanent pacemaker surgery as appropriate.

Suggested references

Abbott. (2019). Resources and frequently asked questions. Retrieved from https://www.heartmate.com/patient/resources-and-faqs

American Heart Association. (2018). What is TAVR. Retrieved from https://www.heart.org/en/health-topics/heart-valve-problems-and-disease/understanding-your-heart-valve-treatment-options/what-is-tavr

American Heart Association. (2020a). *Advanced cardiovascular life support provider manual*. American Heart Association.

American Heart Association. (2020b). *Basic cardiovascular life support provider manual*. American Heart Association.

American Nurse Today. (2017). Caring for patients with a left ventricular assist device. *American Nurse Today, 12*(5). Retrieved from https://www.americannursetoday.com/caring-patients-left-ventricular-assist-device/

Broglio, K., & Eichholz-Heller, F. (2015). Left ventricular assist devices: When the bridge to transplantation becomes the destination. *Journal of Hospice and Palliative Nursing, 17*(5), 374–379. https://doi.org/10.1097/NJH.0000000000000166

Cheng, T. (2014). Is it TAVI or TAVR. *International Journal of Cardiology, 175*(2), 222–223. https://doi.org/10.1016/j.ijcard.2014.05.006

Circulation Foundation: The Vascular Charity. (2018). Endovascular aneurysm repair (EVAR). Retrieved from http://www.circulationfoundation.org.uk/help-advice/abdominal-aortic-aneurysm/endovascular-aneurysm-repair-evar

Eagleton, M., Follansbee, M., Wolski, K., Mastracci, T., & Kuramochi, Y. (2016). Fenestrated and branched endovascular aneurysm repair outcomes for type II and III thoracoabdominal aortic aneurysms. *Journal of Vascular Surgery, 63*(4), 930–942.

Ellis, M., Farrell, D., Pena, H., Kettle, M., Johnson, T., & Rudolph, A. (2018). Barriers to early extubation after cardiac surgery. *American Journal of Critical Care, 27*(3), e9–e10.

Joseph, C., Garrubba, M., Smith, J., & Melder, A. (2018). Does the use of a pulmonary artery catheter make a difference during or after cardiac surgery? *Heart Lung and Circulation, 27*(8), 952–960. https://doi.org/10.1016/j.hlc.2018.02.004

Kofler, M., Schachner, T., Reinstadler, S., Stastny, L., Dumfarth, J., Wiedemann, D., Feuchtner, G., Friedrich, G., Bonatti, J., & Bonaros, N. (2017). Comparative analysis of perioperative and mid-term results of TECAB and MIDCAB for revascularization of anterior wall. *Innovations, 12*(3), 207–213.

Leininger, S. (2018). Blood glucose management for reducing cardiac surgery infections. *Critical Care Nursing Quarterly, 41*(4), 399–406. https://doi.org/10.1097/CNQ.0000000000000227

Nakagawa, S., Garan, A., Takayama, H., Takeda, K., Topkara, V., Yuzefpolskaya, M., Lin, S. X., Colombo, P. C., Naka, Y., & Blinderman, C. D. (2018). End of life with left ventricular assist device in both bridge to transplant and destination therapy. *Journal of Palliative Medicine, 21*(9), 1284–1289. https://doi.org/10.1089/jpm.2018.0112

New Heart Valve. (2019). Take control of your options. Learn if TAVR is right for you. Retrieved from https://newheartvalve.com/tavr-treatment/is-tavr-right-for-you/?gclid=EAIaIQobChMI6YbXpoPk3wIVAoTICh0ncAHUEAAYAiAAEgKqA_D_BwE

Ramos Dos Santos, P., Aquaroni Ricci, N., Aparecida Bordignon Suster, É., de Moraes Paisani, D., & Dias Chiavegato, L. (2017). Effects of early mobilisation in patients after cardiac surgery: A systematic review. *Physiotherapy, 103*(1), 1–12.

Society for Vascular Surgery. (2018). Endovascular repair of abdominal aortic aneurysms. Retrieved from https://vascular.org/patient-resources/vascular-treatments/endovascular-repair-abdominal-aortic-aneurysms

University of California, San Francisco, Department of Surgery. (2018). Endovascular aneurysm repair. Retrieved from https://surgery.ucsf.edu/conditions–procedures/endovascular-aneurysm-repair.aspx

Waugaman, S., VanNortwick, C., Dionne, H., Whitmore, E., & Bradley, L. (2015). Early mobilization in cardiac surgery patients decreases complications, length of stay, and readmission. *Critical Care Nursing, 35*(2), e24–e25.

Appendix and index

1. During systole, the ventricles contract. This causes:
    A. all four heart valves to close.
    B. all four heart valves to open.
    C. the AV valves to close and the semilunar valves to open.
    D. the AV valves to open and the semilunar valves to close.

Answer: C. During systole, the pressure is greater in the ventricles than in the atria, causing the AV valves (the tricuspid and mitral valves) to close. The pressure in the ventricles is also greater than the pressure in the aorta and pulmonary artery, forcing the semilunar valves (the pulmonic and aortic valves) to open.

2. The pressure the ventricular muscle must generate to overcome the higher pressure in the aorta refers to:
    A. stroke volume.
    B. contractility.
    C. preload.
    D. afterload.

Answer: D. Afterload is the pressure the ventricular muscle must generate to overcome the higher pressure in the aorta to get the blood out of the heart.

3. When you hear the term "valvular regurgitation," what do you know is occurring inside the heart?
    A. The blood is flowing from the right atrium to the right ventricle.
    B. The blood is flowing from the right ventricle to the pulmonary artery.
    C. The blood is flowing from the right ventricle to the right atrium.
    D. The blood is flowing from the mitral valve to the left ventricle.

Answer: C. Regurgitation refers to backward flow of blood; in this case, the blood is trying to reverse its direction and return or flow back to the atrium.

4. When evaluating the cardiovascular condition, we evaluate the amount of blood pumped out by the heart in 1 minute. This is also referred to as:
    A. preload.
    B. afterload.
    C. contractility.
    D. cardiac output.

Answer: D. Cardiac output refers to the amount of blood the heart is able to pump out in 1 minute. The cardiac output is usually expressed in liters per minute and provides information on the heart's ability to work as a pump.

5. The diastole phase of the cardiac cycle occurs when:
    A. the ventricles contract increasing pressure into the aorta.
    B. the mitral and tricuspid valves close.
    C. pulmonic and aortic valves open.
    D. the ventricles relax and empty decreasing pressure in the aorta.

Answer: D. Diastole refers to the "relaxation" of the ventricles, thereby decreasing the pressure in the pulmonary artery and aorta.

6. When listening to heart sounds, you can best hear S_1 at the:
    A. base of the heart.
    B. apex of the heart.
    C. aortic area.
    D. second intercostal space to the right of the sternum.

Answer: B. S_1 is best heard at the apex of the heart.

7. You're auscultating for heart sounds in a 3-year-old girl and hear an S_3. You assess this sound to be:
    A. a normal finding.
    B. a probable sign of heart failure.
    C. a possible sign of atrial septal defect.
    D. a probable sign of mitral stenosis.

Answer: A. Although an S_3 can indicate heart failure in an adult, it's a normal finding in a child.

8. When grading arterial pulses, a 1+ grade indicates:
    A. bounding pulse.
    B. increased pulse.
    C. weak pulse.
    D. absent pulse.

Answer: C. A 1+ pulse indicates weak pulses and is associated with diminished cardiac perfusion.

9. When assessing a patient for jugular vein distention, you should position them:
    A. sitting upright.
    B. lying flat on their back.
    C. lying on their back, with the head of the bed elevated 30° to 45°.
    D. lying on their left side.

Answer: C. Assessing jugular vein distention should be done when the patient is in semi-Fowler position (head of the bed elevated 30°–45°). If the patient lies flat, their veins will be more distended; if the patient sits upright, the veins will be flat.

10. Capillary refill time is normally:
    A.   less than 15 seconds.
    B.   7 to 10 seconds.
    C.   4 to 6 seconds.
    D.   1 to 3 seconds.

Answer: D. Capillary refill time that lasts longer than 3 seconds is considered delayed and indicates decreased perfusion.

11. The recommended maximum daily dietary sodium intake is:
    A.   2,300 mg per day.
    B.   3,300 mg per day.
    C.   4,000 mg per day.
    D.   5,000 mg per day.

Answer: A. Sodium intake should be limited to 2,300 mg or less per day.

12. What is the recommended amount of exercise for decreasing the risk of CVD?
    A.   30 minutes of moderate physical activity 1 day per week
    B.   1 hour of low-impact activity 2 days per week
    C.   30 minutes of moderate physical activity 3 days per week
    D.   30 minutes of moderate physical activity most days of the week

Answer: D. Engaging in moderate physical activity for at least 30 minutes per day on most days of the week decreases the risk of developing CVD and also lessens the risk of developing hypertension and diabetes.

13. The National Cholesterol Education Program recommends routine screenings for abnormal lipid levels:
    A.   every 5 years beginning at age 40.
    B.   every 5 years beginning at age 20.
    C.   every 10 years beginning at age 30.
    D.   every 10 years beginning at age 20.

Answer: B. The National Cholesterol Education Program recommends screening for abnormal lipid levels every 5 years beginning at age 20.

14. Which test provides the best means of standardizing measurement of PT to monitor oral anticoagulant therapy?
    A.   Plasma thrombin time
    B.   INR
    C.   PTT
    D.   Activated bleeding time

Answer: B. The INR is the best means of standardizing measurement of PT to monitor anticoagulant therapy.

15. Cardiac enzyme levels are monitored in the patient with chest pain for which reason?
    A. Serial measurement of enzyme levels reveals the extent of cardiac damage and helps monitor healing progress.
    B. Cardiac enzymes help identify the area of myocardial damage.
    C. Decreasing enzyme levels help to estimate the recovery time for the patient with myocardial damage.
    D. Cardiac enzyme results will reveal if the patient is truly having chest pain.

Answer: A. Serial enzymes indicate whether cardiac damage is occurring.

16. TEE combines ultrasonography with which other procedure?
    A. Electrocardiography
    B. Endoscopic retrograde cholangiopancreatography
    C. Endoscopy
    D. Sigmoidoscopy

Answer: C. In TEE, ultrasonography is combined with endoscopy to provide a better view of the heart's structures.

17. A noninvasive method of evaluating blood flow is:
    A. duplex ultrasonography.
    B. venography.
    C. angiography.
    D. cardiac catheterization.

Answer: A. Duplex ultrasonography evaluates blood flow in the major blood vessels of the arms, legs, abdomen, and extracranial cerebrovascular system through use of high-frequency sound waves and a handheld transducer.

18. For a patient with symptom-producing sinus bradycardia, appropriate nursing interventions include establishing IV access to administer:
    A. atropine.
    B. anticoagulants.
    C. a calcium channel blocker.
    D. digoxin.

Answer: A. Atropine is standard treatment for sinus bradycardia.

19. Treatment for symptom-producing sick sinus syndrome includes:
    A. beta-adrenergic blockers.
    B. ventilatory support.
    C. pacemaker insertion.
    D. synchronized cardioversion.

Answer: C. A pacemaker is commonly used to maintain a steady heart rate in patients with sick sinus syndrome.

20. The treatment of choice for a patient with ventricular fibrillation is:
    A. defibrillation.
    B. transesophageal pacing.
    C. synchronized cardioversion.
    D. digoxin administration.

Answer: A. Patients with ventricular fibrillation are in cardiac arrest and require defibrillation.

21. The term *pulseless electrical activity* refers to a condition in which there's:
    A. a ventricular rate exceeding 100 beats/minute.
    B. asystole on a monitor or rhythm strip.
    C. an extremely slow heart rate but no pulse.
    D. electrical activity in the heart but no actual contraction.

Answer: D. Pulseless electrical activity is electrical activity without mechanical contraction. The patient is in cardiac arrest, with no blood pressure or pulse.

22. In type I second-degree AV block, the PR interval:
    A. varies according to the ventricular response rate.
    B. progressively lengthens until a QRS complex is dropped.
    C. remains constant despite an irregular ventricular rhythm.
    D. can't be determined.

Answer: B. Progressive lengthening of the PR interval creates an irregular ventricular rhythm with a repeating pattern of groups of QRS complexes. Those groups are followed by a dropped beat in which the P wave isn't followed by a QRS complex.

23. In atrial flutter, the key consideration in determining treatment is the:
    A. atrial rate.
    B. ventricular rate.
    C. configuration of the flutter waves.
    D. PR interval.

Answer: B. If the ventricular rate is too fast or too slow, cardiac output will be compromised. A rapid ventricular rate may require immediate cardioversion.

Matchmaker

24. Match each of the arrhythmias shown with their correct name.

_____ A. VF

_____ B. Atrial fibrillation

_____ C. VT

1. —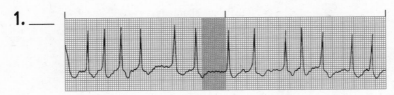

2. —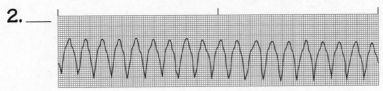

3. —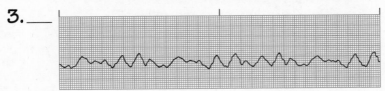

Answer: 1. B, 2. C, 3. A

Able to label?

25. Label each component of the normal arterial waveform shown here.

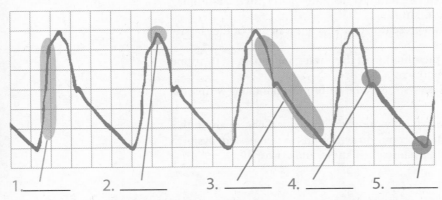

1._____   2._____   3._____   4._____   5._____

Answer: 1. Anacrotic limb, 2. Systolic peak, 3. Dicrotic limb, 4. Dicrotic notch, 5. End diastole

Matchmaker

26. Match the abnormal arterial waveforms shown to their possible causes.

1.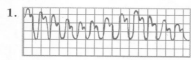

2.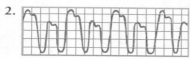

3.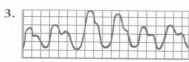

4.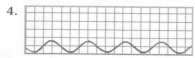

5.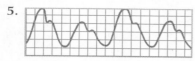

6.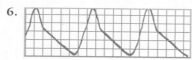

A. Pulsus paradoxus

B. Ventilator

C. Pulsus alternans

D. Ventricular bigeminy

E. Aortic stenosis

F. Overdamped waveform

Answer: 1. B, 2. D, 3. A, 4. F, 5. C, 6. E

27. Which of the following statements is true about an acute MI?
   A. There should be no relief from the pain with the administration of nitrates.
   B. Females can present with an MI without any of the classic symptoms.
   C. A typical presentation of the chest pain is pain in the upper back or abdomen.
   D. Troponin assays should be within normal range with serial testing.

Answer: B. Females typically present with atypical chest pain in the case of an MI. The more common symptoms in females are dyspnea, sweating, palpitations, nausea, weakness, and syncope.

28. Which patient should be screened for an abdominal aortic aneurysm?
    A. A 30-year-old male with a history of alcohol use disorder
    B. A 62-year-old female with a history of hypertension
    C. A 67-year-old male who quit smoking cigarettes twenty years ago
    D. An 81-year-old male with a history of atrial fibrillation

Answer: C. Because a AAA is usually asymptomatic until it is too late, male patients with a current or former history of smoking should be screened for a AAA once between the ages of 65 and 75.

29. Signs and symptoms of right-sided heart failure include:
    A. paroxysmal nocturnal dyspnea.
    B. unilateral calf erythema and swelling.
    C. a heave or lift over the chest.
    D. anasarca.

Answer: D. Anasarca is a late sign of right-sided heart failure. Paroxysmal nocturnal dyspnea or waking suddenly at night with shortness of breath is a sign of left-sided heart failure. Option B is a sign of a DVT. Bilateral edema of the lower extremities is a sign of right-sided heart failure. Option C is a sign of pulmonary hypertension.

30. Which intervention should the nurse use to prevent a DVT in a patient on strict bed rest after surgery?
    A. Apply heat to the affected area.
    B. Apply cold to the affected area.
    C. Apply antiembolic stockings and graduated compression to the lower extremities.
    D. Provide oxygen therapy as ordered.

Answer: D. Oxygen is used to prevent DVTs for patients on bed rest. Heat is used in the treatment of superficial and deep vein thrombosis. Cold is used initially after an IV infiltration.

31. Which valvular disorder increases with advanced age due to atherosclerosis?
    A. Mitral stenosis
    B. Aortic stenosis
    C. Mitral regurgitation
    D. Aortic regurgitation

Answer: B. Aortic stenosis is caused by growing calcifications from advanced age and atherosclerosis. The calcification on the valve leaflets makes them stiff and difficult to open and close causing an ejection "click" sound on auscultation.

32. The nurse is providing discharge instructions to a patient who is newly diagnosed with essential hypertension. Which statement by the nurse is correct?
    A. "Your sodium intake should be no more than 2,500 mg per day."
    B. "There is no excuse for not taking your blood pressure medications."
    C. "Do not smoke, drink caffeine, or exercise thirty minutes prior to checking your BP at home."
    D. "Herbal remedies that help you to lose weight are safe and effective."

Answer: C. Smoking, drinking caffeinated beverages, and physical activity will cause a false elevation of the BP. The recommended daily sodium intake for patients with hypertension is 1500 mg. BP medications have several unpleasant side effects, which may cause the patients to stop their medications. Maintain an open and supportive dialogue and present the patient concerns to the healthcare provider for treatment plan options. Herbal weight loss supplements can have stimulants, which will raise BP.

33. What's the most common site of injury from blunt chest trauma?
    A. Aorta
    B. Left ventricle
    C. Superior vena cava
    D. Right ventricle

Answer: D. Because of its location directly behind the sternum, the right ventricle is the most common site of injury from a blunt chest trauma.

34. What's the immediate goal of treatment for cardiac tamponade?
    A. Relieving pain
    B. Alleviating anxiety
    C. Improving mobility
    D. Relieving intrapericardial pressure

Answer: D. The goal of treatment is to relieve intrapericardial pressure and cardiac compression by removing accumulated blood or fluid.

35. Emergency treatment of hypovolemic shock includes:
    A. administration of antibiotics.
    B. administration of IV fluid or blood products.
    C. relief of pain.
    D. administration of vasodilators.

Answer: B. Emergency treatment relies on prompt and adequate fluid and blood replacement to restore intravascular volume and to raise systolic blood pressure and maintain it above 90 mm Hg. Rapid infusion of normal saline or lactated Ringer's solution and, possibly, albumin or other plasma expanders may expand volume adequately until blood is available.

36. Which measures should be performed immediately following a CABG?
    A. Ambulation, 12-lead ECG, and clear liquid diet
    B. Vital signs, cardiac rhythm, and pulse oximetry
    C. Vital signs, cardiac rhythm, and clear liquid diet
    D. 12-lead ECG, vital signs, and ambulation

Answer: B. Immediately following a CABG, the patient's vital signs should be obtained, their cardiac rhythm evaluated, and a pulse oximetry reading obtained to assess oxygenation.

37. What are the signs of hemodynamic compromise?
    A. Hypotension, decreased cardiac output, and shock
    B. Tachycardia, hypertension, and increased urine output
    C. Shock, diaphoresis, and increased cardiac output
    D. Bradycardia, hypertension, and decreased urine output

Answer: A. Signs of hemodynamic compromise include hypotension, decreased cardiac output, and signs of shock (cool, clammy skin; decreased urine output; initially tachycardia and then bradycardia).

38. What's an important teaching point for the patient receiving a heart transplant?
    A. They will need to stay indoors during the winter months.
    B. They will need to take immunosuppressants for at least 6 months following surgery.
    C. They will be at risk for life-threatening infections because of the medications they will be taking.
    D. After 6 weeks, they will no longer be at risk for rejection.

Answer: C. After a heart transplant, the patient is treated with monoclonal antibodies and potent immunosuppressants. The resulting immunosuppression places the patient at risk for life-threatening infection.

39. In a life-threatening situation, which pacemaker is the best choice?
    A. Permanent pacemaker
    B. Transcutaneous pacemaker
    C. Transvenous pacemaker
    D. Epicardial pacemaker

Answer: B. A transcutaneous pacemaker provides quick and effective pacing, but it's used only until a healthcare provider can institute transvenous or permanent pacing.

40. What's a nonsurgical alternative to coronary artery bypass surgery?
    A. PTCA
    B. VAD
    C. ICD
    D. MIDCAB

Answer: A. PTCA offers a nonsurgical alternative to coronary artery bypass surgery. Performed in the cardiac catheterization laboratory under local anesthesia, PTCA doesn't involve a thoracotomy, so it's less costly and requires shorter hospitalization. Patients can usually walk the next day and return to work in 2 weeks.

Scoring

⭐⭐⭐   If you answered all 40 questions correctly, fantastic! You put your whole heart into studying this book.

⭐⭐   If you answered 32 to 39 questions correctly, nice work!

⭐   If you answered fewer than 32 questions correctly, no worries. Now that you've assessed your risk, you can go back and review.

INDEX

Note: Page numbers followed by f indicate figures, t indicates tables and b indicates boxes.